Human Drug Metabolism

Human Drug Metabolism

An Introduction

Michael D. Coleman
Aston University, Birmingham

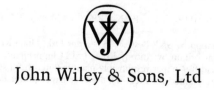

John Wiley & Sons, Ltd

Other Wiley Editorial Offices

John Wiley & Sons Inc., 111 River Street, Hoboken, NJ 07030, USA

Jossey-Bass, 989 Market Street, San Francisco, CA 94103-1741, USA

Wiley-VCH Verlag GmbH, Boschstr. 12, D-69469 Weinheim, Germany

John Wiley & Sons Australia Ltd, 33 Park Road, Milton, Queensland 4064, Australia

John Wiley & Sons (Asia) Pte Ltd, 2 Clementi Loop #02-01, Jin Xing Distripark, Singapore
129809

John Wiley & Sons Canada Ltd, 22 Worcester Road, Etobicoke, Ontario, Canada M9W 1L1

Wiley also publishes its books in a variety of electronic formats. Some content that appears in
print may not be available in electronic books.

Library of Congress Cataloging-in-Publication Data

British Library Cataloguing in Publication Data

A catalogue record for this book is available from the British Library

ISBN-13 978-0-470-86352-7 (H/B)   ISBN-13 978-0-470-86353-4 (P/B)

Typeset in 10¹/₂/12¹/₂ pt Sabon by SNP Best-set Typesetter Ltd., Hong Kong
Printed and bound in Great Britain by Antony Rowe Ltd., Chippenham, Wilts
This book is printed on acid-free paper responsibly manufactured from sustainable forestry in
which at least two trees are planted for each one used for paper production.

For Mark, Carol and Devon

Contents

Preface

'Throw physic to the dogs; I'll none of it' exclaims the eponymous Macbeth in Act 5, Scene 3, in one of Shakespeare's shortest and most violent plays. This response to the lack of efficacy and severe toxicity of early seventeenth-century therapeutics unfortunately has some resonance today. Despite the spectacular advances made in the last 50 years, many medicines in practice are neither beneficial nor safe. Indeed, increasing numbers of patients are dying as a result of their treatment, rather than their condition. There are many reasons for our inability to eradicate 'iatrogenic' (literally, physician induced) disease; these might include pharmacological interactions or factors relating to the patient's condition. However, the metabolism of drugs by the patients' own systems can have a powerful influence on the success of treatment.

This book is intended to provide a basic grounding in human drug metabolism, although it is useful if the reader has some knowledge of biochemistry, physiology and pharmacology from other sources. In addition, a qualitative understanding of chemistry can illuminate many facets of drug metabolism and toxicity. Although chemistry can be intimidating, I have tried to make the chemical aspects of drug metabolism as user-friendly as possible.

Regarding the layout of the book, Chapter 1 uses the idea of the therapeutic window to outline how both efficacy and toxicity are dependent on drug concentration, which is in turn linked to the rate of drug removal from the system. Biological systems actively eliminate small xenobiotic (foreign) molecules and how quickly this happens is a strong determinate of treatment outcome. Chapter 2 tries to put the metabolism of drugs in the context of other biological processes. Human metabolizing systems must synthesize endogenous molecules, inactivate them when their purpose is served and defend the body from foreign molecules. Drugs fit into the latter category and are treated by biological systems as foreign and unwelcome. Chapter 3 outlines how human metabolizing systems have availed themselves of highly specialized metabolizing enzymes of bacterial and eukaryotic origin, particularly cytochrome P450s. Phase I, the initial, mainly oxidative, phase of metabolism, begins the process of the conversion of lipophilic drugs to easily excreted water-soluble metabolites. The chapter considers the remarkable flexibility and capability of these oxidative enzymes. Chapter 4 reveals the mechanisms whereby the presence of some drugs can induce a massive adaptive increase in the metabolizing capability of cytochrome P450s. The threat to clinical drug efficacy posed by the resulting acceleration of drug removal from the body is outlined in a number of drug classes. By contrast, the inhibition of drug-metabolizing systems described in Chapter 5 is shown to cause life-threatening drug accumulation in a very short space of time. The mechanisms of cytochrome P450 inhibition are explained in the context of the main pharmacological features of enzyme inhibition. Chapter 6 illustrates the companion processes for Phase I, which are Phases II and III. In Phase II, large hydrophilic molecules are either attached directly to drugs or Phase I metabolites with the object of increasing their water solubility and molecule weight. This process, in concert with Phase III efflux pump systems, facilitates the removal of the metabolites from cells to the urine and the bile. Chapter 7 discusses other factors that influence drug-metabolizing processes, such as genetic polymorphisms, age, gender, diet, alcohol intake and disease. Chapter 8 explains some of the toxicological consequences of xenobiotic metabolism. The roles of cytochrome P450s in the origins of reversible and irreversible effects on the body are discussed. Irreversible events associated with reactive species formation due to cytochrome P450 metabolism include necrosis, immune-related toxicity and cancer.

At the end of the book, in Appendix A, there is a brief discussion of the role of drug metabolism in the commercial development of new therapeutic agents. The increasing popularity of illicit drugs makes it interesting to include some background on the metabolism of some major drugs of abuse in Appendix B, although it does include clinically useful agents such as opiates. Many readers of this book will be studying for formal examinations of some type, so some accumulated general advice on the preparation for examinations is supplied in Appendix C. Appendix D contains a brief list of cytochrome P450 substrates, inhibitors and inducers, and finally there is a list of suggested reading for those interested in a deeper, more detailed knowledge of the subject.

Whilst no human effort is without error and this book is no exception, it is hoped that it will facilitate understanding of the impact of metabolizing systems on drug therapeutic outcomes. All of us eventually participate in healthcare in some capacity, if not professionally, then as patients. Therefore, it is our duty to constantly update our therapeutic knowledge to liberate the full potential of the many remarkably effective drugs currently available.

I am very grateful to Mr Graham Smith for drawing the detailed figures. I would like to acknowledge the support and encouragement of my wife Clare, as well as my mother Jean, during the writing process and I very much hope you, the reader, find this book useful.

M.D. Coleman, D.Sc.

1 Introduction

1.1 Therapeutic window

Introduction

It has been said that if a drug has no side effects, then it is unlikely to work. Drug therapy labours under the fundamental problem that usually every single cell in the body has to be treated just to exert a beneficial effect on a small group of cells, perhaps in one tissue. Although drug-targeting technology is improving rapidly, most of us that take an oral dose are still faced with the problem that the vast majority of our cells are being unnecessarily exposed to an agent that at best will have no effect, but at worst will exert many unwanted effects. So all drug treatment is a compromise between positive and negative effects in the patient. The process of drug development weeds out agents that have seriously negative actions and usually releases onto the market drugs that may have a profile of side effects, but these are relatively minor within a set concentration range where the drug's pharmacological action is most effective. This range, or 'therapeutic window' is rather variable, but it will give some indication of the most 'efficient' drug concentration. This means the most beneficial pharmacological effects for the minimum side effects.

The therapeutic window (Figure 1.1) may or may not correspond exactly to active tissue concentrations, but it is a useful guideline as to whether drug levels are within the appropriate range. Sometimes, a drug is given once only and it is necessary for drug levels to be within the therapeutic window for a relatively brief period, perhaps when paracetamol is taken for mild analgesia. However, the majority of drugs require repeated dosing in time periods which range from a few days for a course of antibiotics, to many years for anti-hypertensives and antithyroid drugs. During repeated intermediate and long-term dosing, drug levels may move below or above the therapeutic window due to events such as patient illness, changes in diet or co-administration of other drugs. Below the lowest concentration of the window, it is likely that the drug will fail to work, as the pharmacological effect will

Human Drug Metabolism, Michael D. Coleman
© 2005 John Wiley & Sons, Ltd

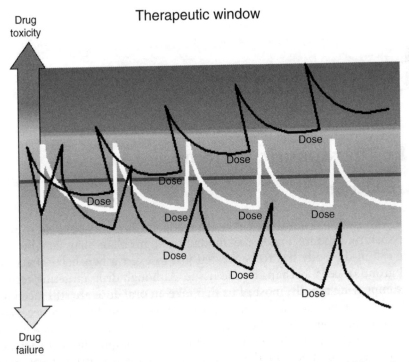

Figure 1.1 The 'therapeutic window', where drug concentrations should be maintained for adequate therapeutic effect, without either accumulation (drug toxicity) or disappearance (drug failure)

be too slight to be beneficial. If the drug concentration climbs above the therapeutic window, an intensification of the drug's pharmacological actions will occur. If drug levels continue to rise, irreversible damage may occur which is usually described by the word 'toxicity'. To some extent, the therapeutic window is unique to every patient, as there is such huge variation in our sensitivities to the pharmacological actions of the drug (pharmacodynamic sensitivity). This book is concerned with what systems influence how long the drug stays in our bodies.

Whether drug concentrations stay in the therapeutic window is obviously related to how quickly the agent enters the blood and tissues prior to its removal. When a drug is given intravenously, there is no barrier to the entry of the drug, which can thus be easily and quickly adjusted to correspond with the rate of removal, so drug levels can be maintained within the therapeutic window. This is known as 'steady state', the main objective of therapeutics. The majority of drug use is by other routes such as oral or intramuscular rather than intravenous, and there will be a considerable time lag as the drug is absorbed from either the gastro-intestinal tract (GIT) or the muscle, so achieving drug levels within the therapeutic window is a slower, more 'hit and miss' process. The result from repeated oral dosing is a rather crude peak/trough pulsing, or 'sawtooth' effect which you can see in the diagram (Figure 1.1). This should be adequate provided that the peaks and troughs remain within the confines of the 'therapeutic window'.

Therapeutic index

Drugs vary enormously in their toxicity and the concentrations at which one drug might cause potentially lethal effects might be 10 or 100 times lower than a much less toxic drug. A convenient measure for this is the 'therapeutic index'. This has been defined as the ratio between the lethal or toxic dose and the effective dose which shows the normal range of pharmacological effect:

$$\text{Therapeutic index (TI)} = \frac{\text{Lethal dose}}{\text{Effective dose}}$$

In practice, a drug (such as digoxin) is listed as having a narrow TI if there is less than a twofold difference between the lethal and effective doses, or a twofold difference in the minimum toxic and minimum effective concentrations. Back in the 1960s, many drugs in common use had narrow TIs. Drugs such as barbiturates could be toxic at relatively low levels. Over the last 30 years, the drug industry has aimed to replace this type of drug with agents with much higher TIs. This is noticeable in drugs used for depression. The risk of suicide is likely to be high in a condition that takes some time (often weeks) to respond to therapy. When the tricyclic antidepressants (TCAs) were the main treatment option, these relatively narrow TI drugs could be used by the patient to end their lives. However, more modern drugs such as the SSRIs have much higher TIs, so the risk of the patient using the drugs for a suicide attempt is virtually removed. However, there are many drugs (including the TCAs to a limited extent), which remain in use that have narrow or relatively narrow TIs (e.g. phenytoin, carbamazepine, valproate, warfarin). Therefore the consequences of accumulation of these drugs are much worse and happen more quickly than drugs with high TIs.

Changes in dosage

If the dosage exceeds the rate of the drug's removal, then clearly drug levels will accumulate and depart from the therapeutic window towards toxic levels. If the drug dosage is too low, levels will fall below the lowest threshold of the window and the drug will fail to work. If a patient is established at the correct dose that does not change, then this is the oral version of 'steady state'. So theoretically, the drug should remain in its therapeutic window for as long as it is necessary to take it unless other factors change this situation.

Changes in rate of removal

The patient may continue to take the drug at the correct dosage, but drug levels may drop out of, or exceed, the therapeutic window. This could be linked with redistribution of the drug between bodily areas such as plasma and a particular organ, or protein binding might fluctuate; however, the major factor in the maintenance of drug levels within the therapeutic window is the rate of removal and/or inactivation of the drug by bodily processes.

1.2 Consequences of drug concentration changes

If there are large changes in the rate of removal of a drug, then this can lead *in extremis* to severe problems in the outcome of the patient's treatment: the first is drug failure, the second is drug toxicity (Figure 1.2). These extremes and indeed all drug effects are related to the blood concentrations of the agent in question.

Drug failure

Although it might take nearly a decade and huge sums of money to develop a drug that is highly effective in the vast majority of patients, the drug can of course only exert an effect if it reaches its intended target in sufficient concentration. There may be many reasons why sufficient concentrations cannot be reached. Drug absorption may have been poor, or it may have been bound to proteins or removed much more rapidly from the target area than it can enter. This situation of drug 'failure' might occur after treatment has first appeared to be successful, where a patient becomes stabilized on a particular drug regimen, which then fails due to the addition of another drug or chemical to the regimen. The second drug causes the failure by accelerating of the removal of the first from the patient's system, so drug levels are then too low to be effective. The clinical consequences of drug failure can be serious for both for the patient and the community. In the treatment of epilepsy, the loss of effective control of the patient's fits could lead to injury to themselves or others. The failure of a contraceptive drug would lead to an unwanted pregnancy and the failure of an antipsychotic drug would mean hospitalization for a patient at the very least. For the community, when the clearance of an antibiotic or antiparasitic drug is accelerated, this causes drug

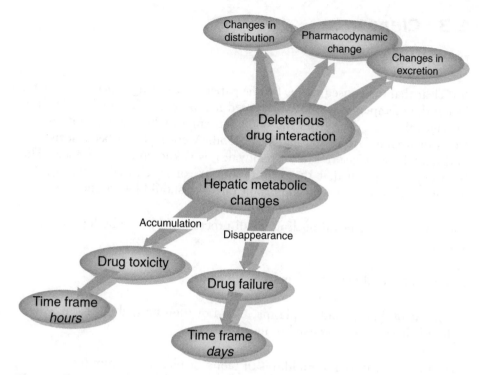

Figure 1.2 Consequences of drug interactions in terms of metabolic changes and their effects on drug failure and toxicity

levels to fall below the minimum inhibitory concentration, thus selecting drug-resistant mutants of the infection. Therapeutic drug failure is usually a gradual process, where the time frame may be days before the problem is detected (Figure 1.2).

Drug toxicity

If a drug accumulates for any reason, either by overdose or by a failure of drug removal, then serious adverse reactions will result. A reduction in the rate of removal of the drug from a system (often due to administration of another drug), will lead to drug accumulation. Toxicity can be an intensification of a drug's therapeutic action, or an unrelated damaging effect on a tissue or organ system. If the immunosuppressive cyclosporine is allowed to accumulate, severe renal toxicity can lead to organ failure. Excessive levels of anticonvulsant and antipsychotic drugs cause confusion and drowsiness, whilst the accumulation of the antihistamine terfenadine, can lead to lethal cardiac arrhythmias. In contrast to drug failure, drug toxicity may occur much more rapidly, often within hours rather than days.

1.3 Clearance

Definitions

It is clear that the consequences for the patient when drug concentrations fall below the therapeutic window or exceed it can be life threatening. The rate of removal of the drug from the body determines whether it will disappear from, or accumulate in the patient's blood. A concept has been devised to understand and measure rate of removal; this is known as 'Clearance'. This term does not mean that the drug disappears or is 'cleared' instantly. The definition of clearance is an important one that should be retained:

Clearance is the removal of drug by all processes from the biological system.

A more advanced definition could be taken as:

A volume of fluid (could be plasma, blood or total body fluid) from which a drug is irreversibly removed in unit time.

Clearance is measured in millilitres of blood or plasma per min (or litres per hour) and is usually taken to mean the 'clearance' of the drug's pharmacological effectiveness, which resides in its structure. Once the drug has been metabolized, or 'biotransformed', even though only a relatively trivial change may have been effected in the structure, it is no longer as it was and this metabolite, or metabolites, often exert less, or even no therapeutic effect. Even if they still have some therapeutic effect, metabolites (products of biotransformation) are usually removed from the cell faster than the parent drug and they will be excreted in urine and faeces. There are exceptions where metabolites are as effective as the parent drug (some tricyclic antidepressants, such as desipramine and morphine glucuronides), and there are metabolites that are strangely even less soluble in water and harder to excrete than the parent compound (acetylated sulphonamides), but in general, the main measure of clearance is known as total body clearance, or sometimes, systemic clearance:

$$Cl_{total}$$

This can be regarded as the sum of all the processes that can clear the drug. Effectively, this means the sum of the liver and kidney contributions to drug clearance, although the lung and other organs can make some contribution.

For a drug like atenolol, which unusually does not undergo any hepatic metabolism, or indeed metabolism by any other organ, it is possible to say that:

$$Cl_{total} = Cl_{renal}$$

So renal clearance is the only route of clearance for atenolol, in fact it is 100 per cent of clearance.

For paracetamol and for most other drugs, total body clearance is a combination of hepatic and renal clearances:

$$Cl_{total} = Cl_{hepatic} + Cl_{renal}$$

For ethanol, you will probably already be aware that there are several routes of clearance, hepatic, renal and the lung, as breath tests are a well-established indicator of blood concentrations.

$$Cl_{total} = Cl_{hepatic} + Cl_{renal} + Cl_{lung}$$

Once it is clear what clearance means, then the next step is to consider how clearance occurs.

Means of clearance

In absolute terms, to clear something away is to get rid of it, to remove it physically from the system. The kidneys are mostly responsible for this removal, known as elimination. The kidneys cannot filter large chemical entities like proteins, but they can remove most smaller chemicals, depending on size, charge and water solubility. The filtrate eventually reaches the collecting tubules that lead to the ureter and the bladder. As the kidney is a lipophilic (oil-loving) organ, if it filters lipophilic drugs or toxins, these can easily leave the urine in the collecting tubules and return to the surrounding lipophilic tissues and thence back to the blood. So the kidney is not efficient at clearing lipophilic chemicals.

The role of the liver is to use biotransforming enzymes to ensure that lipophilic agents are made water soluble enough to be cleared by the kidney. So the liver has an essential but indirect role in clearance, in that it must extract the drug from the circulation, biotransform (metabolize) it, then return the water-soluble product to the blood for the kidney to remove. The liver can also actively clear or physically remove its metabolic products by excreting them in bile, where they travel through the gut to be eliminated in faeces. Bacterial effects on this process can lead to the reabsorption of the metabolite or parent drug into the gut, a process known as enterohepatic recirculation.

The liver has an impressive array of enzymatic systems to biotransform drugs, toxins and other chemical entities to more water-soluble products. However, the ability of the liver to metabolize a drug can depend on the structure and physicochemical characteristics of the agent, so some drugs are easy for it to clear and some are difficult.

1.4 Hepatic extraction and intrinsic clearance

High extraction drugs

Hepatic extraction is a useful term to measure how easily the liver can process, or metabolize, a given drug or toxin. The term 'hepatic extraction' effectively means the difference between the drug level in blood that enters the liver (100 per cent) and the amount that escapes intact and unmetabolized (that is, 100 per cent minus the metabolized fraction).

Extraction is usually termed E and is defined as the extraction ratio, or

$$\text{Extraction ratio} = \frac{\text{Concentration } \textit{entering} \text{ the liver} - \text{Concentration } \textit{leaving} \text{ the liver}}{\text{Concentration } \textit{entering} \text{ the liver}}$$

For a high extraction drug ($E > 0.7$), the particular enzyme that metabolizes this drug may be present in large amounts and drug processing is very rapid. This often happens if the drug is very similar in structure to an endogenous agent, which is normally processed in great quantity on a daily basis. In the case of a high extraction drug, the inbuilt, or 'intrinsic' ability of the liver in metabolizing the drug means that the only limitation in the liver's ability to metabolize this type of drug is its rate of arrival, which is governed by blood flow.

So in the case of a high clearance drug, where the liver's intrinsic ability to clear it is very high:

$$Cl_{\text{hepatic}} = Q \text{ (liver blood flow)} \times \text{Extraction ratio } E$$

i.e.

$$Cl_{\text{hepatic}} = QE$$

So, basically, hepatic clearance is directly proportional to blood flow:

$$Cl_{\text{hepatic}} \; \alpha \; Q$$

Liver blood flow does not normally vary that much, so the drugs are extracted and processed at a fairly even rate. The only time blood flow to the liver falls is in old age or end-stage cirrhotic alcoholism. Normally, for any given drug, there is equilibrium between protein-bound and free drug. In effect, high extraction drugs are cleared so avidly, that the free drug disappears into the metabolizing system and the bound pool of drug becomes exhausted. The amount of free drug in the blood will be very low.

Examples of high extraction drugs include pethidine, metoprolol, propranolol, lignocaine and verapamil.

You might see the term 'intrinsic clearance' which reflects the inbuilt ability of the liver to remove a drug; high extraction drugs have a high intrinsic clearance. As mentioned above, the only limitation in clearance for these drugs is how much drug the blood can deliver. If blood flow was to be infinite, then hepatic clearance would be the same as intrinsic clearance.

Low extraction drugs

On the opposite end of the scale ($E < 0.3$), some drugs are cleared slowly, as the metabolizing enzymes have some difficulty in oxidizing them, due to stability in the structure, or the low capacity and activity of the metabolizing enzymes. The enzymes may also be present only in very low levels. These drugs are considered to be low intrinsic clearance drugs, as the inbuilt ability of the liver to remove them is relatively low.

If a low extraction drug is strongly protein bound, then the liver essentially cannot get at the drug, as the affinity of drug for the protein is much greater than the liver's affinity for the drug. The drug is thus liable to stay bound and the amount of drug actually cleared by the liver really depends on how much unbound or free drug there is in the blood. This means that:

$$Cl_{\text{hepatic}} \propto Cl_{\text{intrinsic}} \times \text{fraction unbound}$$

So clearance is proportional to the ability of the liver to metabolize the drug ($Cl_{\text{intrinsic}}$) and the amount in the plasma that is actually available for metabolism as free (unbound to protein) drug. This means that if the low intrinsic ability of the liver falls any further, there will be a greater increase in plasma levels than would happen with a highly extracted drug.

Examples of low extraction drugs are phenytoin, paracetamol, diazepam, naproxen and metronidazole.

1.5 First pass and plasma drug levels

Clearance is thus the removal of drug from all tissues and usually the liver is seen as the major force in the clearance of drugs. However, this is an oversimplification, as other tissues can clear drugs and in the real world of a drug entering the body, the gut makes a significant contribution to clearance (Figure 1.3). To be absorbed from the gut, the drug must pass through the gut wall and enter the hepatic portal circulation, which leads directly to the liver. Even before the drug has crossed the gut cells, it can be pumped back out of the gut wall into the lumen by efflux proteins and metabolized by

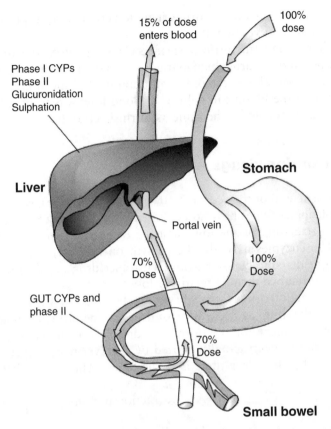

Figure 1.3 The 'first pass' of an orally dosed highly cleared drug showing the removal of drug by the gut and liver, leading to relatively low levels of drug actually reaching the circulation

various enzymes in the gut wall cells. In the case of some drugs, this can account for a high proportion of the dose before it reaches the liver. The fraction of the original dose left then enters the liver and by the time the liver has extracted the drug (especially if it is a high extraction drug), most of the dose has been inactivated. This process, where an oral dose is metabolized by various systems, is termed 'first pass'.

In some drugs, the vast majority of the dose is lost before it reaches the systemic circulation. The amount that actually reaches the plasma can be measured and the amount that was dosed is also known, so an equation can be produced which gives us how much enters the system. This is known as the 'bioavailability' of the drug and is termed F. It can be defined as

$$F = \frac{\text{Total amount of drug in the systemic circulation after oral dosage}}{\text{Total amount of drug in the systemic circulation after intravenous dose}}$$

Highly extracted drugs are often stated to have a 'poor bioavailability'. This means that the oral dose required to exert a given response is much larger than the intravenous dose. If the bioavailability is 20 per cent, then you might need about five times the intravenous dose to see an effect orally.

Changes in clearance and plasma levels

Considering an extreme example, if the intravenous dose of a poorly bioavailable (F = 20 per cent) narrow TI drug X was 20 mg and the usual oral dose was 100 mg, it is clear that if the whole oral 100 mg were to reach the plasma, the patient would then have plasma levels far in excess of the normal intravenous dose, which could be toxic or fatal. This could happen if the first pass effect was reduced or even completely prevented by factors that changed the drug's clearance.

Similarly, if the clearance of the drug was to be accelerated, then potentially none of the 100 mg would reach the plasma at all, so causing lack of efficacy and drug failure.

1.6 Drug and xenobiotic metabolism

From the therapeutic point of view, it is essential to ensure that drug concentrations remain within the therapeutic window and neither drug failure, nor drug toxicity, occur in the patient. To understand some of the factors related to drug metabolism that can influence the achievement of these aims, there are several important points to consider over the next few chapters of this book.

- What are the metabolic or biotransformational processes that can so dramatically influence drug concentrations and therefore drug action?

- How do these processes sense the presence of the drugs and then remove these apparently chemically stable entities from the body so effectively?

- What is the effect of illness, genetic profile and other patient circumstances on the operation of these processes?

- How can these processes of removal of a drug lead to toxicity?

- What were these processes originally designed to achieve and what is their endogenous function?

The next chapter considers the last point and illustrates that in a subject usually termed 'drug metabolism', modern drugs are newcomers to an ancient, complex and highly adaptable system that has evolved to protect living organisms, to control instruction molecules and carry out many physiological tasks.

2 Drug Biotransformational Systems – Origins and Aims

2.1 Biotransforming enzymes

John Lennon once said 'Before Elvis, there was nothing.' Biologically, this could be paraphrased along the lines of 'Before bacteria, there was nothing.' Although life on this planet has left traces suggesting that it began around 1000 million years ago, it is likely that bacteria appeared much earlier and had a far more hostile environment to endure than we do at present. Bacteria would have had to survive above and below the earth in exceedingly harsh conditions in terms of corrosive/reactive chemicals, heat and lack of oxygen. The phenomenal growth and generation rates of bacteria enabled them to evolve very rapidly enzyme systems to establish their basic structural features and to make sufficient energy to survive. Cell structures eventually settled around the format we see now, a largely aqueous cytoplasm bounded by a predominantly lipophilic protective membrane. Although the membrane does prevent entry and exit of many potential toxins, it is no barrier to other lipophilic molecules. If these molecules are highly lipophilic, they will passively diffuse into and become trapped in the membrane. If they are slightly less lipophilic, they will pass through it into the organism. So aside from 'housekeeping' enzyme systems, some enzymatic protection would have been needed against invading molecules from the immediate environment. Among the various molecular threats to the organism would have been the waste products of other bacteria in decaying biomass, as well as various chemicals formed from incomplete combustion. These would have included aromatic hydrocarbons (multiples of the simplest aromatic, benzene) that can enter living systems and accumulate, thus deranging useful enzymatic systems and cellular structures. Enzymes that can detoxify these pollutants such as aromatics are usually termed 'biotransforming enzymes'.

Human Drug Metabolism, Michael D. Coleman
© 2005 John Wiley & Sons, Ltd

2.2 Threat of lipophilic hydrocarbons

Living organisms that cannot rid themselves of lipophilic aromatic and non-aromatic hydrocarbons accumulate them to high levels. This happens with oysters to their detriment, but not with mudskippers, which can remove them from their systems. The majority of living organisms including ourselves now possess some form of biotransformational enzyme system and these were effectively 'stolen' from bacteria over millions of years. The main biotransformational protection against aromatic hydrocarbons is a series of enzymes so named as they absorb UV light at 450 nm when reduced and bound to carbon monoxide. These specialized enzymes were termed cytochrome P450 monooxygenases or sometimes oxido-reductases. They are often referred to as 'CYPs' or 'P450s'. They may have evolved at first to accomplish reductive reactions in the absence of oxygen and they retain this ability. The main function of these monoooxygenases is to carry out oxidations. These enzymes are part of a family whose functional characteristics are reminiscent of a set of adjustable spanners in a tool kit. All the CYPs accomplish their functions using the same basic mechanism, but each enzyme is adapted to dismantle particular groups of chemical structures. It is a testament to millions of years of 'research and development' in the evolution of CYPs, that perhaps 50 000 or more man-made chemical entities enter the environment for the first time every year and the vast majority can be oxidized by at least one form of CYP.

2.3 Cell communication

Signal molecule design

At some point in evolution, single-cell life forms began to coalesce into multi-cell organizations, allowing advantages in influencing and controlling the cells' immediate environment. Further down this line of development, groups of cells differentiated to perform specialized functions, which other cells would not then need to carry out. At some point in evolution, a dominant cellular group will have developed methods of communicating with other cell groups to coordinate the organisms' functions. Once cellular communication was established, other cell groups could be instructed to carry out yet more specialized development. In more advanced organisms, this chain of command and control has two main options for communication: either by direct electrical nervous impulse or instruction through a chemical. Neural impulse control is seen where the sympathetic nervous system influences the adrenal gland by direct innervation. For an instructional chemical such as a hormone (from the Greek meaning to urge on) to operate, its unique shape must convey information to a receptor, where the receptor/molecule complex is capable of activating the receptor to engage its function. An instructional molecule must possess certain features to make it a viable and reliable means of communication. Firstly, it must be stable and not spontaneously change its shape and so lose the ability to dock accurately with its receptor. Secondly, it must be relatively resistant to reacting with various other cell enzymes or chemicals it might contact, such as proteolytic enzymes on the cell surface or in the cytoplasm. Finally, it must be easily manufactured in large amounts with the components of the molecule being readily available. It is immediately obvious that the pharmaceutical industry uses the same criteria in designing its products that often mimic that of an endogenous molecule. The final feature of an instruction molecule is that it must also be *controllable*. It is no use to an organism to issue a 'command' that continues to be slavishly obeyed long after the necessity to obey is over. This is wasteful at best, and at worst seriously damaging to the organism which will then carry out unnecessary functions which cost it energy and raw materials which should have been used to address a current, more pressing problem. The chemical instruction must be controlled in a period that is appropriate for its function. Thus it might be necessary for it to operate for seconds, minutes, hours or days.

There are contradictions in this approach; the formation of a *stable* molecule which will be easily and quickly disposable. To make a stable compound will cost energy and raw materials, although to dismantle it will also cost the organism. It all hinges on for what purpose the instruction molecule was designed. For changes that are minute by minute, second by second, then perhaps a protein or peptide would be useful. These molecules that can retain information by their shape are often chemically stable, although the large numbers of various protease and other enzymes present at or around cell membranes mean that their half-lives can be exceedingly short. This allows fine control of a function by chemical means, as rate of manufacture can be adjusted to necessity given that the molecule is rendered non-functional in seconds.

Lipophilic hydrocarbons as signal molecules

Unlike short-term modulations of tissue function, processes like the development of sexual maturity require long-term changes in tissue structure as well as function, and these cannot be achieved through direct neural instruction. Chemical instruction is necessary to control particular genes in millions of cells over many years. To induce these changes, hormone molecules need to be designed and assembled to be stable enough to carry an instruction (the shape of the molecule) and have the appropriate physicochemical features to reach nuclear receptors inside a cell to activate specific genes.

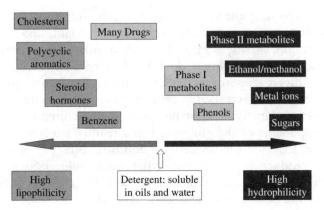

Figure 2.1 The lipophilicity (oil loving) and hydrophilicity (water loving) of various chemical entities that can be found in living organisms

Lipophilic hydrocarbon chemicals have a number of advantages as signalling molecules. Firstly, they are usually stable, plentiful and their solubility in oils and aqueous media can be chemically manipulated. This sounds surprising given that they are generally known to be very oil soluble and completely insoluble in water. However, those enzymes we inherited from bacteria such as CYPs, have evolved to radically alter the shape, solubility and stability of aromatic molecules. This is in effect a system for 'custom building' stable instructional small molecules, which are easiest to make if a modular common platform is employed which is the molecule cholesterol. From Figure 2.1 you can see the position of cholesterol and other hormones in relation to oil and water solubility, relative to a detergent, which is amphipathic, i.e. soluble in oil and water. The nearest agents with a detergent-like quality in biological systems are bile salts, which use this ability to break large fat droplets into smaller ones to aid absorption.

Cholesterol itself is very soluble in lipids and has almost zero water solubility so it requires a sophisticated transport system to move it around the body. Although a controversial molecule for its role in cardiovascular disease, it has many vital functions such as the formation of bile acids as well as maintenance of cell membrane fluidity. This latter function shows that cholesterol itself is so lipophilic that it is trapped in membranes. However, steroid hormones built on the cholesterol 'platform' are much less lipophilic than their parent molecule so they do not get trapped in lipid-rich areas, although from Figure 2.1 it is clear they are still not water-soluble. Highly lipophilic pollutant molecules like large polycyclic hydrocarbons are trapped within membranes and fatty tissue. Steroid hormones are synthesized so that they move through the circulation bound to the appropriate carrier molecule and then they can leave the blood to enter cells without being trapped within membranes.

They can then progress through the cytoplasm, binding various sensor molecules associated with the nucleus. Thus, their information is conveyed intact to instruct the cell. Once the stable steroid platform has been built by CYPs and served its purpose, the final link in the process is the use of various other CYPs to ensure the elimination of these molecules. The complete synthesis and degradation system is fully adjustable according to changing circumstances and can exert a remarkably fine control over steroid molecules. Such is the efficiency of this system that early human contraception studies showed that after an oral dose of oestradiol-17β, systemic bioavailability was virtually zero.

2.4   Potential food toxins

As living organisms developed in complexity and their diets expanded to include many types of plants and animals, it was clearly necessary to evolve a system that would protect an organism from food toxins. This process was probably greatly accelerated by the evolution of land animals from their seagoing ancestors. Diets rich in plant material led to the consumption of high numbers of lipophilic agents with long half-lives, including many aromatic-based compounds. To counter this, it has been suggested that plants evolved chemical defence agents like toxic alkaloids to avoid being eaten. Aside from direct lipophilic toxins, more long-term threats to animals in this regard would be the large number of plant hormone-like chemicals, such as phytoestrogens. Animals and humans can have enough problems regulating their own hormone levels to ensure timely and appropriate reproduction and maintenance of reproductive tracts, without exogenous hormones deranging function, just because the organism prefers a diet rich in hormone-laden plants. It is now clear that oestrogen receptors will bind and function in response to a wide variety of chemicals. This is mainly because large numbers of molecules have an aromatized ring in a similar orientation to a steroid. Regarding diet, there are so many oestrogens and other female hormones in some foods that diet alone has been successfully used to control the menopause in women as an alternative to drug therapy. There are commercial sources of plant oestrogens that are sufficiently potent to be marketed as human breast size enhancers that actually work. It is also clear that long-term exposure to inappropriate hormone levels can lead to cancer in vulnerable tissues such as the endometrium, breasts and ovaries. CYPs are a major defence against such unwanted molecules and they actively protect us from exogenous hormone-like molecules. Interestingly, the fact that plant phytoestrogen breast enhancers and other hormone 'mimics' do exert effects in humans indicates that these agents partially thwart CYP systems, as they are not easy to metabolize and inactivate rapidly enough to prevent interference in human hormone balances.

As has been mentioned, plants synthesize many protective toxin-like agents, but in a harsh environment, to be able to consume such plants without

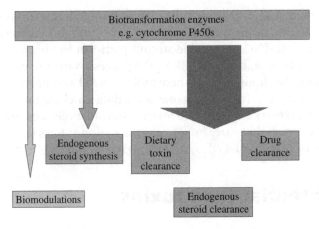

Figure 2.2 Various functions of biotransformational enzymes, from assembly of endogenous steroids, modulation of various biological processes as well as the clearance of drugs, toxins and endogenous steroids

toxicity provides an animal with a significant advantage in its survival prospects. CYPs have also evolved to protect us from such molecules, such as coumarin anticoagulants in some plants. If these cannot be quickly rendered safe and eliminated, severe haemorrhaging can result. However, agents such as mycotoxins can use our own CYPs to cause lethal toxicity and carcinogenicity (Chapter 8). Figure 2.2 illustrates the varying roles of CYPs in living systems.

2.5 Sites of biotransforming enzymes

Aside from their biotransformational roles in steroid biosynthesis and drug/toxin clearance, CYPs carry out a wide array of metabolic activities that are essential to homeostasis. This is not surprising, as they are found in virtually every tissue. The main areas are the liver and gut that have the highest concentrations of biotransformational capability. These CYPs are mainly concerned with the processing and clearance of large amounts of various endogenous and exogenous, or 'xenobiotic', chemicals. The CYPs and other metabolizing systems in organs such as the lung and kidney make relatively little contribution to the overall clearance of a drug, but are relevant in the formation of toxic species from drugs and xenobiotics. In addition, other CYPs have been shown to have highly specific biomodulatory roles that are distinct from high volume chemical oxidation. The brain is a good example of this; CYPs are often found in particular areas, rather than universally distributed. They are found at very low levels, often less than 2 per cent of hepatic P450 levels. Their central nervous system (CNS) role involves catalysing specific neural functions by regulating endogenous entities such as neurosteroids, rather than larger-scale chemical processing. A number of CYPs are also engaged in the regulation of vascular tone through arachidonic acid metabolism in the periphery as well as the brain. Many new functions of these enzymes have only been recently found and it is likely that hundreds more CYP-mediated endogenous functions remain to be discovered.

2.6 Biotransformation

Role of the Liver

Drugs, toxins and all other chemicals can enter the body through a variety of routes. The major route is through the digestive system, but chemicals can by-pass the gut via the lungs and skin for example. Although the gut metabolises many drugs, the liver is the main biotransforming organ and the CYPs and other metabolising enzymes reside in the hepatocytes. These cells must perform two essential tasks at the same time. They must metabolise all substances absorbed by the gut whilst also metabolising all agents already present (from whatever source) in the peripheral circulation. This would not be possible through the conventional way that organs are usually supplied with blood from a single arterial route carrying oxygen and nutrients, leading to a capillary bed that becomes a venous outflow back to the heart and lungs. The circulation of the liver and the gut have evolved anatomically to solve this problem by receiving a conventional arterial supply and a venous supply from the gut *simultaneously* (Figure 2.3); all the blood eventually leaves the organ through the hepatic vein towards the inferior vena cava.

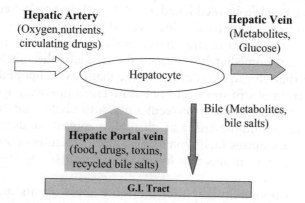

Figure 2.3 The hepatocytes can simultaneously metabolise xenobiotics in the circulation and those absorbed from the gut through their dual circulation of venous and arterial blood. Metabolites escape in the hepatic vein for eventual renal excretion, whilst biliary metabolites reach the gut

The hepatic arterial blood originates from the aorta, and the venous arrangement is known as the hepatic portal system, which subsequently miniaturises inside the liver into *sinusoids,* which are capillary blood-filled spaces. This capillary network effectively routes everything absorbed from the gut direct to the hepatocytes, which are bathed at the same time in oxygenated arterial blood. Metabolic products can leave the hepatocytes through the hepatic vein or by a separate system of *canalicali,* which ultimately form the bile duct, which leads to the gut. So, essentially, there are two blood routes into the hepatocytes and one out, which ensures that no matter how a xenobiotic enters the body, it will be presented to the hepatocytes for biotransformation.

Aims of biotransformation

Although you can see some of the many functions of CYPs and other biotransformational enzymes (Figure 2.2), it is essential to be clear on what they have to achieve with a given molecule. Looking at many endogenous substances like steroids and xenobiotic agents, such as drugs, all these compounds are mainly lipophilic. Drugs often parallel endogenous molecules in their oil solubility, although many are considerably more lipophilic than these molecules. Generally, drugs, and xenobiotic compounds, have to be fairly oil soluble or they would not be absorbed from the GI tract. Once absorbed these molecules could change structure and function of living systems and their oil solubility makes these molecules rather 'elusive', in the sense that they can enter and leave cells according to their concentration and are temporarily beyond the control of the living system. This problem is compounded by the difficulty encountered by living systems in the removal of lipophilic molecules. As previously mentioned in section 1.3, even after the kidney removes them from blood by filtering them, the lipophilicity of drugs, toxins and endogenous steroids means that as soon as they enter the collecting tubules, they can immediately return to the tissue of the tubules, as this is more oil-rich than the aqueous urine. So the majority of lipophilic molecules can be filtered dozens of times and only low levels are actually excreted. In addition any high lipophilicity molecules like insecticides and fire retardants might never leave adipose tissue at all (unless moved by dieting or breast feeding, which mobilizes fats). Potentially these molecules could stay in our bodies for years. This means that for lipophilic agents:

- The more lipophilic they are, the more these agents are trapped in membranes, affecting fluidity and causing disruption at high levels;

- If they are hormones, they are exerting an irreversible effect on tissues that is outside normal physiological control;

- If they are toxic, they can potentially damage endogenous structures;

- If they are drugs, they are also free to exert any pharmacological effect for a considerable period of time.

The aims of a biotransformational system are to assemble endogenous molecules and then clear these and related chemicals from the organism. These aims relate to *control* for endogenous steroid hormones (assembly and elimination), as well as *protection*, in the case of highly lipophilic threats, like drugs, toxins and hormone 'mimics'. Metabolizing systems have developed mechanisms to control balances between hormone synthesis, and clearance provides a dynamic equilibrium for the organism to finely control the effects of potent hormones such as sex-steroids. These systems also adapt to the presence of drugs and act to eliminate them.

Task of biotransformation

Essentially, the primary function of biotransforming enzymes such as CYPs is to 'move' a drug, toxin or hormone from the left-hand side of Figure 2.1 to the right-hand side. This means making very oil-soluble molecules highly water-soluble. This sounds impossible at first and anyone who has tried to wash his or her dishes without using washing up liquid will testify to this problem. However, if the lipophilic agents can be structurally altered, so changing their physicochemical properties, they can be made to dissolve in water. Once they are water-soluble, they can easily be cleared by the kidneys into urine and they will be finally excreted.

Phases I–III of biotransformation

Most lipophilic agents that invade living systems, such as aromatic hydrocarbons, hormones, drugs and various toxins, vary in their chemical stability, but many are relatively stable in physiological environments for quite long periods of time. This is particularly true of polycyclic aromatics. This means that a considerable amount of energy must be put into any process that alters their structures. This energy expenditure will be carried out pragmatically. This means that some molecules may require several changes to attain water solubility, such as polycyclics, whilst others such as lorazepam, only one. The stages of biotransformation are usually described as 'Phases' I, II and III. Phase I metabolism mainly describes oxidative CYP reactions, but non-CYP oxidations such as reductions and hydrolyses are also sometimes included in the broad term 'Phase I'. This has been highlighted as rather arbitrary and inconsistent and it is recommended that it is more accurate to refer to a particular process specifically, rather than using the loose term 'Phase I'.

The term 'Phase II' describes generally conjugative processes, where water-soluble endogenous sugars, salts or amino acids are attached to xenobiotics or endogenous chemicals. The very term 'Phase II' suggests that 'Phase I' processes must necessarily occur prior to conjugative reactions with a molecule. Although this does often happen, conjugation also occurs directly without prior 'preparation' by oxidative processes. The products of 'Phase II' are also strongly associated with detoxification and high water solubility. This is not always the case either and it is important to realise that some conjugative 'Phase II' processes can form either toxic species, or metabolites even less water-soluble than the parent drug. The more recent term 'Phase III' describes the system of efflux pumps that excludes water-soluble products of metabolism from the cell to the interstitial fluid, blood and finally the kidneys. The efflux pumps can also exclude drugs as soon as they are absorbed from the gut, as well as metabolites. Although the Phase I–III terminology remains popular and thus is sometimes used in this book, it is important to recognise the limitations of these terms in the description of many processes of biotransformation.

Biotransformation has a secondary effect, in that there is so much structural change in these molecules that pharmacological action is often removed or greatly diminished. Even if the metabolite retained some potential pharmacodynamic effects, its increased polarity compared with the parent drug means that the Phase III systems are likely to remove it relatively quickly, so diminishing any effects it might have exerted on the target tissue.

The use of therapeutic drugs is a constant battle to pharmacologically influence a system that is actively undermining the drugs' effects by removing them as fast as possible. The three phases of metabolism thus clear a variety of chemicals from the body into the urine or faeces, in the most rapid and efficient manner. The phases of metabolism also sense and detect increases in certain lipophilic substances and the systems increase their capability to respond to the increased load. The next chapter will outline how Phase I CYP-mediated systems achieve their aim of converting stable lipophilic agents to water-soluble products.

3 How Oxidative Systems Metabolize Substrates

3.1 Introduction

It is essential for living systems to control lipophilic molecules, but as mentioned earlier, these molecules can be rather 'elusive' to a biological system. Their lipophilicity means that they may be poorly water-soluble and may even become trapped in the first living membrane they encounter. To change the physicochemical structure and properties of these molecules they must be conveyed somehow through a medium that is utterly hostile to them, i.e. a water-based bloodstream, to a place where the biochemical systems of metabolism can physically attack these molecules.

3.2 Capture of lipophilic molecules

Virtually everything we consume, such as food, drink and drugs that are absorbed by the gut, will proceed to the hepatic portal circulation. This will include a wide physicochemical spectrum of drugs, from water-soluble to highly lipophilic agents. Charged, or water-soluble agents (if they are absorbed) may pass through the liver into the circulation, followed by filtration by the kidneys and elimination. The most extreme compounds at the end of the lipophilic spectrum will be absorbed with fats in diet via the lymphatic system and some will be trapped in membranes of the gut. The majority of predominantly lipophilic compounds will eventually enter the liver. As mentioned in the previous chapter, the main functional cell concerned with drug metabolism in the liver is the hepatocyte. In the same way that most of us can successfully cook foodstuffs in our kitchens at high temperatures without injury, hepatocytes are physiologically adapted to carry out millions of high-energy, potentially destructive reactive biochemical processes every second of the day without cell damage occurring. Indeed, it could be argued that hepatocytes have adapted to this function to the point that they are biochemically

Human Drug Metabolism, Michael D. Coleman
© 2005 John Wiley & Sons, Ltd

the most resistant cells to toxicity in the whole body – more of those adaptations later.

In the previous chapter it was outlined how the circulation of the liver and gut were adapted to deliver xenobiotics to the hepatocytes. The next task is 'subcellular', that is to route these compounds to the CYPs themselves inside the hepatocytes. To attract and secure highly physicochemically 'slippery' and elusive molecules such as lipophilic drugs requires a particular subcellular adaptation in hepatocytes, known as the smooth endplasmic reticulum (SER; Figure 3.1). You will be aware of the rough endoplasmic reticulum (RER) from biochemistry courses, which resembles an assembly line where ribosomes 'manufacture' proteins. Regarding the SER, an analogy for this organelle's structure is like the miles of tubing inside a cooling tower in a power station. The most lipophilic areas of the SER are the walls of these irregular tubing-like structures, rather than the inside (lumen). The drugs/toxins essentially flow along inside the thickness of the walls of the SER's tubular structure (Figure 3.1) straight into the path of the CYP monooxygenases. This is a highly lipophilic environment in a lipid-rich cell within a lipid-rich organ, so in a way, it is a 'conveyor belt' along which lipophilic molecules are drawn along once they enter the liver for two reasons. Firstly, their lipophilicity excludes them from the aqueous areas of the cell and secondly, the CYPs metabolize them into more water-soluble agents. This 'repels' the metabolites from the SER, so they leave and enter the lumen, so creating and maintaining a concentration gradient, which causes the lipophilic agents to flow towards the P450s in the first place.

3.3 Cytochrome P450s classification and basic structure

CYPs belong to a group of enzymes which all have similar core structures and modes of operation. Although these enzymes were discovered in 1958, despite vast amounts of research we still do not know exactly how they work or the many fine details of their structure. Currently, CYPs are classified according to their amino acid sequence homology, that is, if two CYPs have 40 per cent of their amino acid structure in common they are assumed to belong to the same 'family'. Overall, there are over 70 CYP families, of which around 17 have been found in humans. The families are numbered, such as CYP1, CYP2, CYP3, etc. Subfamilies are identified as having 55 per cent sequence homology; these are identified by using a letter and there are often several subfamilies in each family. So you might see CYP1A, CYP2A, CYP2B, CYP 2C, etc. Finally, individual 'isoforms', which originate from a single gene, are given a number, such as CYP1A1, CYP1A2, etc.

The amino acid sequences of many bacterial, yeast and mammalian enzymes are now well known and this has underlined the large differences

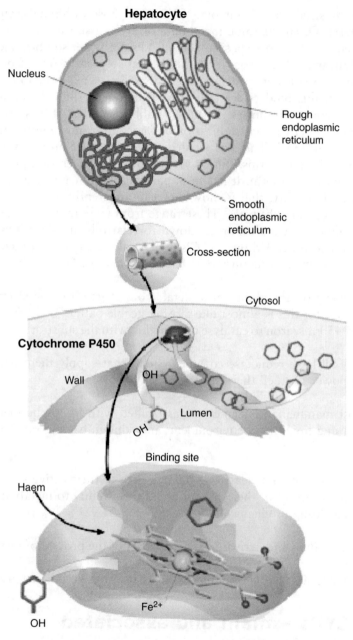

Figure 3.1 Location of CYP enzymes in the hepatocyte and how lipophilic species are believed to approach the enzymes active site

between the structures of our own CYPs and those of animals, eukaryotes and bacteria. Often the same metabolite of a given substance will be made by different CYPs across species. Some CYPs are water-soluble, such as the yeast P450cam, which was crystallized relatively early on, affording the opportunity to study it in detail. As mammalian CYPs function in a lipid environment, this renders crystallization exceedingly difficult. However, by making certain compromises, in 2000 a rabbit CYP (2C5) was crystallized, followed in 2003 by the crystallization of some of the most important human CYPs, 2C9 and 3A4. This has yielded a great deal of information on the structure of these isoforms, but as yet the complete operating procedure of these enzymes is not clear. It has been particularly difficult to determine the key to their flexibility; that is, how they can apparently recognize and bind so many groups of substrates. These range from large molecules such as the immunosuppressant cyclosporine, down to relatively small entities such as ethanol and acetone. Although CYPs in general are capable of metabolizing almost any chemical structure, they have a number of features in common:

- They exploit the ability of a metal, iron, to gain or lose electrons. An analogy for this is almost like a rechargeable battery in a children's toy. All P450s use iron to catalyse the reaction with the substrate (Figure 3.1).

- They all have reductase enzyme systems that supply them with reducing power to 'fuel' their metabolic activities.

- Most mammalian enzymes are associated with lipophilic membranes, exist in a lipid 'microenvironment' and contain haem groups as part of their structures.

- They all contain at least one binding area in their active site, which is the main source of their variation and their ability to metabolize a particular group of chemicals.

- They all bind and activate oxygen as part of the process of metabolism.

- They are all capable of reduction reactions that do not require oxygen.

3.4 CYPs – main and associated structures

Hydrophobic pocket

It is useful to take the trouble to visualize a CYP isoform in three dimensions in such a way that you could somehow approach and travel into the CYP with a TV camera, like one of those underwater exploration documentaries on the

Titanic. This really helps in understanding how structure relates to function in these enzymes. As you approach the enzyme from the outside, you would see an expanse of a protein framework of many hundreds of amino acid residues. You would spot the entrance to the enzyme, known as the access channel. This is designed to ensure that the substrate does not bind or become retarded on its way through to the enzyme active site, a term which can be taken to mean the area where the substrate binds as well as where metabolism takes place. Your camera would then proceed down the channel to the site where the substrate is bound, which is sometimes known as the hydrophobic 'pocket', although not all P450 substrates are entirely hydrophobic. The hydrophobic pocket consists of many amino acid residues that can bind a molecule by a number of means, including weak van der Waals' forces, hydrogen bonding, as well as other interactions between electron orbitals of phenyl groups, such as 'pi-pi bond stacking'. This provides a grip on the substrate in a number of places in the molecule, preventing excessive movement.

There are two ingenious aspects to this process that are particularly striking. The first is how the enzyme has evolved to orient a particular type of substrate in the direction that presents the most vulnerable and therefore most easily oxidized part of the molecule. The second is how the enzyme does not bind the molecule so strongly that it cannot be released easily, but it is secure enough to be metabolized by the oxidizing portion of the enzyme. This latter process is influenced by the change in structure of the molecule caused by the CYP that makes it more polar and usually less likely to bind to the CYP. It is useful to bear in mind that enzymes such as neural acetyl cholinesterase have had millions of years to evolve around metabolizing one substrate, acetylcholine, which never changes. However, CYPs have evolved to metabolize successfully a vast array of exogenous as well as endogenous substrates; indeed, CYPs already have the capability to metabolize virtually any one of the millions of man-made molecules synthesized for the forseeable future.

Haem moiety

Returning to the CYP enzyme structure, below the hydrophobic pocket, on the 'floor' of the enzyme, is the haem structure, which is also known as ferriprotoporphyrin-9 (F-9; Figure 3.2). The F-9 is the highly specialized lattice structure that supports a CYP iron molecule, which is the core of the enzyme. This is the area of the enzyme where the iron will catalyse the oxidation of part of the xenobiotic molecule. This part of the CYP is basically the same for all CYP enzymes; indeed, F-9 is a convenient way of positioning and maintaining iron in a number of other enzymes, such as haemoglobin, myoglobin and catalase. The iron is normally secured by attachment to five other molecules; in the horizontal plane, four of them are pyrrole nitrogens, whilst the fifth group, a sulphur atom from a cysteine amino acid residue holds the iron in a vertical plane. This is known as the 'pentacoordinate' (five-position) state

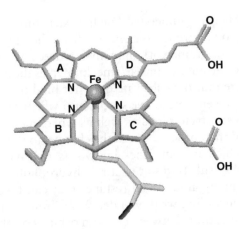

Figure 3.2   Main structural features of ferriprotoporphyrin-9, showing the iron anchored in five positions (pentacoordinate form). The cysteinyl sulphur is holds the iron from below

and could be described as the 'resting' position, prior to interaction with any other ligand (Figure 3.2).

The pentacoordinate state appears to show iron bound tightly to the sulphur and below the level of the nitrogens. When the iron binds another ligand, it is termed 'hexacoordinate' and iron appears to move 'upwards' and draws level with the nitrogens to bind a water molecule which is hydrogen bonded to a threonine amino acid residue that is located just above the iron, which is linked with proton movements during operation of the enzyme. The F-9 is held in place by hydrogen bonding and a number of amino acid residues, particularly an argenine residue, which may also stabilize the F-9 molecule. The iron is crucial to the catalytic function of CYP enzymes, and the process whereby they oxidize their substrates requires a supply of electrons, which is carried initially by NADPH. The electrons are carried to the CYP by the 'fuel pump' of the system, the NADPH CYP reductase enzyme complex.

NADPH cytochrome P450 reductase

This is a separate enzyme and not part of mammalian CYPs but it is closely associated with the CYP. NADPH reductases are found in most tissues, but they are particularly common in the liver. The expression of this enzyme is mainly under the control of the active thyroid hormone, triiodothyronine. The reductase is a flavoprotein complex, which consists of two equal components, FAD (flavin adenine dinucleotide) and FMN (flavin mononucleotide). Although in tissues, NADH (used in oxidative metabolic reactions) can be plentiful, FAD has evolved to discriminate strongly in favour of NADPH, which fuels reductive reactions. NADPH is formed by the con-

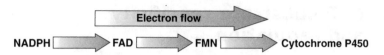

Figure 3.3 CYP reductase uses NADPH to provide electrons for CYP-mediated metabolic processes

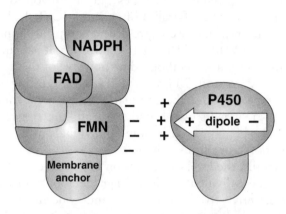

Figure 3.4 Position of CYP reductase in relation to CYP enzyme and the direction of flow of electrons necessary for CYP catalysis

sumption of glucose by the pentose phosphate pathway in the cytoplasm. This oxidative system, which can consume up to 30 per cent of the glucose in the liver, produces NADPH to power all reductive reactions related to CYPs, fatty acid and steroid synthesis, as well as the maintenance of the major cellular protectant thiol, glutathione (Chapter 8).

Hepatic NADPH reductase can be seen as the 'fuel pump' for the CYP it serves (Figure 3.3). It uses NADPH to supply the two electrons necessary for the cycling of the CYP. As CYPs run continuously like a machine tool, a constant flow of electrons is necessary to maintain CYP metabolism.

The reductase is embedded next to the CYP in the SER membrane and operates as follows: FAD is reduced by NADPH, which is then released as NADP+ (Figure 3.4). FAD then carries two electrons as $FADH_2$ that it passes on to FMN, forming $FMNH_2$, which in turn passes its two electrons to the CYP. In the lung, these enzymes have a toxicological role, as they mediate the metabolism of the herbicide paraquat, which occasionally features in accidental and suicidal poisonings. The reduction of paraquat by the enzyme leads to a futile cycle that generates vast amounts of oxidant species, which destroy the non-ciliated 'Clara' cells of the lung leading to subsequent death several days later. To date there is still no known antidote to paraquat poisoning and it is an agonizing and drawn-out method of suicide. These enzymes are also implicated in the reduction of nitroaromatic amines to carcinogens (Chapter 8).

3.5 CYP substrate specificity and regulation

The design of the access channel and hydrophobic pocket are the keys to the flexibility of these enzymes, and certainly the pockets vary hugely within the main families of CYPs. Aside from CYPs that are involved in steroid production, there are three main families of enzymes (CYP 1, 2 and 3) and 11 individual CYP enzymes that are expressed in a typical human liver (CYPs 1A2, 2A6, 2B6, 2C8/9/18/19, 2D6, 2E1 and 3A4/5). It is believed that 9 out of 10 drugs in use today are metabolized by only five of these isoforms; *CYPs 1A2, 2C9, 2C19, 2D6* and *3A4/5*. CYP2E1 is interesting mostly from a toxicological perspective and the internal regulation of small hydrophilic molecules. Each CYP has its own broad substrate 'preferences', and in some cases they may not be expressed in some individuals at all, or in very low levels (CYP2D6 polymorphisms; Chapter 7).

However, generally, the level of expression of any given CYP and therefore the capability of the individual to clear drugs metabolized by that isoform is almost always sensitive to substrate type and concentration. Increases in certain substrate levels, known as inducers, lead to a dynamic increase in CYP expression in the liver, lung and kidneys, a process known as induction (Chapter 4). Inducers are often lipophilic and/or quite bulky molecules that accelerate the clearance of all other drugs cleared by the particular induced CYP. This process can lead to the inducer causing its own and co-administered drug plasma levels to fall below the therapeutic window. An exception to this process is CYP2D6, which cannot be induced in this fashion. CYP2D6 is the most studied 'polymorphic' isoform of CYPs, as a varying proportion of patients (depending on ethnic group) express an abnormally low level of 2D6. This means that these 'poor metabolizers' cannot easily clear 2D6 substrates and the drugs accumulate, leading to toxicity in some cases. There are several polymorphisms in CYPs that have varying toxicological and pharmacological impact on patients (Chapter 7). The main human families of CYPs have been extensively studied over the last 15 years and a summary of what is known of these enzymes is given below. In Appendix D, a more extensive list of substrates, inhibitors and inducers of the main clinically relevant human CYPs can be found.

3.6 Main human CYP families

CYP 1A series

CYP 1A1

This isoform binds and oxidizes planar aromatic, essentially flat molecules. These compounds are multiples of benzene, such as naphthalene (two benzenes), and what are usually termed polycyclic aromatic hydrocarbons (PAHs) that are many benzene molecules in chains. Interestingly, it is 'non-constitutive' in the liver, i.e. it is not normally expressed or found in the liver. This is probably because its natural function is not needed in the liver and an individual would not normally be exposed to large amounts of planar aromatic hydrocarbons that might accumulate in the liver. However, the enzyme is found in other tissues, such as the lung, where aromatics are more frequently encountered from traffic pollution and smoking. Smokers exhibit high levels of this CYP in their lungs and this is linked with effects of the epoxides CYP1A1 can form from PAHs. These products vary in their stability and the most reactive, such as those from benzpyrene derivatives, are carcinogenic. There is also some evidence of higher levels of CYP1A1 in breast cancer sufferers. Although CYPs have evolved to clear potential threats to the organism, CYP1A1 is polymorphic (Chapter 7) and can appear to be more of a threat than a protection, as it is often expressed in high levels in the vicinity of carcinogenesis.

CYP1A2

This originates from a gene on chromosome 15 in humans and it is linked with oestrogen metabolism, as it is capable of oxidizing this series of hormones. Increased levels of this enzyme are also associated with colon cancer. 1A2 oxidizes planar aromatic molecules that contain aromatic amines, which its relative CYP1A1 does not. 1A2 orientates aromatic amines, some of which are quite large, in such a way as to promote the oxidation of the amine group. Consequently, this enzyme is able to metabolize a variety of drugs that resemble aromatic amines: these include caffeine, β-naphthylamine (a known carcinogen) and theophylline. The enzyme is also capable of oxidizing several tricyclic antidepressants. It tends to be inhibited by molecules that are planar, and possess a small volume to surface area ratio. It is blocked by the methylxanthine derivative furafylline.

CYP2 series

Around 18–30 per cent of human CYPs are in this series, making it the largest single group of CYPs in man. They appear to have evolved to oxidize various sex hormones, so their expression levels can differ between the sexes. As with many other CYPs, they are flexible enough to recognize many potential toxins such as drugs.

CYP2A6

This was originally of interest as it is responsible for the metabolism of nicotine to cotinine, as well as the further hydroxylation of cotinine. More recently, the polymorphisms (absence of the expression of the enzyme in a small proportion of patients: Chapter 7) associated with this CYP have indicated that it has a role in smoking behaviour. 2A6 comprises up to 10 per cent of total liver CYP content and is the only CYP that clears coumarin to 7-hydroxycoumarin, which has been used as the major marker for this CYP for many years. Methoxalen (an antipsoriatic agent) is a potent mechanism-based (Chapter 5) inhibitor of 2A6, as is grapefruit juice, although it is also weakly inhibited by imidazoles (e.g. ketoconazole). 2A6 has toxicological significance, in that it oxidizes carcinogens such as aflatoxins, 1,3 butadiene (Chapter 8) and nitrosamines. It tends to have a small role in the metabolism of a number of drugs and mutagens, but it is often difficult to determine how large a contribution 2A6 is making in the metabolism of these substrates. This CYP is clinically inducible by anticonvulsants such as phenobarbitone and the antibacterial rifampicin, although a number of other drugs may also induce it.

CYP2B6

This originates from a gene found on chromosome 19, although it is less well known than many other CYPs, partly due to a lack of experimental inhibitors. The 2B series have been extensively investigated in animals, but 2B6 is the only 2B form found in man. Antibodies generated towards this isoform have shown that it is likely to be found in all human livers and not subject to sex differences, but it has been suggested that there is a polymorphism in less than 5 per cent of Caucasians. This isoform will oxidize amfebutamone (bupropion), mephenytoin, some coumarins, cyclophosphamide and its relatives, as well as methadone. It is inducible by rifampicin, phenobarbitone and the DDT substitute pesticide methoxychlor. This pesticide acts as an endocrine disruptor when it is oxidized to pro-oestrogenic metabolites by a number of human CYPs including CYP2B6. It has also been observed that CYP2B6 hydroxylates at highly specific areas of molecules, particularly close to methoxy groups, which suggests that it may have a biosynthetic role in the assembly of specific endogenous molecules.

CYP2C8

This originates on chromosome 10 and is one of four CYP2C isoforms (the others are CYP2C9, 18 and 19) which comprise about 18 per cent of total CYP content which share 80 per cent amino acid sequence identity, although CYP2C8 is the most unusual of the four and is of interest for its metabolism of the anti-cancer agent taxol, verapamil, cerivastatin (now withdrawn), amodiaquine and rosiglitazone. Although 2C8 is similar in structure to 2C9, it differs catalytically concerning several drugs, metabolizing tolbutamide more slowly than 2C9, but clearing trans-retinoic acid more efficiently. Warfarin is cleared by CYP2C9 to a 4-hydroxy metabolite, whilst 2C8 forms a 5-hydroxy derivative. The different binding orientations of substrates such as diclofenac that both 2C9 and 2C8 metabolize are related to differences between the hydrophobicity and geometry of the respective binding sites. CYP2C8 can be inhibited by quercetin, the glitazone drugs, gemfibrozil and diazepam in high concentrations, although it is inducible by rifampicin and phenobarbitone. This CYP is also thought to be polymorphic (Chapter 7).

CYP2C9

The recent crystallization of CYP2C9 has informed a great deal about its structure as related to function. It has evolved to process relatively small, acidic and lipophilic molecules, although no basic amino acid residues have been found in the active site to attract and bind acidic molecules. It is thought that the design of the access channel may be responsible for this enzyme's preference for acidic molecules. There are a large number of substrates for this CYP, which include tolbutamide, dapsone and warfarin. The active site is large and it appears that there is more than one place where drugs can bind. With warfarin, there appears to be a primary recognition site, which is too far from the catalytic area of the enzyme (the iron) for the drug to be metabolized. It has been suggested that the events of the catalysis of the substrate automatically promote binding of the next substrate molecule, possibly through allosteric mechanisms. Sulphafenazole is a potent inhibitor of this polymorphic enzyme and it is inducible by rifampicin and phenobarbitone.

CYP2C19

This is also inducible and differs by only around 10 per cent of its amino acids from 2C9, but it does not oxidize acidic molecules, indicating that the active sites and access channels are subtly different. CYP2C19 metabolizes omeprazole, a common ulcer medication. CYP2C19 is inducible (rifampicin) and polymorphisms in this gene exist and there is a higher incidence of poor metabolizer phenotypes in Asians (23 per cent) vs Caucasians (3–5 per cent). This means that parent drug can accumulate in poor metabolizers, leading to toxicity (Chapter 7). Tranylcypromine acts as a potent inhibitor of 2C19.

CYP2D6

This is responsible for more than 70 different drug oxidations. This enzyme is non-inducible, but is strongly subject to polymorphisms (Chapter 7), with around 7–10 per cent of Caucasians expressing poorly, or even non-functioning enzyme. Since there may be no other way to clear these drugs from the system, poor metabolizers may be at severe risk from adverse drug reactions. Quinidine inhibits this enzyme. Relatively little is found in the gut, and it comprises about 2–4 per cent of the CYPs in human liver. There are several groups of drugs that are metabolized by CYP2D6, these include:

- antiarrhythmics: (flecainide, mexiletine);

- TCAs, SSRI and related antidepressants: (amitriptyline, paroxetine, venlafaxine, fluoxetine);

- antipsychotics: (chlorpromazine, haloperidol);

- beta-blockers: (labetalol, timolol, propanolol, pindolol, metoprolol);

- analgesics: (codeine, fentanyl, meperidine, propoxyphene).

CYP2E1

This comprises around 7 per cent of human liver P450 and is unusual as a mammalian CYP in that it oxidizes small heterocyclic agents, ranging from pyridine through to ethanol, acetone and other small ketones (methyl ethyl ketone). Ethanol and acetone are strong inducers of this isoform. Many of its substrates are water-soluble and it is often implicated in toxicity, as the metabolites it forms can be highly reactive and toxic to tissues. It is responsible for the oxidation of paracetamol, which will be dealt with in Chapter 8. There is a polymorphism associated with this gene that is more common in Chinese people. The mutation correlates with a two-fold increased risk of nasopharyngeal cancer linked to smoking. This is the second CYP isoform that may be related to smoking-induced cancers (see 1A1/2 above). Many sulphur-containing agents block this enzyme, such as carbon disulphide, diethyl dithio carbamate and antabuse.

CYP3 series

CYP3A4 and 3A5

These are virtually indistinguishable and present in roughly equal proportions in most individuals. These CYPs are responsible for the metabolism of more than 120 drugs. 3A4 has also been crystallized and details of its active site are under intense investigation. CYP3A4 comprises around 28 per cent of our total P450s. Indeed, the colour of a healthy liver with normal blood flow is actually partly due to this enzyme. It is also found in our intestinal walls in considerable quantity. Its major endogenous function is to metabolize steroids, but its active site is so large and flexible that a vast array of different molecules can undergo at least some metabolism by this enzyme The three-dimensional structure of 3A4 has been modelled using crystallographic analysis of several bacterial P450s, which emphasizes the closeness of our enzymes to those of the 'original owners', so to speak. CYP3A4 seems to resemble a bacterial CYP, BM-3 the most, but there are similarities with other bacterial CYPs that can metabolize erythromycin. It is clear that the human enzyme has a much larger active site compared with bacterial enzymes, which underlines its evolution to oxidize such a wide variety of substrates. As with CYP2C9, there is an access channel and a large active site with many points of potential hydrophobic binding. Binding studies with steroids and erythromycin again show the similarities with other CYP enzymes across various species. CYP3A4/5 are inducible through anticonvulsants, St John's Wort, phenytoin and rifampicin.

CYP3A4 *binding characteristics*

Before CYP crystal structures were available, the active sites were studied through a combination of mutagenesis and binding studies. Using bacterial or insect cell expression systems, human genes that expressed CYP3A4 were damaged by the use of mutagens in areas coding for specific amino acids that corresponded to the active site of the enzyme. This would, of course, change the binding characteristics of the damaged enzyme. Information gained from these studies shows that this enzyme binds more than one substrate at a time, in a similar manner to CYP2C9. On one level, if both substrates are the same, the process of one molecule being metabolized would allosterically adjust the mobility of the molecule on its binding site, making it easier or more difficult for it to be oriented for oxidation, thus modulating the process of CYP function. This is termed a 'homotropic' effect. This multi-site binding is yet more complex; studies with flavonoids have shown that they can bind at one place in the active site and at the same time stimulate the metabolism of a different type of molecule (PAHs) in another area of the active site. This simultaneous binding at two distinct but adjacent areas of the same broad site also is thought to be responsible for the inhibitory effects of one compound on the metabolism of another, which is termed a 'heterotropic' effect. Testosterone metabolism is partially competitively inhibited by erythromycin. Whilst in another chapter it will be explained how the amount of CYPs present in the liver is a response to substrate pressure (Chapter 4), it is now clear that there is a high degree of sophistication in control of function of all CYPs in various tissues as well as the liver. This is especially important in the liver, where fine-tuning of steroid levels is necessary in response to changes in menstrual cycles or pregnancy in women, as well as spermatogenesis formation in men, where various steroid molecules are required to maintain different levels relative to each other at specific times in the cycles. This allosterically based process of multi-site internal regulation of CYP function is just one of the mechanisms whereby hormone metabolism is controlled. The role of xenobiotics in this process, as you can imagine, is potentially exceedingly complex. It is also apparent how easily drugs or toxins can disrupt hormone regulatory processes.

As has been mentioned, the range of substrates that can be oxidized by CYP3A4 runs from bulky molecules such as cyclosporin A (molecular weight 1202), to small phenolics such as paracetamol. That a molecule of fungal origin such as cyclosporine can be easily and rapidly metabolized by CYP3A4, underlines the evolution of these enzymes to cope with the possibility of the ingestion of exogenous toxin molecules in the diet of humans.

Other substrates include: codeine (narcotic), diazepam (tranquillizer), erythromycin (antibiotic), lidocaine (anaesthetic), lovastatin (HMGCoA reductase inhibitor, a cholesterol-lowering drug), taxol (cancer drug), warfarin (anticoagulant).

Azole antifungal agents, such as ketoconazole and fluconazole, as well as anti-HIV agents such as ritonavir, inhibit CYP3A4. Due to the importance of this enzyme in the endogenous regulation of steroid metabolism, any inhibition can have serious consequences in the form of disruption of hormone control and more immediately, marked changes to the clearance of drugs metabolised by this CYP.

3.7   Cytochrome P450 catalytic cycle

Having established the multiplicity and flexibility of these enzymes, it should be a relief to learn that all these enzymes essentially function in the same way. Although CYPs can carry out reductions, their main function is to insert an oxygen molecule into a usually stable and hydrophobic compound. Many textbooks present this cycle, but it appears intimidating due to the many details involved. However, it is important to understand that there are only five main features of the process whereby the following equation is carried out:

$$\text{Hydrocarbon (---RH)} + O_2 + 2 \text{ electrons} + 2 \text{ H}^+ \text{ ions gives:}$$
$$\text{alcohol (---ROH)} + H_2O$$

1. Substrate binding

2. Oxygen binding

3. Oxygen scission (splitting)

4. Insertion of oxygen into substrate

5. Release of product

Substrate binding

The first step, as covered in the previous section, is the binding and orientation of the molecule. This must happen in such a way that the most vulnerable part of the agent must be presented to the active site of the enzyme, the iron, so the molecule can be processed with the minimum of energy expenditure and the maximum speed. The iron is in the ferric form when the substrate is first bound:

$$Fe^{3+}-RH$$

Once the substrate has been bound, the next stage is to receive the first of two electrons (in the form of NADPH) from CYP reductase, so reducing the iron:

$$Fe^{2+}-RH$$

Oxygen binding

The next stage involves the iron/substrate complex binding molecular oxygen from the lungs.

$$Fe^{2+}-RH$$
$$|$$
$$O_2$$

You will note that oxygen does not just exist as one atom. It is much more stable when it is found in a molecule of two oxygen atoms, O_2. Indeed, oxygen is almost never found in nature as a single atom as its outer electron orbitals only have 6 instead of the much more stable 8 electrons. To attain stability, two oxygen molecules will normally covalently bond so sharing 4 electrons, so this gives the same effect as having the stable 8 electrons. So to split an oxygen molecule requires energy, but this is like trying to separate two powerful electromagnets – the oxygen will tend to 'snap back' immediately to reform O_2 as soon as it is separated. So two problems arise: first, how to apply reducing power to split the oxygen and second, how to prevent the oxygen reforming immediately and keeping the single oxygen atom separate long enough for it to react with the vulnerable hydrocarbon substrate.

Oxygen scission (splitting)

To split the oxygen molecule into two atoms firstly requires a slow rearrangement of the $Fe^{2+} O_2$ complex to form

$$Fe^{3+} RH$$
$$|$$
$$O_{2-}$$

The next stage is the key to whether the substrate will be oxidized or not. This is the rate-limiting step of the cycle. A second electron from NADPH via the CYP reductase feeds into the complex and forms

$$\begin{array}{l} Fe^{3+}\ RH \\ | \\ O^2_2 \end{array}$$

or

$$\begin{array}{l} Fe^{3+}\ RH \\ | \\ O\text{--}O_{2-} \end{array}$$

As this stage of the process is so rapid it is not feasible to detect experimentally, so the most likely pathway has been worked out which corresponds to what is possible and what actually happens in terms of the products, which we can measure. Certainly an oxygen atom with two spare electrons is a very attractive prospect to two hydrogen atoms and water is formed, leaving a single oxygen atom bound to the iron of the enzyme. This solves the two problems described above; the oxygen molecule has been split, but it cannot just 'snap back' to form an oxygen molecule again, as water is stable and takes an oxygen molecule away from the enzyme active site.

Insertion of oxygen into substrate

The remaining oxygen is temporarily bound to the iron in a complex, which is sometimes termed a 'perferryl' complex (below).

$$\begin{array}{l} (Fe\text{---}O)^{3+} \\ | \\ RH \end{array}$$

There is also evidence to suggest that the perferryl complex is not the only way oxygen is bound to the iron. The group FeO_2^+ (peroxo-iron) form has also been suggested to take part in some CYP reactions.

The perferryl is thought to be the main method of oxygen binding to the CYP and it is exceedingly reactive and can activate the substrate by either removing hydrogen (hydrogen abstraction) or an electron (e.g. from nitrogen atoms) from part of the substrate molecule. These steps are not necessarily in that order and multiple electron or abstractions can take place. It is apparent that the hydrogen abstraction part of the process takes longer than the subsequent processes and is thought to be the 'rate-limiting step' in the oxidation process. The hydrogen to be removed will be closest to the carbon to be oxidized. The abstracted hydrogen is then bound to the perferryl complex. This leaves the carbon with a spare electron, which makes it a reactive radical, as seen below. The substrate, i.e. the carbon atom, has been activated which makes sense as it is now much more likely to react with the hydroxyl group.

$$(Fe—OH)^{3+}$$
$$|$$
$$R^{\cdot}$$

The final stage is the reaction between the newly created hydroxyl group and the carbon radical, yielding the alcohol, as seen below. The entry of the oxygen atom into the substrate is sometimes called the 'oxygen rebound' reaction.

$$Fe^{2+} \quad and \quad ROH$$

Release of product

The whole CYP catalytic process is as rapid as it is violent and often analogies for CYP function are equally dramatic, likening CYPs to blowtorches, or nailguns. Once the substrate has been converted to a metabolite, it has changed both structurally and physicochemically to the point that it can no longer bind to the active site of the CYP. The metabolite is thus released and the CYP isoform is now ready for binding of another substrate molecule. It is important to break down the function of CYPs to separate stages, so it can be seen how they operate and overcome the inherent problems in their function. However, students often find the catalytic cycle rather daunting to learn and can be intimidated by it. It is much easier to learn if you try to understand the various stages, and use the logic of the enzyme's function to follow how it overcomes the stability of substrate and oxygen by using electrons it receives from the adjacent reductase system to make the product. A simplified cycle is shown on Figure 3.5. As more research is carried out, fine details may change in the cycle, but the main features, the substrate binding, option for reduction, oxygen binding and activation, perferryl complex formation, abstractions of hydrogen or electrons and finally substrate release are well established.

3.8 Real-life operations

The detailed processes on how living systems operate are sometimes focused on at the expense of a global understanding of how these systems might

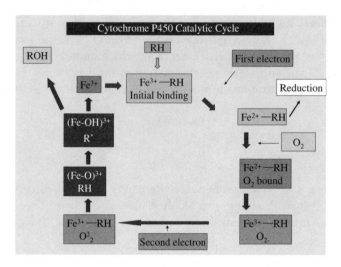

Figure 3.5   Simplified scheme of cytochrome P450 oxidation

operate in the tissue. It is useful to try to visualize how CYPs process massive numbers of molecules from hydrophobic to at least partially hydrophilic products every second. If you visualize just one hepatocyte, and imagine the smooth endoplasmic reticulum, with its massive surface area, with vast numbers of CYP and reductase molecules embedded in its tubing, then you can see how the liver can sometimes metabolize the majority of drugs and endogenous substrates in a given volume of blood in just one passage through the organ.

3.9   How CYP isoforms operate *in vivo*

Illustrative use of structures

Most textbooks at this point show a large number of chemical reactions that highlight how CYP isoforms metabolize specific drugs/toxins/steroids, etc. Many students might not have studied chemistry or may struggle with it as a subject and particularly dislike chemical structures. This is probably due to many reasons, not least because many structures can require some considerable effort to learn. However, simple basic components of drug molecules can be used to illustrate how CYP enzyme systems operate at the molecular level, and if you study the diagrams it should not be to difficult to eventually see a molecule in a way that approaches how a CYP enzyme might 'see' it.

Primary purposes of CYPs

As mentioned before, CYP isoforms have evolved to:

- Make a molecule less lipophilic (and often less stable) as rapidly as possible,

- Make some molecules more vulnerable to conjugation.

The first step is the binding of the substrate. As you will have seen, individual CYPs bind groups of very broadly similar chemical structures. This is partly achieved by the size of the molecule. For example, the entrance to CYP2C9 is not wide enough to bind part of a large molecule like cyclosporine, so this molecule is virtually excluded from all the CYPs, except the one with the largest entrance and binding site, CYP3A4. The molecule then enters the enzyme and binds to perhaps more than one site prior to presentation to the active site. The CYPs metabolize molecules that broadly conform to the characteristics of their binding sites. The process of binding the molecules is intended to orient them in such a way as to present the most vulnerable functional groups for metabolism.

Role of oxidation

CYP metabolism is almost always some form of oxidation, which can achieve their main aims. Oxidizing a molecule can have three main effects on it, as follows.

Increase in hydrophilicity

Forming a simple alcohol or phenol is often enough to make a molecule soluble in water so it can be eliminated without the need for any further metabolic input.

Reduction in stability leading to structural rearrangement

Obviously some chemical structures are inherently less stable than others and any prototype drugs that are unstable and have the potential to react with cellular structures are weeded out in the drug discovery process. However, the process of CYP-mediated metabolism, where a stable drug is structurally changed, can form a much more reactive and potentially toxic product (Chapter 8). A very young child hitting objects randomly with a piece of metal will not be able to discern the difference between an inert object and a extremely dangerous one (electrical equipment or an explosive device). In the same way, a molecule may be bound and metabolized by CYPs, irrespective of the impact these processes may have on the stability and potential toxicity of the product. There is a risk that the new molecule may be very reactive and dangerous indeed. Biological systems have anticipated this risk through the evolution of many conjugation systems that attenuate the reactivity of these agents (Chapter 6). Usually, the risk pays off and a molecule can be quite radically changed in terms of its physicochemical properties without problems: for example, a lipophilic functional group might be oxidized to an alcohol, which may be so unstable that it breaks off. This has the dual advantage of removing a lipophilic structure that leaves the molecule more hydrophilic (see the oxidation of terfenadine). It can also pave the way for Phase II metabolism of the molecule.

Facilitation for conjugation

Many oxidative metabolites are much more vulnerable than their parent molecules to reaction with water-soluble groups such as glucuronic acid and sulphates. Once a conjugate is formed, this vastly increases water solubility and Phase III transport systems will remove it from the cell and into the blood.

Summary of CYP operations

A sculptor was once asked how he would go about sculpting an elephant from a block of stone. His response was 'knock off all the bits that did not look like an elephant'. Similarly, drug-metabolizing CYPs have one main imperative, to make molecules more water-soluble. Every aspect of their structure and function, their position in the liver, their initial selection of substrate, binding, substrate orientation and catalytic cycling, is intended to accomplish this relatively simple aim.

With experience, you should be able to look at any drug or chemical and make a reasonable stab at suggesting how a CYP enzyme might metabolize it. It is important to see these enzymes not as carrying out thousands of different reactions, but as basically carrying out only two or three basic operations on thousands of different molecules every second.

3.10   Aromatic ring hydroxylation

Nature of aromatics

Large, highly lipophilic, planar and stable molecules with few, if any, vulnerable functional groups look to be a difficult proposition to metabolize

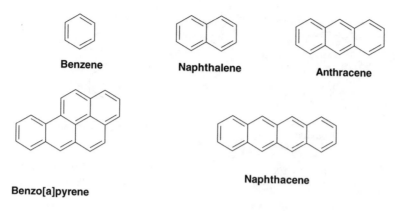

Benzene

Naphthalene

Anthracene

Naphthacene

Benzo[a]pyrene

Figure 3.6   Some aromatic hydrocarbon molecules

(Figure 3.6). Indeed, if there are any aliphatic groups, or non-aromatic rings associated with an aromatic molecule, these will often be attacked rather than the aromatic group. The ring hydroxylation of amphetamines is the exception to this. Polycyclic hydrocarbons are not easy to clear and they are perceived by living systems as a potent threat. This is reflected in the elaborate expression system (Ah/ARNT; next Chapter) which modulates the non-constitutive isoform CYP1A1, which has evolved to deal with them, which is highly effective. These include molecules such as those shown in Figure 3.6. The simplest aromatic is benzene and this can be oxidized by CYP1A1 eventually to phenol, which is more reactive, but more water-soluble than benzene and vulnerable to sulphation and glucuronidation during Phase II metabolism.

The oxidation of benzene

There are several intermediates formed during the oxidation of benzene (Figure 3.7). The two main routes are the cyclohexadienone and an epoxide; in the presence of water both stages will rearrange to form the phenol. During this process, the hydrogen atom close to the oxygen will sometimes be moved around on the ring, or even lost. This is known as the NIH shift.

Epoxidation is defined chemically as a reaction where an oxygen atom is joined to an unsaturated carbon to form a cyclic, three-membered ether. Epoxides are also known as arene oxides and vary enormously in their stability. This stability of an epoxide depends on the electron density of the double bond being oxidized: the higher the density, the more stable the epoxide. So epoxides of varying stability can be formed on the same molecule, due to differences in electron densities. This is apparent in benzpyrene. The anticonvulsant carbamazepine forms a number of epoxides and the 10,11 derivative is stable enough to be pharmacologically active, whilst bromobenzene 3,4 epoxide's half-life in blood is less than 14 seconds. Generally, arene oxides form phenols or diols in the presence of water (as does carba-

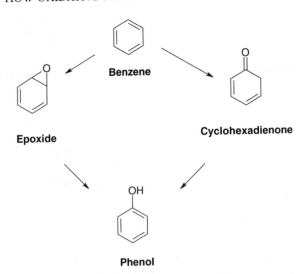

Figure 3.7   Main pathways of benzene hydroxylation

mazepine 10,11 epoxide), although the cytosolic enzyme epoxide hydrolase is present to accelerate this process.

The phenols and diols are usually substrates for sulphation or glucuronidation. Although the process of aromatic hydroxylation is difficult to achieve and the phenolic product is more hydrophilic, the structural features of the larger polycyclics mean that this process can lead to the formation of unstable carcinogenic reactive intermediates.

3.11   Alkyl oxidations

The saturated bonds of straight chain aliphatic molecules are very stable; indeed, they can be even harder to break into from the thermodynamic point of view than aromatic rings, whilst molecules with unsaturated bonds are the easiest to oxidize. Straight chain aliphatic molecules are easier to oxidize if they have an aromatic side chain. Alkyl derivatives are generally oxidized by the routes briefly described below.

Saturated alkyl groups

The oxidation of a saturated alkyl group can lead to the alcohol being inserted in more than one position (Figure 3.8). The 'end' carbon group of the molecule is sometimes called the 'omega' group and the oxidation can result in this group being turned into an alcohol (omega oxidation) or alternatively, the penultimate group (omega minus one).

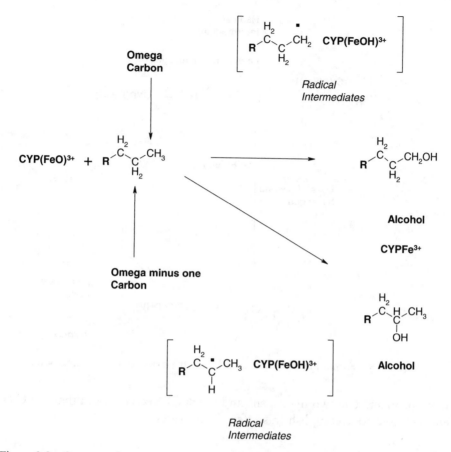

Figure 3.8 Omega and omega minus one carbon oxidation of aliphatic saturated (single bond) hydrocarbons by CYP isoforms

During the oxidation of saturated molecules (Figure 3.8) the CYP will operate as described in section 3.7, abstracting a hydrogen and causing the carbon molecule to form a radical. The carbon radical and the hydroxyl group then react to form the alcohol. Even though alkanes like hexane are very simple structures, they can be metabolized to a large number of derivatives (see 'Pathways of alkyl metabolism').

As well as the formation of alcohols, CYP isoforms can desaturate carbon–carbon double bonds to single unsaturated bonds (Figure 3.9). This process can occur alongside alcohol formation and is a good example of a CYP-mediated process that leads to quite considerable rearrangement of the molecule's structure. The first hydrogen is abstracted by the CYP isoform and may leave the FeO^{3+} complex, allowing it to grab a second hydrogen. The highly unstable adjacent carbon radicals rearrange to form an unsatu-

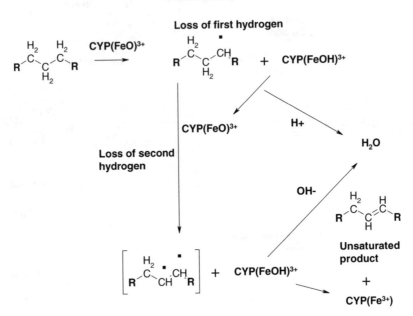

Figure 3.9 Formation of unsaturated bonds from a saturated starting point

rated product. The two hydrogens and the single oxygen atom that the CYP enzyme used to accomplish this effect form water.

Unsaturated alkyl groups

Unsaturated or double bonds are more electron-rich than saturated bonds, and as mentioned earlier, this makes them easier to oxidize and several possible products can be formed (Figure 3.10). These include an epoxide called an 'oxirane', as well as two carbonyl derivatives, or aldehydes, which can split the molecule.

Pathways of alkyl metabolism

A good example of where these pathways can lead is the complex metabolism of an otherwise apparently simple molecule, hexane (Figure 3.11). This hydrocarbon was once used as a volatile component of several adhesive mixtures, which were extensively applied in the leather and shoe industries. If you want an adhesive or paint to dry or cure quickly, the volatility of the carrier solvent is crucial. This makes the adhesive or paint easier to apply in

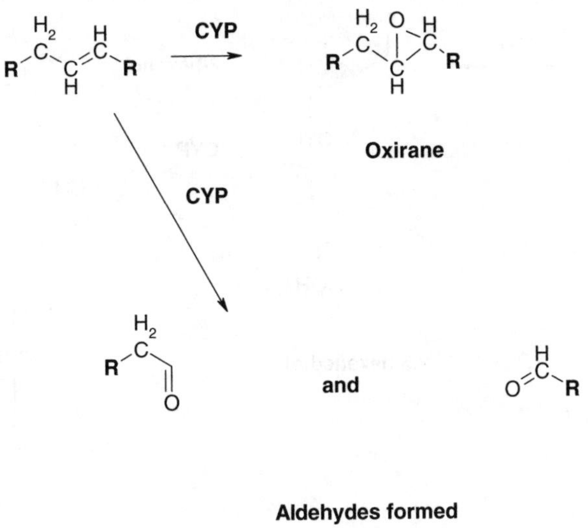

Oxirane

Aldehydes formed

Figure 3.10 Metabolism of unsaturated alkyl groups

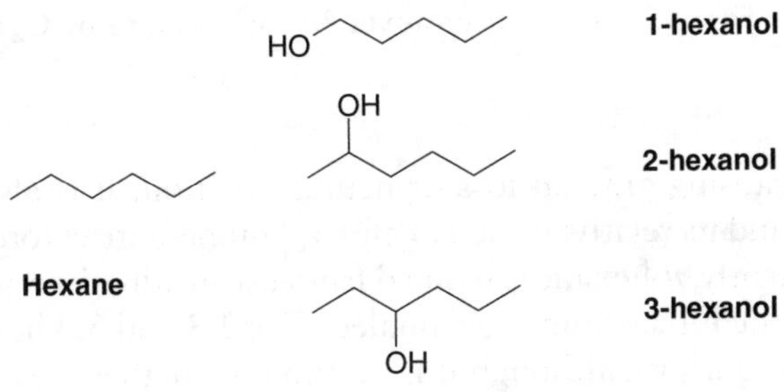

1-hexanol

2-hexanol

Hexane

3-hexanol

Figure 3.11 Oxidation of hexane to hexanols

a mass production setting. However, it was gradually realized that many people who used hexane-based adhesives in the leather industry were suffering from damage to the peripheral nervous system, known as peripheral neuropathy. This was a progressive effect and was traced to the hexane itself. In humans, hexane is cleared at first to several hexanols, which is logical, as a volatile, water-insoluble and highly lipophilic agent capable of causing intoxication will be a strong candidate for rapid clearance to an albeit only slightly water-soluble alcohol.

The 2-hexanol derivative undergoes further oxidative metabolism, initially to a diol, the 2,5 derivative (Figure 3.12), which can undergo further CYP isoform-mediated (probably by 2E1) oxidation to a di-ketone which is the 2,5 hexanedione derivative. This compound is unusual in that it is a specific neurotoxin. It disrupts neural cells by interfering with microtubule formation in

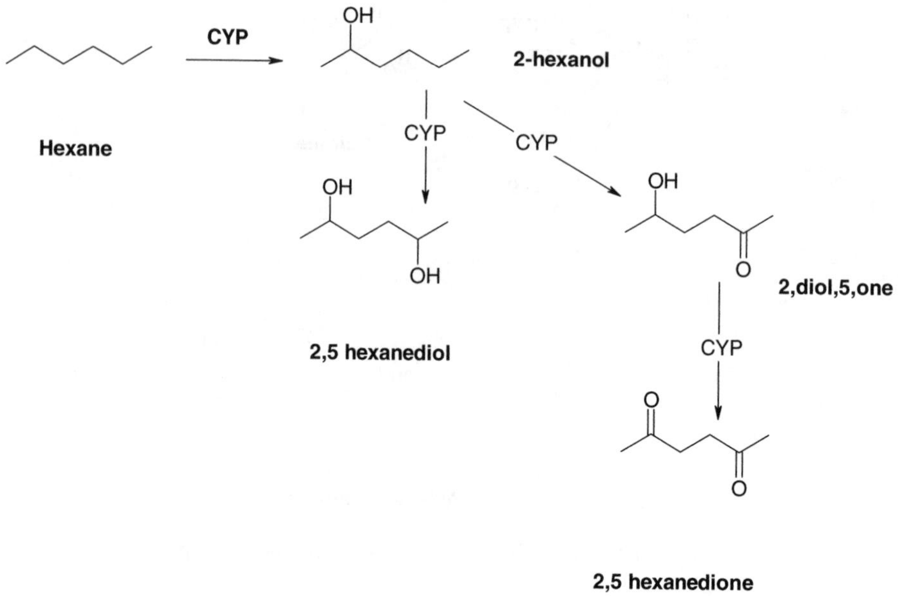

Figure 3.12   Formation of the neurotoxin 2,5 hexanedione by CYP oxidations

neural fibres, causing gradual loss of neural function. It is also cytotoxic to neuronal cells and its relatives, the 2,3 and 3,4 diones, are cytotoxic to cell cultures. Consequently, *n*-hexane is banned from use in adhesives and should only be used where the fumes cannot be inhaled. The 2,3 and 3,4 hexanediones are used as food colourings, although it is unknown whether they can be formed in human liver. Several isomers of hexane have been used as substitutes for hexane, although the potential neurotoxicity of adhesives that use volatile alkanes should never be underestimated.

3.12 'Rearrangement' reactions

The use of oxidation as a tool to rearrange molecules to less lipophilic products has the added benefits of unmasking other vulnerable groups and making the products simpler to conjugate. There are several CYP-mediated oxidations that have this effect on molecules.

Dealkylations

Alkyl groups, especially bulky ones, are very lipophilic and often are attached to drugs through 'hetero' atoms, i.e. nitrogens, oxygens and sulphurs. It makes sense to remove the alkyl group, leaving the hetero group vulnerable

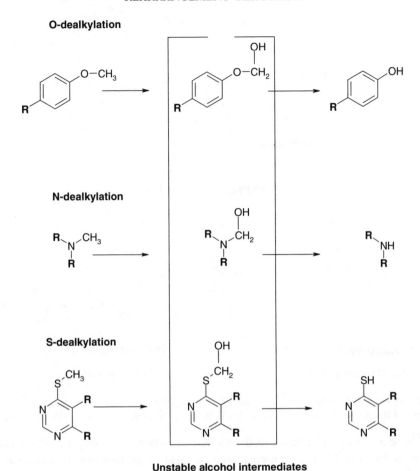

O-dealkylation

N-dealkylation

S-dealkylation

Unstable alcohol intermediates

Figure 3.13 Rearrangement reactions caused by the CYP-mediated oxidation of an alkyl group leading to the formation of a more water-soluble product, which is also more vulnerable to Phase II. The 'waste products' of the reactions are usually small aldehydes or ketones

for conjugation with glucuronides or sulphates (Figure 3.13). The quickest way to remove the alkyl group is to oxidize it to an alcohol. This should be a win–win situation, whether the product is stable or unstable, the alcohol (called a carbinolamine in the case of N-dealkylation) is usually unstable and splits off, forming an aldehyde. This reveals a less lipophilic heteroatom 'handle' for conjugation. If the alcohol is stable, then the drug is still more hydrophilic than it was and that might be a Phase II target also. With substituted aromatic compounds it is easier for the CYP to oxidize an alkyl substituent group than the ring. Another result of dealkylation can be the splitting of a large lipophilic molecule into two smaller more hydrophilic ones (Figure 3.14).

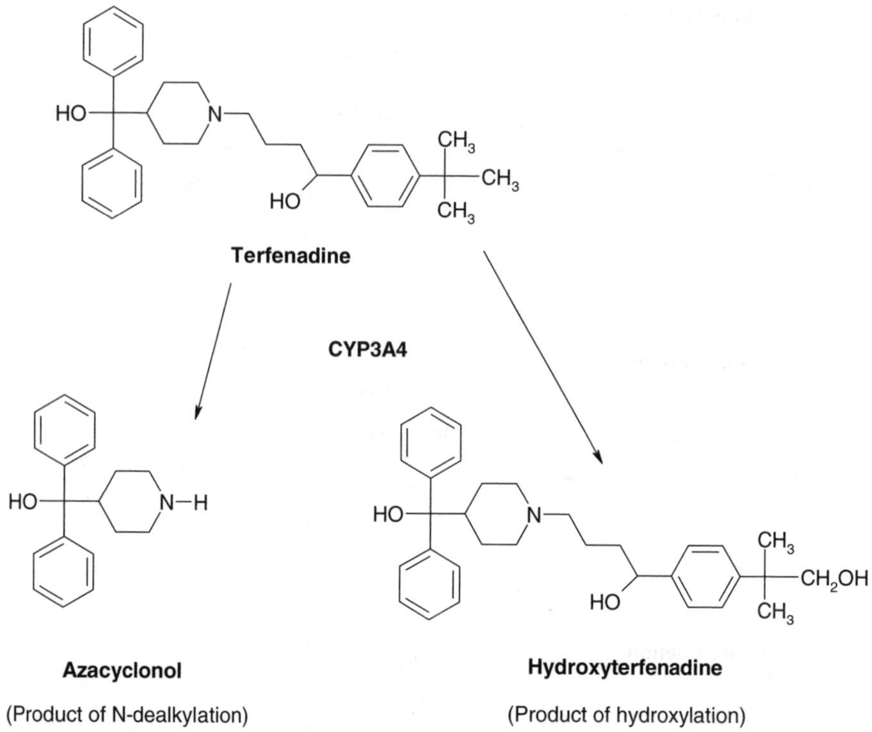

Figure 3.14 Metabolism of terfenadine: essentially the same oxidation reaction applied in two different areas of the molecule leads to vastly different effects on the structure

There are many examples of drugs that undergo this type of dealkylation. Imipramine, the TCA, is demethylated to form desmethyl imipramine, which also has pharmacological potency and is usually known as desipramine. The removal of one methyl group may not make much difference to the lipophilicity of a large molecule, although it may change its pharmacological effects. More than one alkyl group may have to be removed to make the compound appreciably less lipophilic. On the other hand, the N-dealkylation reaction of the antihistamine terfenadine has a much more dramatic effect (Figure 3.14). The oxidation of the alkyl group adjacent to the nitrogen causes an unstable alcohol to be formed, which splits away, taking half the molecule with it. Virtually the same reaction of alkyl oxidation at the other end of the parent molecule results in a stable alcohol that is then oxidized to a carboxy derivative, which is known as fexofenadine and is not metabolised further. It is less toxic than the parent drug (Chapter 5).

N-dealkylations mechanisms

N-dealkylation is only part of the picture of the metabolism of how CYPs can oxidize heteroatoms. Before N-dealkylation occurs, CYPs have the option

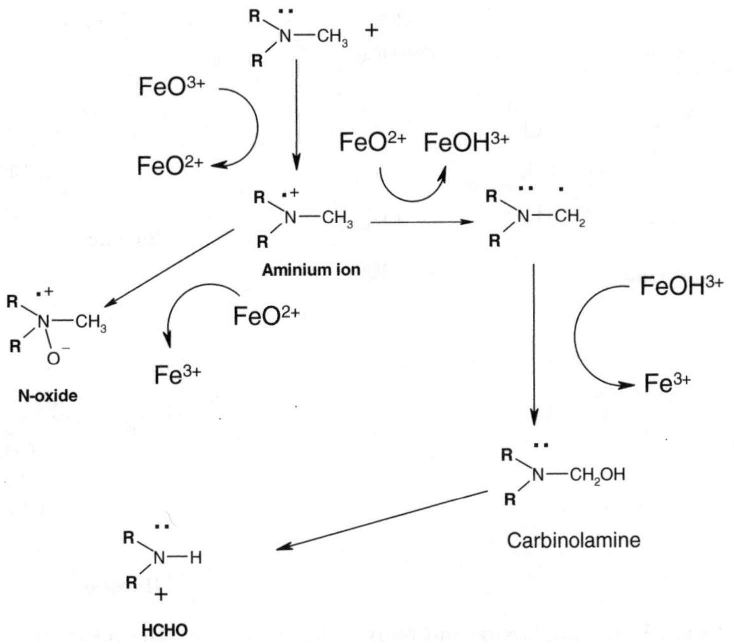

Figure 3.15   Pathways of CYP-mediated N-oxidation and N-dealkylation

of oxidizing the substituted nitrogen itself to form an N-oxide (Figure 3.15). If N-oxide formation does not occur, then N-dealkylation can proceed. Again, this is a 'win–win' process, as N-oxides are more water-soluble than the parent drug. Generally, flavin monooxygenases (next section) are credited with the majority of N-oxidations, but it has become apparent that CYPs can also accomplish them. Whether N-oxide formation or dealkylation occurs is dependent on factors such as the surrounding groups on the molecule and the CYP itself. The mechanism of N-oxidation and N-dealkylation is now believed to differ slightly from the majority of CYP-mediated hydrogen abstractions/oxygen rebound reactions. It begins with the CYP perferryl complex abstracting one of the nitrogen's lone pair of electrons (Figure 3.15), forming an aminium ion (N^+). Once this has been created, either the oxygen reacts with the N^+ giving the N-oxide, or the perferryl complex can abstract a hydrogen from one of the adjacent carbons forming a carbon radical. The reaction then proceeds as with most CYP oxidations, where the hydroxyl group bounces off the haem iron to react with the carbon radical to make the (usually unstable) alcohol, or carbinolamine. Chlorpromazine and the TCAs can undergo N-oxidation or N-dealkylations, as well as sulphoxide formation (Figure 3.16).

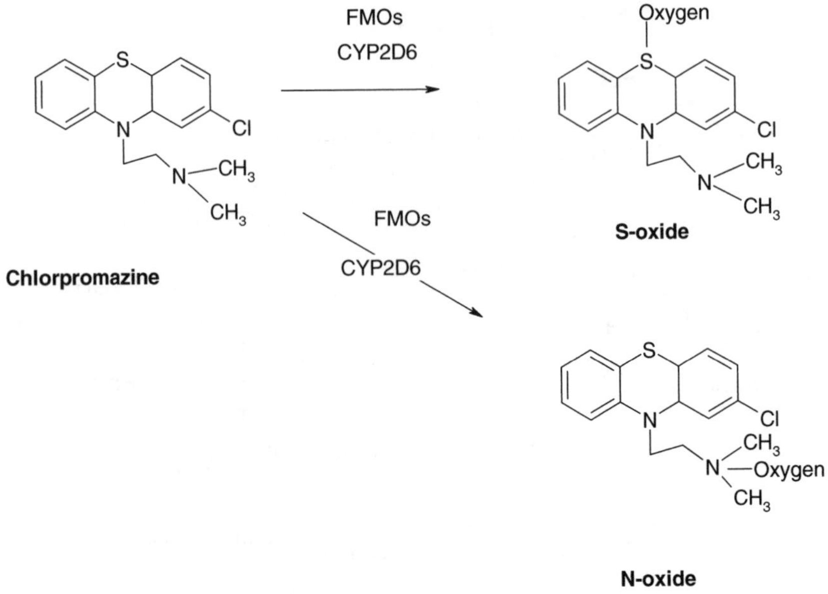

Figure 3.16   Sulphoxide and N-oxide formation with chlorpromazine

Heteroatom nitrogen and sulphur oxidations (flavin monooxygenases)

Alongside the CYPs, other cellular systems can accomplish oxidations of endogenous molecules and so are often widespread in many tissues. Flavin monooxygenases (FMOs) are found in the liver, kidney and lung. They use NADPH and oxygen to catalyse similar reactions to CYPs, and they oxidize nucleophiles such as nitrogen, sulphur and phosphorus in various drugs and xenobiotics and form their respective oxides. The enzymes operate by using NADPH to bind to flavin adenine dinucleotide (FAD) and the FAD/NADP+ complex then binds oxygen, forming peroxide. The substrate is oxidized during the process of conversion of a hydroperoxyflavin to a hydroxyflavin. FMOs have an approximate molecular weight of 60 000 and appear in five different families; expression is specific to species and tissue. The human kidney contains high levels of FMO1, but not FMO3. These enzymes metabolize tertiary amines to form N-oxides in drugs such as TCAs (imipramine), as well as morphine, methadone and meperidine.

As with chlorpromazine, several other molecules undergo N-oxidation, such as 2,4, diaminopyrimidine antiparasitics (trimethoprim and pyrimethamine) that can form 1 and 3 N-oxides.

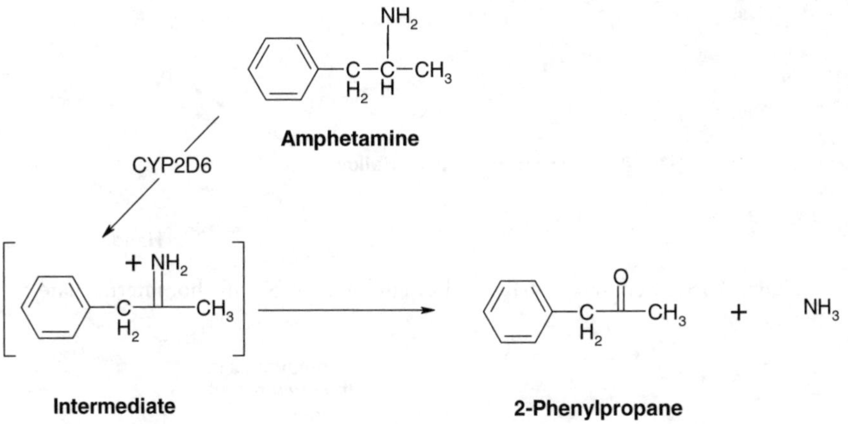

Figure 3.17 Oxidative deamination of amphetamine

Deaminations

Amine groups in drugs can be primary, secondary or tertiary. Primary amines can be removed completely thorough conversion of the carbon—nitrogen single to a double bond, where the nitrogen loses an electron. Via a hydrogen atom from water, ammonia is formed with a ketone product. This is one of the fates of amphetamine (Figure 3.17). More amphetamine metabolism can be found in Appendix B.

Dehalogenations

Using the same basic tool, oxidation to an alcohol, it is possible for CYPs to remove halogens (chloride, bromide or fluoride) from molecules, forming a ketone and a halogen ion. A number of volatile general anaesthetics are subject to this route of metabolism. The adjacent carbon to the halide is oxidized to a short-lived alcohol, which causes the movement of electrons towards the halogen, which dissociates (Figure 3.18).

3.13 Other oxidation processes

Primary amine oxidations

Primary amines found in sulphonamides and sulphones can be metabolized to hydroxylamines and their toxicity hinges on these pathways (Figure 3.19 and see Chapter 8). The hydroxylamines formed are often reactive and

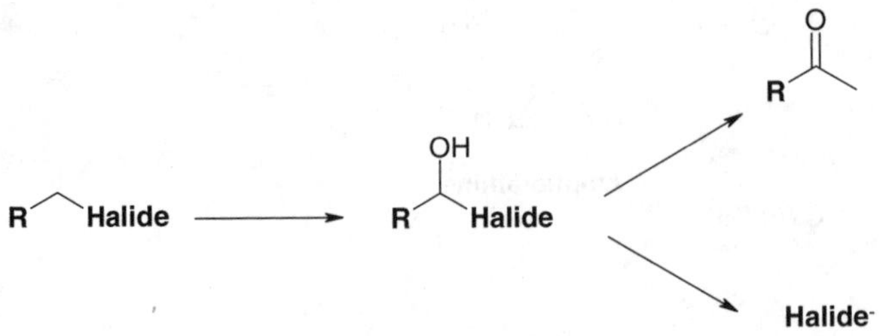

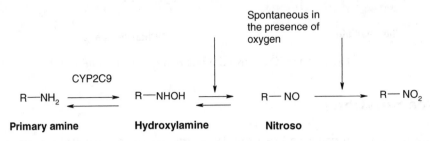

Figure 3.18   Removal of halides through an unstable alcohol intermediate

Figure 3.19   Primary amine oxidation

although they can be stabilized by glutathione (GSH) and other cellular antioxidants, they can spontaneously oxidize in the presence of oxygen to nitroso and then nitro-derivatives. The nitro forms are usually stable, but are vulnerable to reductive metabolism that drives the process shown in Figure 3.19 in the opposite direction. Secondary amines can also be oxidized to hydroxylamines.

Oxidation of alcohol and aldehydes

Although CYP2E1 is induced by ethanol, the vast majority of ethanol clearance (90 per cent) is normally by oxidation to acetaldehyde by another group of enzymes, the alcohol dehydrogenases ADH's, unless the individual is a heavy drinker or alcoholic. These enzymes are found in the cytoplasm and they are NAD$^+$ dependent zinc metalloenzymes. They form NADH from NAD+ in the process of alcohol oxidation. There are five classes of ADH isoforms. Class I (ADH1, ADH2, ADH3) isoforms have a high affinity for ethanol and can be blocked by pyrazoles. Classes II and III are more suited to the metabolism of longer chain alcohols and cannot be blocked by pyrazole.

Aldehydes are formed from many reactions in cells, but they are oxidized to their corresponding carboxylic acid by several enzyme systems, including aldehyde dehydrogenase ALDH's, xanthine oxidase and aldehyde oxidase.

These enzymes are detoxifying, as many aldehydes, such as formaldehyde, are cytotoxic by-products of CYP and other oxidative reactions. Of the three aldehyde dehydrogenase classes, two are relevant to alcohol metabolism. Class I is found in the liver cytosol and specializes in acetaldehyde. Class II ALDHs are found in the liver and kidney mitochondria and metabolize acetaldehyde and several other substrates.

Monoamine oxidase (MAO)

Yet another important oxidative enzyme system that processes endogenous and exogenous substrates is monoamine oxidase (MAO), which exists in two isoforms, MAO A and MAO B. Both are found in the outer membrane of mitochondria in virtually all tissues. They have evolved to become two separate enzymes with similar functions and they originate from different genes in man. They use FAD as a cofactor and are capable of oxidizing a very wide variety of endogenous biogenic amines as well as primary, secondary and tertiary xenobiotic amines. They accomplish their removal of amine groups through an initial reductive half-reaction, followed by an oxidation half-reaction. The reductive half oxidizes the amine and the FAD is reduced. The second half of the process involves the use of oxygen to reoxidize the FAD, leaving hydrogen peroxide and an aldehyde as products. Clorgyline blocks MAO A, whilst deprenyl is a potent inhibitor of MAO B. In the 1960s, irreversible MAO inhibitors were used as antidepressants, aimed at increasing biogenic amine levels. Unfortunately, they could cause hypertensive crises (sufficient to cause a stroke) through ingestion of other amines, such as tyramine from cheese and a long list of other foods. MAO inhibitors are still used, but only in a minority of patients.

3.14 Reduction reactions

As mentioned earlier, it is likely that CYPs carried out reductions well before they evolved to oxidize, due to the scarcity of oxygen in the early period of the earth's development. There are many other tissue enzymes that reduce drugs and toxins, and these include nitro-reductases as well as keto-reductases. In erythrocytes, NADH and NADPH reductases are also capable of reducing xenobiotics. The main suppliers of electrons for the CYPs themselves are the NADPH hepatic reductases and these enzymes can carry out many reductive reactions. These reactions can have toxicological significance, as nitro groups can be reduced to nitrosoarenes and hydroxylamines and this is thought to be a major pathway towards the carcinogenic effects of aromatic amines (Chapter 8). Other reductive reactions include the reduction of ketones to alcohols.

3.15   Control of CYP metabolic function

Although CYPs appear to be part of an impressive and flexible system for the Phase I clearance of drugs, it is not enough just to process endogenous and xenobiotic molecules at a set rate. Endogenous and exogenous CYP substrates can vary enormously in their concentrations within the body, even on a day-to-day basis. For example, steroid hormone levels must be matched to accomplish specific tasks in narrow time frames, so production and destruction must be under exceedingly fine control. This is apparent during the menstrual cycle and pregnancy. Our exposure to various exogenous chemicals, including drugs, is also variable in terms of concentration and physicochemical properties. As an advertising campaign once said, 'power is nothing without control'. It is essential for the CYP system to be finely controllable to respond to the violent changes in the small-molecular weight chemical presence in cells. This process of CYP induction mentioned briefly earlier will be discussed in detail in terms of mechanism and clinical consequences in the next chapter.

4 Induction of Cytochrome P450 Systems

4.1 Introduction

The aim of drug therapy is to provide a stable, predictable pharmacological effect that can be adjusted to the needs of the individual patient for as long is deemed clinically necessary. The physician may start drug therapy at a dosage that is decided on the basis of previous clinical experience and standard recommendations. At some point, the dosage might be increased if the desired effects were not forthcoming, or reduced if side effects are intolerable to the patient. This adjustment of dosage can be much easier in drugs that have a directly measurable response, such as a change in clotting time. However, in some drugs, this adjustment process can take longer to achieve than others, as the pharmacological effect, once attained, is gradually lost over a period of days. The dosage must be escalated to regain the original effect, sometimes several times, until the patient is stable on the dosage. In some cases, after several weeks of taking the drug, the initial pharmacological effect seen in the first few days now requires up to eight times the initial dosage to reproduce. It thus takes several weeks to create a stable pharmacological effect on a constant dose. In the same patients, if another drug is added to the regimen, it may not have any effect at all. In other patients, sudden withdrawal of perhaps only one drug in a regimen might lead to a gradual but serious intensification of the other drug's side effects. These effects are shown by some illustrative histories, as detailed below.

History 1

After suffering a head trauma in a motorcycle accident, a 22-year-old male was subject to recurrent grande-mal convulsions that were treated with carbamazepine. After starting on 200 mg daily, this dose had to be gradually increased stepwise over four weeks to maintain plasma levels within the therapeutic window to 1200 mg daily.

Human Drug Metabolism, Michael D. Coleman
© 2005 John Wiley & Sons, Ltd

Analysis

Plasma levels were not maintained within the therapeutic window at each dose level for more than a week or so, as carbamazepine clearance appeared to gradually increase, until a dosage was reached where clearance stabilized so that drug levels remained within the therapeutic window.

History 2

A 23-year-old male epileptic was prescribed phenytoin (300 mg/day) and carbamazepine (800 mg/day). The laboratory assays showed that phenytoin was in the therapeutic range, while carbamazepine was undetectable in the plasma. A 50 per cent reduction of the phenytoin dosage allowed the carbamazapine plasma concentrations to rise to therapeutically effective levels.

Analysis

The lack of carbamazepine in the plasma at a dosage which is known to exert a reasonable therapeutic effect in other patients implied that the drug's clearance was much higher than normal, to the point where bioavailability was almost zero. Cutting the phenytoin dosage slowed the high rate of clearance of carbamazepine, allowing plasma levels to ascend to the therapeutic window.

History 3

A 49-year-old male epileptic was prescribed phenytoin at 600 mg/day and carbamazepine at 2000 mg/day. The patient's condition was controlled with minimal side effects for three months. The phenytoin was then abruptly discontinued; within four days, the patient became gradually more lethargic and confused, until one week later hospitalization was necessary. The carbamazepine dosage was reduced to 1200 mg/day and the confusion and sedation disappeared.

Analysis

A stable co-administration of two drugs implies that despite the high dose of carbamazepine, blood levels for both drugs were initially in the therapeutic window. The removal of the phenytoin led to gradual increase in the symptoms of carbamazepine overdose, without any change in the dose. This indicates that carbamazepine blood levels climbed way above the therapeutic window into toxicity. This was caused by a marked, but gradual, fall in carbamazepine clearance when the phenytoin was withdrawn.

History 4

A 64-year-old obese male was prescribed simvastatin 10 mg daily. Over the next three months, lack of clinical response led to a fivefold increase in dosage. He was then admitted to hospital with rhabdomyolysis. On his own initiative he had self-administered St John's Wort, which he discontinued when his mood was sufficiently elevated, around 10 days prior to the toxicity manifesting itself.

Analysis

The statin was not effective unless considerably higher doses than normal were used, indicating that the drug was being cleared at a higher rate than normal. The general practitioner was unaware that the patient was taking St John's Wort extract. The patient abruptly stopped taking the herbal extract and the clearance of the statin gradually fell while the dose did not, so the drug accumulated and exerted toxicity.

History 5

A 47-year-old female was stabilised on phenobarbitone and warfarin and her prothrombin time was optimized by substantial increase over the normal dosage of anticoagualant, although blood levels were within normal limits. Within 10 days of the abrupt withdrawal of phenobarbitone the patient suffered a mild haemorrhage.

Analysis

As a higher than normal dosage of warfarin was necessary to maintain its plasma levels in the therapeutic window in the presence of the phenobarbitone, it suggests that the latter drug was accelerating the clearance of warfarin. Once the phenobarbitone was stopped, this accelerating effect was lost too, leading to accumulation of the warfarin to the point that blood levels rose above the therapeutic window leading to toxicity, in this case an exaggerated therapeutic effect.

History 6

A 55-year-old male being treated for tuberculosis was taking rifampicin (600 mg daily), isoniazid (400 mg daily), ethambutol (200 mg daily) and pyrazinamide (400 mg daily), was also epileptic and was taking carbamazepine (2000 mg daily). The patient decided to stop all medication over the Christmas period to enter his annual seasonal alcohol binge, where he drank heavily for several days. After approximately 13 days, he resumed his drug regimen and before the end of the first day, he was drowsy, lethargic, confused and eventually difficult to wake and was hospitalized. Some of the symptoms of the tuberculosis resumed, such as fever, chills and cough.

Analysis

The patient was suffering from carbamazepine toxicity and very high plasma levels were found on blood analysis. This indicates that the cessation of all drug intakes over the Christmas period of 13 days had led to a marked reduction in the clearance of carbamazepine, and the resumption of his previous high dosage caused drug accumulation and significant CNS toxicity. The absence of pressure of the anti-tuberculosis drugs had also allowed the disease to partially re-establish itself and may well have led to selection of partly drug-resistant forms of the bacteria.

Summary

In all five cases, there are a number of common features:

- Some of the drugs' clearances were not stable until a relatively high dose was employed.

- One drug (or herbal preparation) was able to grossly accelerate the clearance of another agent (s).

- The changes in plasma levels were sufficiently great to either lead to toxicity or total loss of efficacy.

- The toxic effects occurred gradually over days, rather than hours.

- The increase in drug clearance caused by other drugs was fully reversible.

4.2 Causes of accelerated clearance

A number of explanations could be put forward for the effects seen above. There could be changes in absorption of a drug in the presence of another agent, although this is unlikely as most drugs are passively absorbed. Perhaps the renal clearance of the drug could be accelerated in some way; in this context this is also unlikely, as the drug has to be in the plasma before it can be filtered by the kidneys. To enter the circulation from an oral dose, the drugs must pass through the gut, the portal circulation and then the liver itself. In Histories 1 and 2, the clearance of carbamazepine was initially unstable and in the presence of phenytoin, virtually 100 per cent cleared before it reached the circulation.

Since the liver's blood flow does not usually change markedly, then the only way such a large effect on drug levels can occur is that the liver is extracting much more of the drug than usual in the presence of the other drug. This acceleration of drug metabolism as a response to the presence of certain drugs is known as 'enzyme induction' and drugs which cause it are often referred to as 'inducers' of drug metabolism. The process can be defined as: '*An adaptive increase in the metabolizing capacity of a tissue*'; this means that a drug or chemical is capable of inducing an increase in the synthesis of a specific CYP isoform, which is usually (although not always) the most efficient metabolizer of that chemical.

4.3 Enzyme induction

Types of inducer

There are several drugs and chemicals capable of inducing hepatic metabolism: these include:

- *Anticonvulsants*, such as phenytoin, carbamazepine and phenobarbitone; these induce many CYP isoforms, including 1A2, 2C9, 2C19 and 3A4.

- *Steroids*, such as dexamethasone, prednisolone and various glucocorticoids, induce CYP3A4.

- *Polycyclic aromatic hydrocarbons*; these are found in atmospheric pollution, cigarette smoke, industrial solvents and barbecued meat. These agents include contaminants of foodstuffs and watercourses like dioxins and polycyclic chlorinated biphenyls. These compounds induce the normally non-constitutive CYP1A1 in the liver, as well as CYP1A2, which specializes in polycyclic aromatic amines. Induction of CYP1A1 is also very strong in the lung in smokers and is a standard marker for heavy tobacco use.

- *Antibiotics*, such as rifampicin and griseofulvin, induce most CYPs including 1A2, 2C9, 2C19 and 3A4.

- *Recreational agents*, such as nicotine in tobacco products, is a known inducer of CYP1A2, and heavy alcohol consumption will induce CYP2E1.

- *Herbal remedies*; although more research must be conducted into the various herbs on the market, St John's Wort is the most clinically relevant and investigated (CYP3A4).

Common features of inducers

Looking at the structures of the most potent hepatic enzyme inducers there are apparently few common features. These chemicals range in size from very small and water-soluble (ethanol) to very large and lipophilic (rifampicin). However, inducers are usually lipophilic and contain aromatic groups and consequently, if they were not oxidized, they would be very persistent in living systems. CYP enzymes have evolved to oxidize this very type of agent; indeed, an elaborate and very effective system has also evolved to modulate the degree of CYP oxidation of these agents, so it is clear that living systems regard inducers as a particular threat among lipophilic agents in general.

The process of induction is dynamic and closely controlled. The adaptive increase is constantly matched to the level of exposure to the drug, from very minor almost undetectable increases in CYP protein synthesis, all the way to a maximum enzyme synthesis that leads to the clearance of grammes of a chemical per day. Once exposure to the drug or toxin ceases, the adaptive increase in metabolizing capacity gradually subsides to the previous low level.

4.4   Mechanisms of enzyme induction

Introduction

The process by which enzyme induction occurs has three main requirements:

- The hepatocyte must detect the presence of particular potentially persistent lipophilic drugs and/or toxins and correctly sense their concentration.

- The process of detection is translated into an increase in the appropriate metabolic system within the cell, which is capable of clearing the drug and/or toxin as efficiently as possible.

- Complete (detection and action) system is dynamic and reversible, so it is sensitive to further changes in drug concentration.

It is apparent that the main inducible CYPs, 1A1/1A2, 2C9 and 3A4, employ broadly similar systems whereby they regulate their ability to respond to increases in drug concentration. The exception to this rule seems to be 2E1.

Apart from CYP1A1/1A2 induction, these systems are not fully understood, but enough is known to suggest that the method of induction is closely related to a combination of the CYP's endogenous as well as xenobiotic-responsive functions.

CYP1A1/1A2 induction

Although enzyme induction has been known since the 1960s, it was not until the 1970s that the first steps in understanding how CYP enzyme induction was regulated were taken. This work was carried out with one of the most potent toxins known, dioxin, or TCDD. In the cytoplasm of most cells a receptor complex can be found which consists of a ligand-binding subunit and a heat-shock protein (HSP-90: Figure 4.1). This complex is known as the aryl hydrocarbon receptor, or 'Ah' receptor. TCDD was found to bind to the Ah receptor and the TCDD/Ah complex migrates to the nucleus, leaving the heat-shock protein behind in the cytoplasm. The TCDD/Ah complex enters the nucleus and heterodimerizes with the nuclear protein ARNT and then the complex binds to specific DNA sequences upstream of the CYP1A1

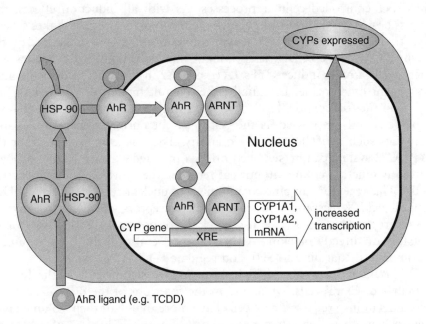

Figure 4.1 Basic mechanism of CYP1A1 and 1A2 induction: the Ah receptor binds the inducer alongside HSP-90, but only the Ah receptor and the inducer cross into the nucleus to meet ARNT and activate the xenobiotic response elements on the DNA to induce expression of the CYP isoforms

or 1A2 genes, which are termed xenobiotic-responsive elements (XRE) or sometimes DREs, or drug-responsive elements.

These sequences are essentially 'switches' which lead to increased transcription and translation of the CYP enzymes. It is thought that the system obeys the law of mass action, so providing there are enough Ah receptors in the cell cytoplasm, then the more TCDD that appears in the cell, will lead to more TCDD/Ah complexes migrating to the nucleus and binding to the DREs, which in turn increase CYP expression. This sensitive system operates constantly and is capable of coordinating a response in terms of increased CYP synthesis, which is capable of eventually clearing (by CYP-mediated oxidation) large amounts of TCDD from the cell.

The Ah and ARNT receptor system is clearly multifunctional, as TCDD induces other enzyme systems as well as CYP1A1/1A2, such as glutathione-S-transferase and aldehyde dehydrogenase; so it is easy to see that exposure to compounds which resemble TCDD will have a significant impact on the concentrations of many other endogenous molecules which are cleared by these enzyme systems.

The Ah/ARNT system is found in virtually all tissues; in mice it appears to be involved with the development of the liver and the immune system, which may be similar to their function in man. Indeed, many of the toxic effects of polycyclic aromatics are thought to be due to their disruption of Ah/ARNT controlled cellular processes. As with all induction effects, this process begins within hours of exposure to the toxin or drug, but takes several days to lead to maximal CYP expression, or maximal induction of the enzyme. As well as TCDD, it is thought that polycyclic hydrocarbons and heterocyclic amines induce CYPs 1A1 and 1A2 in this way, as does the anti-ulcer agent omeprazole. Essentially, the 'default mode' for CYPs 1A1 and 1A2 is in the 'off' or low-level position, so these enzymes are not intended to be constantly expressed as the cell does not normally encounter planar aromatics such as TCDD in any quantity. There is also evidence that the CYP1A1/2 system can be switched off by other agents, such as the 'orphan' (currently function unknown) nuclear receptor, the short heterodimer partner (SHP). This receptor can bind to a number of nuclear receptors such as RXR (retinoic acid X receptor) and several other receptors which control thyroid and oestrogen levels. SHP can also block the response of CYP1A1 to TCDD, probably by directly blocking ARNT. There are also likely to be a number of compounds that bind to SHP and regulate CYP1A1 activity.

CYP1A1/2 induction is of high toxicological significance in the lung in non-ciliated 'Clara' cells, which are in the forefront of the detoxification of pollutants in inspired air. These cells have more than half their volume given over to smooth endoplasmic reticulum (SER) and induction of 1A1/2 by PAHs in tobacco leads to the formation of reactive epoxides, which attack DNA, forming 'adducts' or small PAH-related structures which are covalently bound to DNA and are strongly linked with lung carcinogenicity. It has been suggested that the high state of lung induction of CYP1A1 leads to an increased Clara cell exposure to reactive species of oxygen generated by 1A1 even when it is not metabolizing substrates. This is because 1A1/1A2 are thought to 'leak' reactive oxygen species and this 'drip–drip' effect might make as great a contribution to DNA damage as the aromatic metabolites. CYP1A1 has also been implicated in the metabolism of nitrosamines such as 4-(methylnitrosamino)-1-(3-pyridyl)-1-butanone (NNK). In animal studies, DNA was attacked by the metabolites of this compound resulting in an O^6-methylguanine adduct. Other lung-specific toxins include CYP2E1-activated vinylidene chloride. The likelihood of the development of lung tumours in response to metabolism depends on the amount of carcinogenic species produced, its detoxification and the efficiency of DNA repair mechanisms.

CYP2B6 2C8/2C9 and 3A4

Induction of these CYPs appears to be controlled by a markedly different system from the cytosolic receptor-mediated 1A series (Figures 4.2a and b). Typical inducers of these CYPs include phenobarbitone, primidone, phenytoin and rifampicin. These CYPs are controlled by a nuclear receptor called the 'constitutive androstane receptor' (CAR). The important word here is 'constitutive' which means that CAR constantly mediates CYP expression at

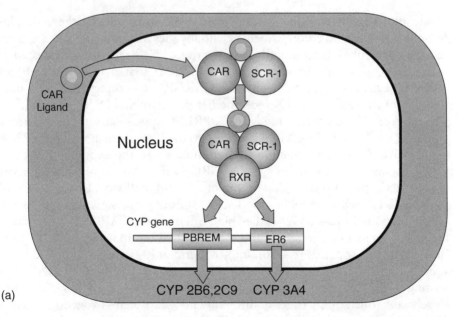

Figure 4.2(a) Possible mechanism of constitutive androstane receptor (CAR)-mediated control of CYP2 series and CYP3A4. CAR and SCR-1 bind the inducer ligand inside the nucleus, bind retinoic acid X receptor (RXR) and activate the CYP expression

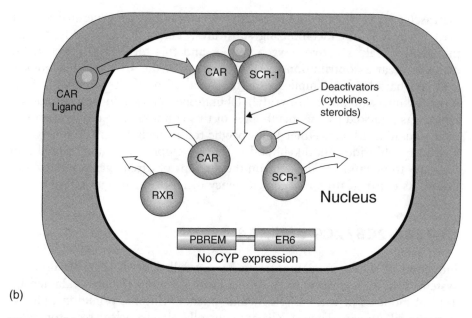

(b)

Figure 4.2(b)   Possible mechanism for the modulation of CAR-ligand activated CYP induction: a series of endogenous deactivators cause break up of the CAR/RXR/SCR-1/ligand complex and induction is switched off

a rate that can be slowed or accelerated by factors outside the cell. This is unlike the Ah receptor, which essentially lies dormant if there are no inducers present to bind it, and the 1A series of CYPs are only expressed at a tiny level, if at all. Another aspect of CAR is that it is linked to a co-activator, called SRC-1. Normally, the CAR/SRC-1 complex will then bind to RXR, or the retinoic acid X-receptor, before it can bind DNA (Figure 4.2a). The CAR/RXR complex binds to PBREM (phenobarbitone-responsive enhancer module) in the CYP2B gene and to the ER6 element of the CYP3A4 gene. PBREM triggers induction by barbiturates. So the expression of these CYPS is constantly managed by CAR/SRC-1, in a way analogous to a car engine with the throttle pressed down around halfway. Deactivators of CAR/SRC-1, such as cytokines and some steroids, can slow or even switch off expression of these CYPS as they bind briefly to the CAR/SRC-1 and cause the SRC-1 element to break off and the CAR will not function, so 'lifting the foot off the throttle (Figure 4.2b). Inducers probably cause CAR to bind SRC-1 even more tightly, thus increasing its effectiveness in binding DNA and leading to the throttle being 'floored'. Thus the expressions of these CYPs are closely controlled by a variety of different endogenous and exogenous agents. This elaborate and sensitive system illustrates the vital day-to-day role of these CYPs in the metabolism of xenobiotics and endogenous chemicals.

CYP2E1 induction

CYP2E1 is of interest from the standpoint of drug metabolism (it oxidizes isoniazid, paracetamol and chlorzoxazone), hepatotoxin activation (paracetamol, carbon tetrachloride, thioacetamide) and carcinogen activation (N-nitrosodimethylamine, benzene, vinyl chloride and trichloroethylene). The major interest in this isoform lies in its induction by such apparently disparate factors as small hydrophilic molecules, such as ethanol, acetone and pyridine, as well as by systemic stresses, such as diabetes and starvation. It is not yet certain exactly how 2E1 is induced, but it appears that more than one mechanism is involved. When animals are exposed to 2E1 inducers, CYP2E1 protein levels are increased up to eightfold, although the CYP2E1 mRNA levels have not been seen to increase. This suggests that 2E1 is not induced like CYP1A1, rather that somehow the regulatory step is after transcription, i.e. at the stage of the actual synthesis of the enzyme at the rough endoplasmic reticulum. Two possible mechanisms have been suggested to account for this; the first is that the presence of the substrate chemically stabilizes the 2E1 protein and makes it functional, when it would normally be poorly or non-functional. The second mechanism suggests that more 2E1 is made in a set time, indicating greater efficiency of translation (Figure 4.3).

The first mechanism implies that in the absence of substrate, considerable effort is being made within the hepatocyte towards the formation of a poorly functional and perhaps even non-functional protein, on the off chance that

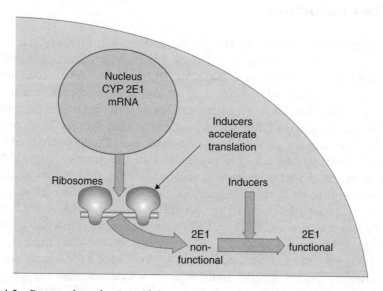

Figure 4.3 Proposed mechanism of CYP2E1 induction: this is partly by acceleration of the translation of the protein as well as a direct effect of the inducer on the structure of the isoform so making it functionally competent

a substrate might appear and then the process would not then be so apparently wasteful. Certainly, when 2E1 is fully induced, the catalytic activity corresponds with the amount of protein present, so it is fully functional at this point.

Why 2E1 might function in such an apparently wasteful way could lie in the specific triggers of its induction and the nature of the chemicals 2E1 is designed to oxidize. Insulin levels fall during diet restriction, starvation and in diabetes; the formation of functional 2E1 is suppressed by insulin, so these conditions promote the increase of 2E1 metabolic capability. One of the consequences of these conditions is the major shift from glucose to fatty acid/tryglyceride oxidation, of which some of the by-products are small, hydrophilic and potentially toxic 'ketone bodies'. These agents could and do cause a CNS intoxicating effect which is seen in diabetics who are hypoglycaemic, they may appear 'drunk' and their breath will smell as if they had been drinking. In the non-diabetic individual who is in a state of starvation, any ketone-mediated intoxication would obviously hamper the search for food, so these molecules must be cleared rapidly. The key factor here is the speed at which these compounds could accumulate – the TCDD mechanism of induction, with its time frame of days, might be too slow to cope with the accumulation of ketone bodies in starvation, so the much quicker 'protein stabilization' system perhaps might be rapid enough to ensure that adequate levels of 2E1 were present to prevent intoxication of the CNS.

CYP3A4 induction

As members of the 3A family are the major P450s in human liver, it is not surprising that they exhibit very broad specificity and are induced by a structurally diverse group of substances. Inducers of 3A4 include steroids, macrolide antibiotics, rifampicin, and imidazole antifungals, barbiturates, and even pesticides, such as organochlorine and organophosphates. The induction process is tailored to species, so animal studies have been less helpful in assessing the possible human enzyme-inducing properties of a novel chemical agent; rifampicin is a potent inducer of human and rabbit 3A enzymes, but it is without effect in the rat. The process by which CYP3A enzymes are induced is still the focus of intense study, however some main steps in the process have emerged. 3A differs from the 1A and 2E control systems, and resembles CYP2B6/2C8/9 series induction/repression with one important difference. With CYP3A4 a sensing receptor does bind the xenobiotic for some time and then activates the gene. Like 2B6/2C8/9, the receptor is nuclear. With CYP3A4 induction, it is believed that the xenobiotic reaches the nucleus and then binds to one of a large family of nuclear receptors (classified as NR1I) called PXR, or the pregnane X receptor. This was so named as it responds to the steroid pregnenolone. PXR is found in the

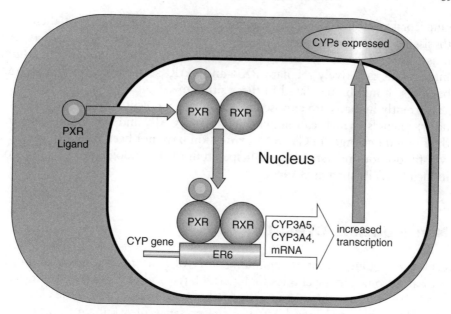

Figure 4.4 Mechanism of CYP3A induction through the pregnane X receptor (PXR) and retinoic acid receptors (RXR)

liver and intestine and may be part of an endocrine signalling pathway, as its function is modulated by many other nuclear receptors as well as cytokines and hormones (Figure 4.4).

PXR is capable of binding and becoming activated by such a diverse group of inducers that it must possess a highly flexible recognition site, which only requires a very poor substrate fit for activation to occur. PXR is also termed a steroid and xenobiotic sensing receptor (SXR). The PXR/substrate complex then binds to another nuclear receptor, the RXR (retinoic acid X receptor). The resultant heterodimer binds to the response elements that are 'upstream' of the human 3A4 gene, known as the ER6 elements (Figure 4.4). It has also been proposed that there is a second xenobiotic response element module (XREM) which is activated either as well as, or instead of, the ER6 elements. Further research will clarify the balance between the two response elemental systems. The expression of CYP3A4 is then upregulated according to the number of 'hits' on the response element system (Figure 4.4).

This process is far from completely understood; it is suggested that RXR as well as other nuclear receptors, such as GR, the glucocorticoid receptor and CAR, are also involved. It is likely that 3A4 can be controlled by CAR as well as PXR, although it appears that PXR is the dominant mechanism of expression control.

The complexity of the regulation of CYPs such as 3A4 will be investigated for many years to come, although the necessity of such systems is understandable as the control of the systemic concentrations of hormones, such as glucocorticoids and steroids, is achieved through the balance of their synthesis and oxidation, so the regulation of steroid-oxidizing CYPs such as 3A4 must be sensitive to systemic threats such as infection and inflammation. Interleukins negatively regulate PXR and CAR, so it is logical that steroid balances should be regulated in these situations.

Currently humans are exposed to many environmental pollutants, such as nonyl phenols, which can activate PXR and CAR, and the implications of the resultant changes in CYP3A4 expression have not been fully explored, as we still do not understand the full spectrum of the endogenous functions of inducible CYPs such as 3A4.

Non-inducible CYPs: CYP2D6

CYP2D6 it is important as the main source of clearance for tricyclic antidepressants, some antipsychotics (haloperidol, risperidone), some beta-blockers and SSRIs. It is not thought to be inducible, and in cases where the clearance of a 2D6 substrate is accelerated in the presence of a known inducer, it is usually because 3A4 has been induced and this isoform is responsible for the increased clearance. CYP2D6 substrates dextromethorphan and mirtazapine clearances are markedly increased by rifampicin and carbamazepine respectively in this way. Interestingly, some studies such as those with the benzodiazepines and citalopram have shown that CYP2D6 activity increases in pregnancy. Whether this is a true induction process remains to be determined.

4.5 Induction – general clinical aspects

From a clinical standpoint, important features of enzyme induction can be summarized:

- The process is relatively slow, i.e. usually days or even weeks;

- The potential changes in drug concentrations can be great enough to cause treatment failure;

- The induction process is usually, but not always, reversible over a similar time frame to its appearance, although reversal can be slower;

- Where a patient is stabilized on a high 'induced' drug dosage, if there is a treatment break of up to several days, drug accumulation and toxicity will occur.

The timescale of the induction process does largely depend on the potency of the inducer. Pentobarbitone causes a marked decrease in nortriptyline blood concentrations within only two days, doubling its clearance. The gradual fall-off in drug levels will lead to a commensurate loss of drug efficacy. Some of the most clinically relevant drug interactions caused by enzyme induction are described below.

Anti-epileptic agents

Drug combinations

In approximately one-third of cases of epilepsy control of the condition can only be achieved with a combination of anticonvulsants, and this leads to potential problems with the induction effects of carbamazepine (2C9, 2C19, 3A4; History 2), phenytoin (1A2, 3A4) and phenobarbitone (1A2, 2C8, 3A4). In a combination of anticonvulsants, co-administered compounds metabolized by these CYP enzymes will have their plasma concentrations significantly reduced. A good example of this is valproic acid, where plasma levels can be reduced by 80 per cent in the presence of phenobarbitone, and by half with phenytoin and nearly 70 per cent with carbamazepine co-administration. Among the second generation of anticonvulsants, drugs such as topiramate and tiagabine are also cleared more rapidly in the presence of inducers.

Drug withdrawal

Problems may arise when the combination of anticonvulsants is changed, or when one drug is completely withdrawn (History 3). The remaining drug plasma levels might rise over the following few days as the inductive effect recedes and clinical signs of an intensification of the pharmacological effect will gradually become apparent. It is most desirable to anticipate this effect by tapering the dosage of the other drugs over days or weeks as appropriate. However, this is not such an easy process, as there is relatively little literature on how long it takes for the effects of standard inducers to fully wear off. There is some evidence that in some drugs it can take longer to disappear than the original onset time. It is better to taper the dose, or the patient might be subject to increased side effects, which they may or may not complain about. Overall, it is important that the drug levels remain within the therapeutic window.

Other drug combinations

Anticonvulsants are co-administered with other CNS modulating drugs, such as antipsychotics, tricyclic antidepressants (TCAs), benzodiazepines and newer agents such as SSRIs. With respect to enzyme induction, anticonvulsants can greatly accelerate the clearance of antipsychotics like haloperidol and benzodiazepines such as midazolam, although temazepam clearance is not dependent on 3A4 and is not affected by inducers of this isoform. CYP3A4 inducers can also accelerate the clearance of some TCAs.

OTC preparations

St John's wort (*hypericum perforatum*) is a freely available over-the-counter antidepressant agent, which has found considerable popularity (History 4). This appears justified, as it has been shown to be clinically effective. Of course, patients are usually unaware that the active component, hyperforin, is one of the most potent activators yet found of the human PXR receptor, leading to induction of CYPs 3A4 and 2C9. Hyperforin itself undergoes extensive metabolism by 3A4 to hydroxylated products. A recent study with this herbal remedy demonstrated that a 14-day course of St John's wort and dosage of a total of 900 mg daily was capable of doubling alprazolam clearance. Many other herbal remedies are available (gingko, ginseng, etc.), although the enzyme-inducing properties of most have not been substantiated. However, commercial and other pressures suggest that these agents are recommended to be taken for long periods of time, so the opportunity for even mild CYP induction is clear. This is potentially a serious problem when a patient terminates their consumption of St John's wort when they have been stabilized on a prescribed dosage regimen of other drugs (History 4). Many patients do not consider herbal remedies as 'drugs' in that they believe that the remedy will not have any side effects, yet somehow exert a strong therapeutic action. In addition, these herbal extracts vary enormously in quality, purity and percentage of the active component, which will all depend on the source and preparation of the extract. It is important that patients are asked if they have taken, or would consider taking, herbal remedies during a drug treatment regimen. This is particularly a problem where a course of conventional antidepressants is embarked upon and the patient's symptoms do not improve quickly. Consequently they may understandably resort to assistance from an herb extract such as hypericum.

Anticoagulant drugs

Anticoagulants such as warfarin are mainly dependent on CYP2C9 for their clearance, with some contribution from 3A4 and 1A2. Inducers of these enzymes will make a substantial reduction in the plasma levels of these drugs and therefore their anticoagulant effects (History 5). There is no substitute for checking the patient's coagulation function to ensure that they remain within the therapeutic window. If an enzyme-inducing drug is withdrawn, there is the danger of accumulation of the anticoagulants, which will lead to haemorrhaging. This situation would be exacerbated if a substitute drug were to be a CYP inhibitor. In that case, anticoagulant drug concentrations would climb so rapidly that the patient's life could be in danger.

Oral contraceptives/steroids

The CYP3A4 inducers can accelerate the clearance of ethinyloestradiol; this is a particular concern with low-dose oral contraceptive preparations. Increasing the contraceptive dose, or a recommendation to use other methods of contraception, may negate this effect. Other prescribed steroids such as corticosteroids will also be cleared more rapidly in the presence of inducers of CYP3A4.

Antiviral/antibiotic drugs

Of the newer anti-HIV antiviral compounds, ritonavir, nevirapine, indinavir and saquinavir are all metabolized by CYP3A4, so it is possible that inducers may affect their clearances *in vivo*. However, this situation is complicated by the fact that for example ritonavir is a potent inhibitor of 3A4 and induces its own metabolism. This induction effect means that at least 14 days' therapy is required before plasma levels stabilize. Potent inducers such as rifampicin do exert some effect on ritonavir plasma levels, but only to a relatively modest (~35 per cent) degree. Any changes in the plasma levels of an antibiotic or antiviral agent can lead to subcurative drug concentrations and a possible selection of resistant variants of the infectious agent, so plasma levels should be closely monitored to ensure minimum inhibitory concentrations (MICs) are exceeded while toxicity is minimized. Certainly abruptly stopping and restarting inducing antibiotics such as rifampicin (History 6) will lead to severe disruption of the clearances of co-prescribed agents and lead to drug levels climbing above the therapeutic window until the inducing effect is re-established. Patient drug tolerance may be severely impaired during this period.

Anti-cancer drugs

Any changes to the plasma levels of antineoplastic agents can have serious repercussions in terms of toxicity and therapeutic effects. A number of these agents are 'pro-drugs' and CYP3A4 activates them to their therapeutic metabolites. Cyclophosphamide is known to cause more toxicity in the presence of 3A4 inducers, and similar effects can be seen with taxol and etoposide. Up to a threefold increase in the clearance of these antineoplastic drugs can be seen in the presence of 3A4 inducers.

5 Cytochrome P450 Inhibition

5.1 Introduction

The previous chapter was mostly aimed at problems associated with drug failure due to enzyme induction. However, when drug clearance is slowed or even stopped for any reason, the consequences are more dangerous and occur much more rapidly compared with enzyme induction. Generally, the pharmacological effects of the drugs will be greatly intensified, leading to a clear manifestation of symptoms in the patient. In drugs with a high therapeutic index, this may not be a problem and the effects of the drug accumulation will be reversible. In narrow therapeutic index drugs, the effects can be lethal in hours. In other cases, a drug may induce a potentially lethal pharmacological effect that is only seen in very high doses, way above the normal range. This effect may or may not have been seen in the initial pre-clinical (animal) toxicity testing of the drug. The following illustrative histories underline the effects of drug accumulation.

History 1

A previously healthy 29-year-old male used terfenadine twice daily for one year to treat allergic rhinitis. The patient drank grapefruit juice two to three times weekly. One day he consumed two glasses of juice, took his terfenadine dose, and then mowed his lawn; within one hour he became ill, collapsed and died. Although usually undetectable, post-mortem terfenadine and terfenadine metabolite plasma levels were reported as 35 and 130 ng/mL respectively. These levels are within range of previously noted arrhythmogenic levels of terfenadine. The individual had no evidence of impaired hepatic function.

Analysis

The presence of grapefruit juice appears to have caused unusually high levels of the parent drug to be present in the patient's plasma. Hence some com-

Human Drug Metabolism, Michael D. Coleman
© 2005 John Wiley & Sons, Ltd

ponent of the juice prevented the clearance of the parent drug, leading to drug accumulation, which led to a fatal cardiac arrhythmia.

History 2

A 67-year-old male patient stabilized on warfarin began to drink cranberry juice twice daily in response to its reported benefits in recurrent kidney infections. Three days after starting to drink the juice, he suffered a fatal stroke. Post-mortem levels of warfarin were 40 per cent higher than previously sampled in this patient.

Analysis

That the patient had been stabilized on warfarin indicates that his clotting time was within acceptable limits and therefore the drug was being cleared at the same rate it was entering the patient's system. The onset of the consumption of cranberry juice coincided with marked accumulation of warfarin, rendering the patient highly vulnerable to haemorrhage, which occurred within the brain and led to death. It was apparent that the cranberry juice had prevented the clearance of warfarin to inactive metabolites.

History 3

A 64-year-old female with a history of depression was stabilized on amitryptiline, 150 mg/day, but without improvement in mood. Her GP added fluoxetine, 40 mg/day, and within three weeks, the patient's symptoms subsided, although one week later, she collapsed at home and was found in a coma by a relative. The patient recovered consciousness two days later and made a full recovery.

Analysis

The addition of fluoxetine to the regime was associated with accumulation of amitryptiline, which led to unconsciousness and could have led to death had she not been discovered. The fluoxetine must have prevented the clearance of amitryptiline.

History 4

A 44-year-old female epileptic was stabilized on carbamazepine but on the advice of a friend started taking a liquorice preparation for stomach problems. Over a period of two days, she became gradually more sedated and confused, until she had difficulty standing up. She was admitted to hospital and recovered within three days.

Analysis

The liquorice extract was taken in considerable amounts and appears to have interfered with the clearance of carbamazepine, leading to drug accumulation and symptoms of toxicity.

History 5

A 55-year-old female stabilized on warfarin suffered from recurrent acid indigestion over the Christmas period and started to self-medicate with over-the-counter cimetidine on the advice of a relative. A few days later, while gardening, the patient noticed that a small cut bled profusely and did not appear to clot for a long period. The patient reported to a hospital accident and emergency room, where her prothrombin time was shown to be excessive. The hospital advised her to use an alternative anti-acid agent and her prothrombin time returned to normal over several days.

Analysis

The excessive anticoagulation was due to a reduction in the clearance of warfarin by cimetidine, which could be averted by the use of low-dose (<400 mg) ranitidine or famotidine, which are not usually associated with changes in warfarin pharmacokinetics. An acceptable proton-pump inhibitor would be lansoprazole, but not omeprazole.

Overall analysis

In these cases:

- The patient was already stabilized on a particular medicine, which suggests that the dosage and clearance are approximately balanced.

- The addition to the regime prevented clearance of the first drug, leading to accumulation and toxicity.

- The toxicity would be predictable as an intensification of the normal pharmacological response, again indicating that drug accumulation was responsible.

- The toxic responses occurred within hours rather than days, after the addition of the drug.

- The toxicity manifests so quickly that death can occur before even the patient realizes what is happening.

- The toxic effects were rapidly reversible once the inhibiting drug was withdrawn.

- The effects can occur in response to the patient's decision to either self-medicate or change their diet routine, without consultation with medical staff, or the effect can occur after medical staff fail to be aware of the potential reaction.

5.2   Inhibition of metabolism – general aspects

In complete contrast to enzyme induction, drug inhibition is not usually a process where a logical adaptive response can be made by the patient's metabolism. The fact that some inhibitors can impair CYP operation for as long as they are administered indicates that the patient's homeostatic systems are not equipped to detect the inhibition effect and cannot quickly respond to the change in the situation within the timescale – it is rather like suddenly blocking the exhaust pipe of a running engine – it will cough and then simply stop. Sometimes, another CYP or metabolizing system may be capable of clearing some of the accumulating drug at higher concentrations. The kidneys may also eliminate some unchanged drug. That the lung can clear some volatile chemicals such as alcohols is exploited in road safety in the detection of drunk drivers. However, if the drug's main route of clearance is a particular CYP in the liver and clearance is mostly dependent on the liver, the resultant accumulation will occur relatively rapidly and toxicity or even death can result.

Essentially, inhibition-based drug reactions are much more potentially clinically serious than induction effects, due to this short timescale and the speed that the patient's clinical situation can change, leading to irreversible damage (such as a stroke or heart attack) within hours of consuming the inhibitor. This is especially problematic in the light of the increasing prevalence of 'polypharmacy', where patients may be taking several pharmacologically active compounds at once.

Another factor is that the inhibitor may arise from a decision the patients make themselves, through the desire to 'self-help', without informing their doctor. It is also possible that a mistake by a medical practitioner could lead to a potent inhibitor reducing the clearance of a potentially toxic drug.

Tissue homeostatic mechanisms in the liver and other tissues can respond to inhibition in certain circumstances, i.e. some form of adaptation to the situation can occur to restore clearance of the usual substrate. This depends on the type of inhibitor and the frequency of dosage and will be discussed later.

5.3 Mechanisms of inhibition

General aspects of inhibition

Enzymes and tissue/cell receptors share similar features. A receptor binds a molecule that then acts like a switch to trigger a cascade of molecules to instruct the cell to perform a function. The molecule must fit the receptor precisely and then trigger the cascade, like a key, which first enters a lock, then is successfully turned to open it. A key that fits and enters the lock, but does not turn it, not only fails to open the door but also prevents the correct key from being fitted. The lock is essentially 'inhibited'.

Although they are highly specialized, CYPs are enzymes like any other in the body and they are inhibited according to the same general principles as other enzymes. How tightly a chemical interacts with a CYP isoform is based on how powerful is the mutual attraction (affinity) between the chemical and the active site of the enzyme.

In the case of CYPs and any enzyme, affinity must be strong enough to ensure the substrate is bound for sufficient time to process it to a product. The quicker this process occurs, the faster the 'turnover' of the enzyme and the more efficient it is. It is useful to try to visualize a CYP isoform, or any other human enzyme for that matter, as a three-dimensional machine tool, or a spot welding machine. The enzyme cycles hundreds of times a second. If any single aspect of substrate binding or processing (oxidation or reduction), followed by product release is prevented, the sequential nature of these events means that the enzyme stops functioning. Another analogy might be an automatic paper stapler in a photocopier. Whatever analogy you might use, it is useful to try to visualize enzymes as dynamic micro machines. Broadly, inhibitors of CYPs may frustrate the enzymes' operating processes in two main ways, with varying impact on drug clearance and the individual enzyme 'health' and survival. At high concentrations, many inhibitors might block several CYP subfamilies, but at lower concentrations, they show more selectivity and their potency in blocking individual isoforms can be measured. Inhibition can occur through four main processes: competitive, non-competitive, uncompetitive and mechanism-based. Which type of inhibition occurs with various drugs can depend on many factors, such as drug concentration and the characteristics of a particular CYP isoform. Many drugs can act as competitive inhibitors with one CYP and non-competitive with others. Many studies with inhibitors of drug metabolism are carried out *in vitro* with human CYPs, either in human liver or in expressed enzyme systems (see Appendix A). These studies do not always reflect what will happen when the drugs are used in patients, but are a reasonable starting point to predict whether a new drug might interfere with the metabolism of another.

Competitive inhibition

This is the simplest form of inhibition, where the substrate (drug) and the inhibitor are very similar in structure and have similar affinities for the same place, i.e. the CYP active site (Figure 5.1). A CYP substrate is normally processed to a different molecule, that is, a metabolite, which then has a much reduced affinity for an active site and is more water-soluble, so it diffuses elsewhere. A competitive inhibitor of a CYP isoform is usually not a substrate and acts like a similar key to the correct key for a doorlock; it may enter and leave the lock freely but does not operate it. As it is not processed into a product, it does not leave the vicinity of the CYP and binds and detaches continually. The CYP might be unable to metabolize the inhibitor, due to particular features of the molecule that might prevent oxidation, but promote binding to the active site. This form of inhibition is common in CYPs and is governed by the law of mass action, which states that the rate of a

Main Types of Enzyme Inhibition

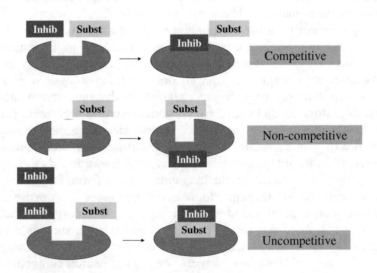

Figure 5.1   Main types of enzyme inhibition that apply to CYP isoforms.

reaction (in this case enzyme binding) is governed by the concentration of the participants. So for CYP metabolism, whichever agent, drug or inhibitor, is in the greatest concentration, then this will occupy the active site. At low inhibitor concentrations more drug can be added to overcome the inhibitory effects. However, as drug levels must be increased to overcome the inhibitor, this effectively means that the drug's affinity falls for the site (K_m increases) in the presence of the inhibitor. Enzymes are often subject to this process of competitive inhibition because it is usually part of the endogenous feedback control mechanism on product formation. This generally involves enzymes that use cellular energy, or are at the junction of several biosynthetic pathways. When high levels of product are formed, these inhibit the substrate, so limiting the enzyme's 'turnover', i.e. when the desired product level is reached. This is rather like a thermostat in a heating system, which automatically maintains a preset temperature irrespective of outside temperatures. This is seen in the regulation of vital endogenous molecules like NADPH and glutathione (GSH) and the process avoids unnecessary use of cellular energy. Although the enzyme is temporarily disabled, it is undamaged and has not cycled or used any reducing power. Mathematically, if a Lineweaver–Burk double reciprocal plot is made of competitive inhibition, the K_m (inverse of the affinity) changes, but the V_{max} does not; in other words, the enzyme will still run at a maximum rate if enough substrate is used, but affinity falls off.

A new drug might be evaluated as a possible inhibitor of a given CYP isoform; if the inhibition of the known CYP substrate yields a Lineweaver–Burk plot as described above, then the new drug is a competitive inhibitor of that CYP and it is likely that the inhibitor is binding the CYP at its active site. There are several examples of competitive inhibitors of CYP isoforms. Indeed, if two drugs of similar affinities are cleared by the same isoform, then competitive inhibition can occur. The major clinically relevant group of competitive inhibitors are the azole antifungal agents.

Azoles

It is not surprising that these agents are potent human P450 inhibitors, as a great deal of money, time and effort was put into designing them as inhibitors of fungal CYPs. They prevent the fungal synthesis of ergosterol, by blocking lanosterol alpha-C_{14}-demethylase, so causing the substrates (14-alpha-methylsterols) to accumulate and this disrupts fungal membranes. Unfortunately, as mentioned in Chapter 2, since all living system CYPs originate from a common bacterial source, inhibition of azole compounds also occurs in human CYPs. Interestingly, this is relatively specific; ketoconazole was initially the most commonly used azole agent and this is a potent competitive inhibitor of CYP3A4, as well as a number of other sex steroid-handling CYPs. This meant that the drug was quite toxic, as it caused a significant fall in testosterone levels in blood, which could lead to feminization of males. This could be seen as the appearance of breasts (gynaecomastia), loss of spermatozoa production and impotence. The female menstrual cycle was also disrupted. These effects, coupled with other toxicity, such as GI tract irritation, nausea, vomiting and occasional severe liver toxicity, propelled the continuing development of these agents to less toxic azoles, which would be more potent therapeutically, but with less human CYP impact. These appeared in the 1990s, in the form of itraconazol and fluconazole, which were followed by the third-generation triazoles, such as voriconazole and posaconazole, which are hundreds of times more potent than ketoconazole as antifungals *in vitro*, but much less inhibitory on human CYPs, although they do still inhibit CYPs 3A4, 2C9 and 2C19. Indeed, the clearance of the anti-rejection drug tacrolimus (CYP3A4 substrate) is probably inhibited by voriconazole. All azoles, including others such as miconazole and clotrimazole, are generally purely competitive inhibitors, due to their lone pair of electrons on the azole nitrogen, which temporarily binds to the haem groups of several CYPs.

Clinically, even the newer azoles can make a marked impact on the clearance of CYP3A4 substrates. In one clinical study the peak plasma concentration of the 3A4 substrate felodipine was increased eightfold and the area under the curve sixfold by the presence of itraconazole. Fluconazole is a much weaker inhibitor of CYP3A4, but can be a potent inhibitor of other CYPs such as 2C19. Fluconazole has been shown to increase the half-life of omeprazole by threefold and its area under the curve (AUC) by a similar value. Other 3A4 substrates, such as midazolam, terfenadine and lovastatin, show similar effects with this azole. Clearly, the impact of the inhibition on the pharmacological effects of these drugs is very strong, with significant potentiation of their particular effects. It is interesting that although the inhibitory action of these drugs is simple and reversible, the clinical effect of this process on other drug effects can potentially be extremely serious. However, in a matter of hours after the withdrawal of the azole, the inhibiting effect is lost and substrate clearance resumes. There appears to be no way that the liver CYP nuclear 'management system' which is seen operating so successfully with enzyme inducers, can overcome the effects of a drug such as ketoconazole when the agent is taken for a long period of time. The serious disruption of steroid metabolism (gynaecomastia again) testifies to this problem. The inhibition appears to be stable for as long as the drug is administered. This has led to attempts to use inhibitors such as ketoconazole and cimetidine to deliberately block the clearance of certain drugs, of which more later.

Non-competitive inhibition

Non-competitive inhibition does not involve the inhibitor and substrate competing for the same active site (Figure 5.1). In non-competitive inhibition, there is another site involved, known as the allosteric site, which is distant from the active site. Once a ligand binds this allosteric site, the conformation of the active site is automatically changed and it becomes less likely to bind the substrate and product formation tails off. This process of allosteric binding is another example of the endogenous control of product formation, perhaps by another product/substrate from a related or similar pathway. The net result is to slow or even halt product formation at the main site, depending on how much allosteric binding occurs. The Lineweaver–Burk plot will show a fall-off in V_{max} (enzyme cannot run at maximal rate) but K_m does not change, that is, the affinity of the substrate for the active site is unchanged.

It has been demonstrated experimentally that many drugs are non-competitive inhibitors of CYP isoforms. This means that the inhibitor is not binding at the active site and must exert some allosteric effect elsewhere. As knowledge of the active site of CYPs is still incomplete, we are still not fully aware as to exactly where these allosteric sites are and where they figure in the control of CYPs. In Chapter 3, it was discussed that CYP3A4 had more than one site available for binding and that various substrates could influence the binding of other substrates, probably connected with hormone metabolism. This potentially provides an hour-by-hour modulation of CYP activity, which is of course necessary during steroidal control of reproductive processes. It is likely that non-competitive inhibition is a result of drugs fitting these allosteric sites within most CYP isoforms and influencing binding of substrates to the main catalytic site. There are several examples of non-competitive inhibitors of CYPs. St John's Wort extract (hyperforin) is a potent inhibitor of CYP2D6 *in vitro*, although it is not known if this occurs significantly *in vivo*. Omeprazole and lansoprazole are non-competitive CYP3A4 inhibitors *in vitro*.

Uncompetitive inhibition

This is an unusual form of inhibition, where the inhibitor binds only to the enzyme/substrate complex (Figure 5.1). This has the effect of stimulating enzyme/substrate complex formation so increasing affinity (fall in K_m), although the enzyme/substrate/inhibitor complex is non-functional, so the V_{max} falls. This appears to be a relatively rare form of inhibition of human CYPs by therapeutic drugs, although some dietary agents such as the flavonoid tangeretin, found in citrous fruits, is an uncompetitive inhibitor of CYP3A4 in human liver microsomes.

Mechanism-based inhibitors

This type of inhibition is outside the normal classification as outlined with competitive, non-competitive and uncompetitive inhibitions. Mechanism

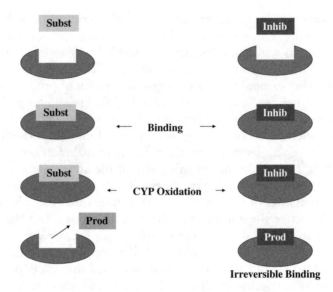

Figure 5.2 Scheme of normal substrate CYP binding (left) and mechanism-based inhibitor on the right, which results in the irreversible binding of product and inactivation of the CYP isoform

based inhibition generally involves the same initial steps as a competitive inhibitor, but then the CYP catalytic cycle proceeds, reducing power is consumed and a metabolite is formed, which then occupies the P450 active site for a far longer period than the usual substrate would (Figure 5.2). Mechanism-based inhibitors could occupy an allosteric site in a CYP and thus act as non-competitive inhibitors; macrolide antibiotics are sometimes classed as non-competitive inhibitors even though they are mechanism-based. The nearest mechanical analogy to a mechanism-based inhibitor would be the incorrect key turning fully in the lock and not opening, followed by difficult extraction of the key, or even the key breaking off in the lock. This form of inhibition can range from delayed product release, all the way to a violently reactive species-mediated damage to the enzyme, leading to the destruction of the active site. There are degrees of mechanism-based inhibition and moderately potent inhibitors such as the macrolides (like erythromycin) are eventually removed from the CYP active site, but do not usually damage the enzyme. However, highly potent mechanism-based inhibitors such as the contents of grapefruit juice, damage the enzyme to a degree that it is non-functional. This latter process is often termed 'suicide' inhibition. Clinically, a competitive inhibitor should wear off after just one or two half-lives, i.e. a few hours to a day or so, depending on a number of factors (inhibitor and substrate dosage, etc.). The most extreme form of mechanism-based inhibition, such as grapefruit juice, norfluoxetine or MDMA-mediated 'suicide' inhibition, destroys the enzyme from one dose of inhibitor and this takes several days to resolve.

The effects of mechanism-based inhibition can be shown very clearly *in vitro*, where the potency of the inhibition is much greater when the CYP enzymes are incubated with NADPH and the compound prior to the addition of the usual substrate. This enables the enzymes to use the reducing power to run the catalytic cycle, which forms the reactive metabolite, which effectively disables the enzyme. The longer this process goes on, the more enzyme is disabled, so the inhibition becomes more potent over time. V_{max} falls and affinity decreases then obviously, no matter how much substrate is added, the inhibition continues, as the law of mass action cannot apply because the inhibitor may well be already covalently bound to most of the CYP sites. If the substrate is present in reasonably high concentrations prior to the appearance of the inhibitor, the substrate can protect the enzyme, although if the inhibitor continues to be present in adequate concentration, this protective effect will eventually be lost. *In vivo*, mechanism-dependent inhibition lasts for days as previously mentioned, although the inhibition is clinically reversible, but as far as the individual enzyme is concerned, irreversible. This is because the clinical effect is consistent with the time taken for more P450 enzyme to be resynthesized to replace the inactivated enzyme. Obviously this will only be clinically reversible if the inhibitor was only dosed once, or over a short period. Mechanism-based inhibition is often summarized as follows:

- The inhibition becomes stronger over time;
- Inhibition does not progress without co-factors (NADPH);
- Presence of substrate slows the rate of inhibition by protecting the CYP;
- After inhibition, intact enzyme cannot be detected by analytical techniques (irreversibly inactivated).

There are many clinically important non-competitive and mechanism-based 'suicide' inhibitors, which vary in the intensity of their inhibition. These include the macrolides (erythromycin, clarithromycin, oleandomycin), HIV protease inhibitors (ritonavir, indinavir, saquinavir, nelfinavir), the SSRIs (e.g. fluoxetine) and finally grapefruit juices. Unfortunately, all these compounds are metabolized by, and eventually inhibit, our major CYP3A4, whilst the illicit amphetamine derivative MDMA irreversibly blocks CYP2D6 (Appendix B).

Grapefruit juice

Although patients have been heroically consuming grapefruit juice for their health for decades, it took until the late 1980s before effects on drug clearance were noted and several more years before it was realized that there could be a major problem with drug interactions (History 1). This led to the regulatory authorities to remove terfenadine from the list of OTC medicines in the UK. The most noteworthy feature of the effect of grapefruit juice is its potency from a single 'dose' which coincides with a typical single breakfast intake of the juice, say around 200–300 ml. Studies with CYP3A substrates such as midazolam have shown that it can take up to three days before the effects wear off, which is consistent with the synthesis of new enzyme. The most interesting aspect is that grapefruit juice was thought not to inhibit hepatic CYP3A4, but gut CYP3A. It is useful to clarify this point. In the mid 1990's it was shown that grapefruit juice did not appear to inhibit the clearance of intravenously dosed drugs, although it would inhibit when the drug was orally dosed. More recently it has been established that *in vitro*, there is no difference in the inhibitory effects of other agents such as azoles (fluconazole and ketoconazole) on CYP3A4 from human gut or liver. So grapefruit juice should be technically capable of blocking hepatic CYP3A4. However, when modest amounts 200–300 mls of average strength juice are consumed, the combination of its irreversible CYP binding and a high gut CYP3A expression, means that virtually none of the inhibitor physically reaches the liver. In 2003, human volunteer studies showed that if the dosage of grapefruit juice is very high, enough inhibitor escapes the gut CYP binding to block hepatic CYP3A4.

It might at first appear unusual that an inhibitor of gut wall metabolism would have such a devastating effect on systemic levels of a drug. However, there are a number of drugs that are subject to a very high gut wall component to their 'first-pass' metabolism (or pre-systemic metabolism); these include midazolam, terfenadine, lovastatin, simvastatin and astemizole. Their gut CYP clearance is so high that if the juice inhibits it, the concentration reaching the liver can increase six- or sevenfold. If the liver normally only extracts a relatively minor proportion of the parent drug, then plasma levels of the drug increase dramatically towards toxicity levels (see section 1.5). This effect is compounded by grapefruit juice-mediated inhibition of efflux pumps such as P-glycoprotein (section 5.4), which normally retard absorption by constantly pumping xenobiotics out of gut cells almost as soon as they enter them.

As has been mentioned, the inhibitor effects of grapefruit juice in high first-pass drugs is particularly clinically relevant as it can occur after one exposure of the juice. Obviously, the higher the pre-systemic metabolism of a drug (low bioavailability) the greater effect the juice is going to show. One interesting characteristic of the grapefruit juice effect is that the plasma half-lives of the drugs do not change, as the liver carries on metabolizing the drugs as usual, provided the grapefruit juice 'dose' is modest.

Summary: drugs that should not be used with grapefruit juice:

- Undergo high pre-systemic (enteric) metabolism;

- Are metabolized by CYP3A;

- Exhibit pharmacological effects in high dose/high plasma levels are life threatening.

Here are some examples of the variable risk of grapefruit juice.

*Drugs that should **not** be taken with grapefruit juice:*
Terfenadine, statins (simvastatin, cerivastatin (withdrawn, 2001),
atorvastatin), amiodarone, astemiszole, buspirone, indinavir, sildinafil,
pimozide, cilostazol, etoposide, saquinavir

Drugs that may be problematic with grapefruit juice:
Benzodiazepines (midazolam, triazolam, diazepam), cyclosporine,
nifedipine, nisoldipine, synthetic opiates (methadone, dextromethorphan),
macrolide antibiotics (erythromycin), carbamazepine, quinine, sertraline,
azole antifungals (Itraconazole), losartan, steroids (prednisolone)

There are several drugs where others in their chemical class are inhibited by
grapefruit juice but they are unaffected:

Fluvastatin, pravastatin, rosuvastatin, loratadine

As to the precise component of grapefruit juice that is responsible for these
effects, there are several agents that have been evaluated. The juice contains
large numbers of flavonoids, which include naringin, a weak CYP inhibitor,
which can be metabolized by gut bacteria to naringenin, which is a more potent
inhibitor. However, it is more likely that the bergamottins (6'7'dihydroxy-
bergamottin and bergamottin itself), a group of furanocoumarins, may be
among the most potent CYP inhibitors in the juice. The 6'7'dihydroxy derivative is much more potent *in vitro* than bergamottin itself. Bergamottins are
also found in Seville orange juice, which can exert similar effects to grapefruit
juice. It appears that however the juice is prepared, either as concentrate, or
canned, as segments or the fruit itself, there is no escape as the inhibitory effects
still occur. It has also been found that a further furanocoumarin, epoxybergamottin, which is present in grapefruit peel, is also a CYP3A4 inhibitor. It has
been suggested that peel contamination might contribute to the inhibitory
effects, or that the epoxybergamottin undergoes hydrolysis to the most potent
CYP3A4 inhibitor in the juice, 6', 7'-dihydroxybergamottin. A number of
other citrous fruits have flavonoid inhibitors also, such as pomelos. The
inhibitors in cranberry juice are not known (Case History 2), however
further research is likely to uncover more potent inhibitors in various juice
extracts.

Seratonin reuptake inhibitors (SSRIs)

SSRIs present a particularly difficult therapeutic problem, in that they are the
current drugs of choice for depression, but adding them to a regimen of
several drugs requires some thought as to the consequences of their considerable inhibitory effects. There are five major SSRIs used in clinical practice:
fluoxetine, paroxetine, citalopram, fluvoxamine and sertraline. Although they
can be potent *in vitro* inhibitors of CYPs such as 2D6, which oxidizes many

TCAs (History 3) and antipsychotics, their *in vivo* effects are not necessarily as potent. It is important to realize that not all the SSRIs are potent inhibitors of drug metabolism *in vivo*, as the doses used for clinical effect are much lower comparatively than those used in *in vitro* studies that show inhibitory effects. The effects of recommended SSRI dosages for depression have been evaluated in patients on TCAs (History 4) such as desipramine, a 2D6 marker. Fluoxetine was the most potent inhibitor, causing a three- to sixfold increase in plasma levels of desipramine; paroxetine caused a three- to fourfold increase, whilst citalpram showed a much less potent effect, which was around a 50 per cent increase. Sertraline and fluvoxamine showed impact on the levels of the TCA.

Fluoxetine (Prozac) is cleared to S-norfluoxetine, and this is among the most potent inhibitors of CYP2D6 *in vitro* and *in vivo*. Essentially, drugs such as TCAs, which have comparatively narrow therapeutic indices, should be used with great care with fluoxetine (History 3). Inhibitor effects will be much worse in patients such as the elderly, who have compromised drug clearance already (Chapter 7). Fluoxetine is a substrate of CYP2D6, so it can even block its own metabolism, making dosage adjustments unusually difficult. Fluoxetine and S-norfluoxetine can also moderately inhibit CYP2C9 and CYP2C19, and clinically they can cause phenytoin, a CYP2C9 substrate, to accumulate dangerously. Although fluoxetine is a weak inhibitor of CYP1A2 and CYP3A4, the clinical significance of such interactions is unclear. Interactions with SSRIs are best documented for 2D6 substrates, although more research is necessary to determine the clinical relevance of their inhibitory effects on other CYPs.

Other mechanism-based inhibitors

Herbal preparations contain some mechanism-based inhibitors of various CYP isoforms and these are capable of making a similar impact on the clearance of prescribed drugs as grapefruit juice. These preparations are often spontaneously adopted by patients on the recommendation of a friend or after reading some form of publicity. Although patients should tell their doctors and health care workers they are taking these substances, they often do not, as they do not feel that it is relevant or important.

Capsaicin

Found in various hot peppers and used as flavourings in spicy foodstuffs. Pepper extracts have been used medicinally to treat many conditions from diabetes to inflammatory diseases. However, capsaicin is oxidized by CYP2E1 to reactive metabolites such as epoxides and phenoxy radicals that irreversibly inhibit the CYP isoform.

Liquorice extract

Contains an isoflavan known as glabridin, which is a potent mechanism-based inhibitor of CYP3A4, although it can competitively inhibit CYP2C9 (History 4).

Extracts have been used in the South Pacific islands for many years for a wide variety of applications, although the kavalactones in the extract, methysticin and dihydromethysticin, are potent inhibitors of most human CYPs *in vitro* with the exception of 2E1. Kava-Kava has been associated with liver damage, from mild toxicity, all the way to liver failure, requiring transplant.

5.4 Cell transport systems and CYP3A inhibitors

Efflux transporters (P-glycoprotein)

Although a great deal of effort is focused on the role of the liver in drug clearance, it is becoming more apparent that the gut wall has a particularly important role to play in the metabolism of drugs. In a recent study in human duodenum, jejunum and liver biopsies, it was found that CYP3A4 levels were three times higher in the gut wall than in the liver. Although inhibition of gut CYP3A by agents such as grapefruit juice should greatly increase bioavailability, this effect can be highly variable, partly due to the effects of such inhibitors on other cellular systems, such as mechanisms of drug cellular transport. P-glycoprotein is a molecular pump system, which is part of the group of ATP-binding cassette transporters (ABC transporters). P-glycoprotein, as well as CYP3A, is strongly expressed in intestinal cells where drugs are absorbed. Indeed, it is found in the apical areas of the human gut wall enterocytes at seven times the activity of liver tissue. As the drug enters the gut cells, the P-glycoprotein system actively pumps it out into the gut lumen again. The combination of the high apical P-glycoprotein and CYP3A4 levels in enterocytes appears to operate as a coordinated response to the threat posed by lipophilic xenobiotics. The effect of pumping the drug out is said to increase the possibility of the drug meeting the CYP on its return journey. The combination clearly retards drug absorption, but does not usually completely prevent it. P-glycoproteins are found in all species and have been the subject of intense interest, as bacteria, protozoa and human cancerous cells all use this system to protect themselves from potential toxic agents by simply pumping out the toxin, be it an antibiotic or an alkylating agent. If P-glycoprotein appears in sufficient quantity to clear the agent as fast as it enters, even potent cytotoxins will exert little or no effect. Attempts to use drugs such as verapamil, to inhibit P-glycoprotein to improve the bioavailability of anticancer agents have not been as effective as predicted, partly due to a lack of specific P-glycoprotein inhibition. This is because many of these inhibitors also block CYP3A isoforms, which impedes the effectiveness of drugs such as cyclophosphamide that depend on CYP3A4 activation to kill tumour cells. Specific P-glycoprotein inhibitors are under development, but there is some scepticism as to whether they will be useful in clinical practice, as efflux pumps are found in most tissues and it may be difficult to target the effect of the inhibitors.

The genes that code for P-glycoproteins have been termed MDR or multidrug resistant genes and their substrate specificity is so wide as to be almost non-specific and has been described as 'fuzzy'. Some studies have suggested that substrates are likely to be lipophilic, with molecular weights greater than 400, to have pKa's greater than 4, and the sum of their nitrogen and oxygen molecules to be greater than or equal to eight. Non-substrates are low in nitrogen and oxygen, less than 400 Mwt and a basic pKa of less than eight.

It is logical to expect that there would be considerable overlap between MDR proteins and CYPs as they are effectively carrying out a similar function using different means, that is, to protect the cell from small lipophilic molecules. If a drug is a potent inhibitor of gut CYP3A, it is often, but not always, capable of blocking P-glycoprotein.

In terms of what is known about P-glycoprotein, an inhibitor such as verapamil or grapefruit juice will increase the bioavailability of other drugs that are substrates for the pump system, such as cyclosporine. The anti-rejection agent tacrolimus has a narrow therapeutic index, so small changes in its bioavailability may have serious clinical effects. Tacrolimus blood levels increase in the presence of pomelo, a citrus fruit related to grapefruit, as this agent is a CYP3A4 and P-glycoprotein substrate.

However, digoxin is a known substrate of P-glycoprotein and it also has a narrow therapeutic index. Inhibitors of P-glycoprotein can certainly elevate digoxin to fatal levels in animal studies, but grapefruit juice does not appear to affect digoxin bioavailability in man, possibly because P-glycoprotein transport does not normally have as much effect on total digoxin availability as it does with other drugs. However, other P-glycoprotein substrates such as atorvastatin are believed to increase the bioavailability of digoxin, possibly by competition for P-glycoprotein transport. Interestingly, atorvastatin is not thought to change the clearances of other 3A4 substrates, i.e. ritonavir, nelfinavir or terfenadine.

To further complicate the picture, there are a series of organic anion-transporting polypeptides, known as OATPs. These transport systems can also be inhibited by grapefruit juice and can reduce the absorption of fexofenadine that is a known OATP substrate.

Overall, the contribution of the multi-factorial complexity of pre-systemic metabolism is still being researched and it is often difficult to establish what contribution cellular transport systems make to bioavailability. Indeed, it is emerging that one of the reasons for the very wide variety of drug bioavailability in modern medicine could be the sheer number of possible inhibitors and substrates that exist for P-glycoprotein in the diet. These range from natural products to food contaminants. Since no two people's diets are identical, the impact of P-glycoprotein modulation on drug absorption may never be fully realized. Efflux transporter systems are discussed again under the heading of Phase III of metabolism, where MDR-type transporters remove conjugated metabolites from the cell using efflux pumps of similar structure and function to P-glycoprotein (Chapter 6).

5.5 Clinical consequences of drug inhibition

Introduction

Although CYP inhibition can be competitive, non-competitive, uncompetitive or mechanism dependent, in clinical practice the main concern is how rapidly the inhibitor causes drug levels to climb towards toxicity and whether the toxic effects can be treated before serious injury or death results. As has been mentioned already, there are a number of major clinical conditions caused by inhibition of drug clearance that can overtake even healthy individuals in a matter of hours. The speed at which these problems can be manifested cannot be overemphasized. Clearly, the best option is prevention:

- Firstly, by ensuring that health care professionals do not make mistakes; if these do occur, someone should immediately 'pick up the ball' and ensure that the mistake is not translated to a potentially fatal prescription that could be handed to a patient.

- Secondly, the patient must be informed about the dangers of some drugs in combination with inhibitors. This should prevent patient intake of both dietary inhibitors and over-the-counter/herbal preparations that could block the metabolism of prescribed drugs.

Torsades des Pointes

Literally translated as 'twisting of the points', this is where a drug blocks the potassium ion channel known as IKr. This leads to the cardiac ventricular QT interval becoming prolonged. The expression QT is described in an ECG wave analysis of the period elapsed between ventricular depolarization and repolarization – this effectively means the time taken for heart muscle to contract and then recover. The recommended treatment for torsades des pointes is to withdraw the suspected causative agent and then administer intravenous magnesium sulphate. If the QT interval increases beyond 0.45 of a second, this leads to ventricular tachycardia, arrhythmia and eventually fibrillation, with total cardiac disorganization and no detectable QRS complex. The patient collapses and the only treatment is rapid defibrillation (History 1). It is most often caused by myocardial infarction, but a significant list of drugs can also trigger it. These include: Amiodarone, sotalol, procainamide, disopyramide, pimozide, (cisapride was withdrawn in 2000 for this reason) and non-sedative antihistamines such as terfenadine and astemizole, TCA's, macrolides, fluoroquinolones and antipsychotics.

Obviously any inhibitor that prevents clearance of these agents could precipitate QT interval prolongation. This has been found to be the case with a number of 3A4 substrates, including amiodarone, pimozide, cisapride, terfenadine and astemizole.

Clearly it is important to avoid any possibility of triggering QT interval problems; for example, terfenadine can be replaced with its active metabolite, fexofenadine (carboxyterfenadine). It has also been suggested that less potent azoles such as fluconazole would be much less of a risk in triggering QT interval change with a CYP3A4 substrate as it is a much less potent inhibitor compared with the other azoles, although it is known to increase cyclosporine plasma levels and is a risk with low therapeutic index 3A4 substrates in general.

Sedative effects

The risk of sedation is obviously less of a problem in the home, rather than perhaps operating heavy machinery with razor-sharp rotating blades. The co-administration of inhibitors with drugs such as the benzodiazepines and others such as buspirone can potentiate their sedative effects markedly. Midazolam is used as a sedative in intensive care units and particularly in children, there is already a large variation in individual clearances, so any inhibition of the metabolism of this drug may cause excessive sedation. The azole inhibitors, in the expected order of severity, can seriously retard midazolam clearance: ketoconazole > itraconazole > fluconazole. The selective serotonin reuptake inhibitor (SSRI) fluoxetine and its principal metabolite, norfluoxetine, are also potent inhibitors of midazolam clearance, and the norfluoxetine derivative is a particularly potent inhibitor of any 3A4 substrate. Fluvoxetine is also a strong 3A4 inhibitor. However, these can be replaced by sertraline or paroxetine that have much less significant inhibitory effects to prevent excessive sedation with benzodiazepines. Co-administration of SSRIs and other 3A4 inhibitors cause accumulation of other 3A4-cleared drugs such as carbamazepine (History 4). In addition to sedation, the effects of high plasma levels of carbamazepine can lead to mental confusion, ataxia (staggering gait) and even unconsciousness.

Muscle damage (rhabdomyolysis)

This is when striated muscle disintegrates and the released myoglobin enters the blood and then the urine, eventually leading to renal failure. Blunt force trauma, some infections, burns, ischaemia, or severe exercise usually cause it. However, it can also occur in response to exposure of some drugs and chemicals. Heroin and solvent abusers can develop it, but it can occur in response to statin treatment. The use of cerivastatin has been curtailed as rhabdomyolysis has occurred when the drug was used with gemfibrozil. It seems that if statin plasma levels rise to high levels, creatine kinase levels are elevated in plasma and this can lead to rhabdomyolysis. The statins have become increasingly important as their cholesterol-lowering effects are a valuable component of the general effort to reduce ischaemic cardiovascular disease. They are seen as quite safe drugs and some statins are now available OTC at relatively low doses. However, simvastatin, lovastatin, atorvastatin and cerivastatin are 3A4 substrates and are vulnerable to elevation of plasma levels in the presence of potent 3A4 inhibitors. This is a particular concern with inhibitors such as grapefruit juice, the azoles and erythromycin. If statin therapy must be continued in the presence of a 3A4 inhibitor, it would be wise to use those which are cleared by other CYPs, such as fluvastatin (CYP2C9) or pravastatin. Patients taking immunosuppressants and those with renal problems are more prone to develop rhabdomyolysis than others and are at particular risk. It is safest to avoid the interaction by substituting non-inhibiting drugs or statins cleared by other CYPs.

Excessive hypotension

As you will, of course, no doubt remember from your pharmacology studies, there are several different drug options in the management of hypertension. This is fortunate, as this condition is very common, sometimes does not respond to therapy and deteriorates with age. This means that antihypertensives of various types are prescribed in vast amounts to older patients, usually for many years. These include CYP3A4 substrates, such as the dihydropyridines (nifedipine, felodipine, nicardipine, and nimodipine). These calcium channel blockers very useful and well tolerated. Nicardipine is more selective for heart vessels, while nimodipine is more effective in cerebral vessels. However, the most common problem with them is excessive vasodilatation that can lead to postural hypotension, dizziness, and headache. They can work too well, to the point where blood pressure is insufficient to force blood through diseased coronary arteries and they can cause reflex tachycardia; these effects can make some forms of angina worse.

Obviously any marked changes in the clearance of these potent drugs could lead to potentially major deleterious changes in cardiovascular function. It is easy to see how the azoles and the macrolide inhibitors could cause severe cardiovascular problems due to non-clearance of dihydropyridines. Their high pre-systemic metabolism means that grapefruit juice would have a particularly potent and possibly life-threatening effect. Interestingly, the lack of gut metabolism of amlodipine makes this agent less susceptible to grapefruit juice interactions. Any antihypertensive agent that is a 3A4 substrate will be liable to cause excessive reductions in blood pressure if they accumulate in the presence of an inhibitor. This is a particularly problematic effect in the case of suicide inhibitors like grapefruit juice and norfluoxetine.

Ergotism

Until the advent of the highly effective group of triptan 5HT agonists, severe migraine sufferers were faced with the prospect of using ergotamine tartrate or suffering the extremely unpleasant pain that this syndrome can inflict. As a migraine sufferer myself, my one experience with ergotamine in 1980 led to a painful effect as if there were wires tightening inside my calf muscles. This took two days to wear off and I still suffered the headache. Ergotamine can also cause severe neural derangement known as 'St Anthony's fire', which sometimes affected people where mouldy flour was used to make bread that contained a considerable dose of ergot alkaloids. Ergotamine is cleared by CYP3A4, so the effects of any inhibitor of this isoform on ergot clearance would lead to an extremely grim series of peripheral and CNS symptoms. Fortunately, the triptans (sumatriptan, naratriptan, zolmatriptan, etc.) are the mainstay of acute migraine treatment and the ergotism problem with CYP3A4 inhibitors should now be very rare.

Excessive anticoagulation

Although a number of new anticoagulants are under development, warfarin remains the most commonly used agent for the treatment of a number of conditions where thrombosis is at high risk, such as those with replacement heart valves, atrial fibrillation and deep venous thrombosis. It is a reflection of the vast patient mortality and morbidity due to cardiovascular disease in developed countries that warfarin is the fourth most commonly prescribed agent in the US alone. Warfarin therapy is closely monitored through its pharmacological effect (prothrombin time and INR; international normalized ratio, usually set at 1.5–3), rather than its plasma levels. The drug is given as a racemic mixture (R and S-isomers) and the S-isomer is more potent than the

R-isomer. The clearance of the drug to hydroxylated metabolites occurs sterioselectively, with 1A2 and 2C19 metabolizing the R-isomer, whilst 2C9 is responsible for the clearance of the more potent S-isomer. Inhibition of 2C9-mediated S-isomer clearance has more impact on warfarin's pharmacological effect than effects on the other CYPs, although they do show some impact. Cimetidine, an inhibitor of 1A2 and 2C19 (Case History 5), is not recommended for concurrent therapy with warfarin, although it is available OTC and thus there is potential for a moderate increase in prothrombin time. Potent CYP2C9 inhibitors, such as some azoles and SSRIs, can cause a major increase in warfarin's half-life and thus dangerously magnify its anticoagulating effects. A number of other drugs can also partially inhibit warfarin metabolism and lead to increases in prothrombin time; these include amiodarone, trimethoprim, isoniazid, sulphamethoxazole (in the bactrim combination with trimethoprim), sulfinpyrazone, propafenone, metronidazole (inhibits S-isomer), some statins and disulfiram.

Warfarin acts by antagonizing the effects of vitamin K, which is necessary for the formation of several clotting factors. A therapeutic dose basically knocks out around half the usual formation of these factors. It is worth noting that changes to warfarin clearance can take some time to be reflected in changes in prothrombin time. This is because the effect of the drug depends on the rate of removal of blood clotting factors that had already been formed before the drug took effect. From an initial dose, it can take up to a day and a half before any change in INR occurs. The drug already has a long half-life (1–3 days) so when a drug increases warfarin's clearance, it will take perhaps 1–2 days before an effect is seen in terms of prothrombin time and this effect will not disappear for a few days. The most serious effects of excessive coagulation are GI tract bleeding and intracranial haemorrhage, both of which can be fatal.

5.6   Use of inhibitors for positive clinical intervention

Introduction

The effects of inhibitors on the concentrations of CYP substrates can be so dramatic that it has occurred to a number of scientists and clinicians to explore various strategies to exploit this effect to provide some form of benefit to the patient. This can take the form of preventing the formation of a toxic metabolite, to modulate hormone levels in cancer chemotherapy, or even to reduce the cost of prescribing an expensive drug. The key factor in this approach is whether the increased burden and risk to the patient of taking another drug in what is effectively an unlicensed application is really beneficial to the patient. As you can imagine, these applications have met with varying levels of success and acceptance and are discussed below.

The use of inhibitors to arrest hormone-dependent tumours

This is by far the most successful clinical application of inhibitors of CYP-mediated metabolism, although the development of these drugs has taken nearly 30 years. Most breast cancers are hormone dependent for their progression, so two treatment strategies can be pursued, one to blockade the receptors (tamoxifen) and the other to prevent the oestrogens being formed from androgenic precursors, such as 4-hydroxyandrostenedione. Unfortunately, the 'ATAC' Trial showed no benefit in combining the two strategies. The main distinguishing characteristic of an oestrogenic molecule to an oestrogen receptor is the aromatized 'A' ring and the androgenic precursor is subject to a series of CYP19 'aromatase'-mediated reactions, rather like a spot-welding robot in car advertisements, which result in the aromatic 'A' ring; the oestrogen is completed by CYP17 that also alters the substituents on the D (far right-hand) ring of the steroid. The first aromatase inhibitor to be useful clinically was aminoglutethimide, which blocked oestrogen formation in peripheral tissues. However, this drug was quite toxic and resulted in haematological problems and agranulocytosis (loss of all neutrophils), which can be fatal.

It was shown in the 1970s that ketoconazole had potential to treat some breast cancers, although it was not pursued due to its hepatotoxicity. A great deal of research into aromatase led to the development of anastrazole (Arimidex®), exemestane (Aromasin®), and letrozole (Femara®). These agents are vastly more potent than aminoglutethimide, although the latter agent is still used in Cushing's syndrome and to control adrenal hormone formation in post-menapausal women. Anastrazole is highly effective in abolishing oestrogen formation, although it does show the side effects expected from loss of oestrogen, such as loss of body strength, nausea and hot flushes. However, it is superior to tamoxifen in hormone sensitive early breast cancer. Interestingly, a new generation of agents has emerged which provide a third strategy to fight hormone-dependent tumours. These oestrogen receptor downregulators are designed to degrade and destroy oestrogen receptors. The most effective of these agents at the time of writing is faslodex.

The use of inhibitors to reduce toxic metabolite formation

There are a number of P450-mediated metabolic reactions which result in short-lived, highly unstable and exceedingly toxic products which are capable of severe toxicity. Some of these agents will be described in detail in Chapter 8. The capacity of CYPs to form potentially toxic metabolites is usually rooted in the oxidation of a metabolized molecule, which, according to its structure, may become highly unstable. Some metabolites are so reactive they destroy the enzyme, which has been seen in 'suicide' inhibitors mentioned earlier. Slightly less reactive metabolites might enter the rest of the hepatocyte and react with protein structures resulting in change in function and eventual necrosis or apoptosis, depending on the rapidity of formation and the reactivity.

Paracetamol-mediated hepatic necrosis

The best example of this is the metabolism of paracetamol in overdose to reactive quinone-imine derivatives. The resulting damage leads to necrosis of the liver. This process is covered in more detail in Chapter 8. It was shown in the 1980s that various inhibitors could slow or prevent the metabolism of paracetamol to its reactive metabolites and several animal studies were carried out to show that this could work clinically. However, this approach never became a clinical reality. Acutely, patients presenting before liver damage was sufficient to cause necrosis could be saved with glutathione (GSH) precursor supplements, such as N-acetylcysteine. After liver damage was too severe, then it would either be transplant time or death. Considering a preventative approach, including an inhibitor in paracetamol tablets could potentially prevent the formation of the toxic metabolite without affecting clearance that much, as 95 per cent of paracetamol clearance is accomplished by sulphation and glucuronidation. However, the main inhibitors of CYP2E1 are mostly sulphur-containing agents and inhibit other enzymes such as alcohol dehydrogenase and aldehyde dehydrogenase. It would not be practical to include a 2E1 inhibitor in paracetamol tablets because as soon as the patient drank any alcohol, they would be violently ill. So the use of a CYP inhibitor to prevent paracetamol-mediated hepatic necrosis is a dead end.

However, another route of inhibition may in the future have some therapeutic value. A small proportion of paracetamol is cleared to a reactive cytotoxic metabolite (NAPQI: Chapter 8) and this can be detoxified by GSH, either directly, or through catalysis by the cytosolic Phase II enzymes, glutathione-S-transferases (GSTs). Studies in knockout mice have shown that in animals where GST pi has been deleted they sustain less hepatoxicity than those with intact enzyme. This is bizarre, as it might be expected that the enzyme would be necessary to catalyse NAPQI clearance to a benign mercapturate. In both knockout and control animals, GSH was depleted, so thiol consumption during detoxification occurs. So it is possible that GST pi depletes GSH in a process that is not relevant to NAPQI clearance. Whatever the role of GST in this experiment, it raises the possibility that future GST inhibitors might prevent hepatotoxicity in the later stages of liver damage in paracetamol overdose and in combination with N-acetyl cysteine, the standard antidote, may rescue those previously doomed to liver failure.

Dapsone-mediated methaemoglobin formation

The sulphone drug dapsone is used in leprosy therapy in the Third World, but is also a useful anti-inflammatory agent in conditions which feature the infiltration of activated neutrophils, such as the skin condition dermatitis herpetiformis (DH). The drug is very effective and will suppress DH symptoms, such as intense pruritus and skin eruptions within hours of dosage. This brings rapid relief from a condition that can make patient's lives intolerable. However, the drug causes methaemoglobin formation, which is due to the CYP2C9-mediated oxidation of the drug to a hydroxylamine (Chapter 8). This particular hydroxylamine is a relatively poor substrate for Phase II glucuronyl transferase and the greater the drug dose, the more hydroxylamine escapes conjugation, enters the circulation and oxidizes haemoglobin to methaemoglobin, which cannot carry oxygen. The more methaemoglobin formed as a percentage of total haemoglobin, the more tissue anoxia occurs; symptoms range from a headache/hangover-like effects at sub 10 per cent levels to hospitalization (nausea, tiredness and breathing problems) at 20 per cent. The standard daily dosage in leprosy of around 100 mg of dapsone usually leads to around the 5–8 per cent level of methaemoglobin and it is just about tolerable to most patients, in the light of the alternative of the progression of the disease. However, with DH, the dosage varies wildly from patient to patient. Some can be fully controlled on 25 mg per week, whilst others must take 400 plus mg of dapsone daily and the condition is only partially suppressed. At this dosage, the patient's quality of life is much diminished by the drug and the only reason to persist with treatment might be a lack of effect of the only other drug alternative (sulphapyridine). Even moderately effective drug therapy with high side effects is better than the recurrence of the disease symptoms.

In rat studies in the late 1980's a number of potential inhibitors were tested for their ability to retard or arrest dapsone-dependent methaemoglobin formation. Piperonyl butoxide, an insecticide and broad CYP inhibitor, was effective, as was cimetidine, although ketaconazole and methimizole were not. Although it was known then that animal and human CYPs were not the same, the main families of CYPs were still being unravelled. These animal studies were reinforced by *in vitro* work with human liver microsomes, which again showed that cimetidine could be effective. This work led to volunteer studies that showed that cimetidine on a single dose would reduce hydroxylamine formation. Multiple dose studies in animals were also promising and a clinical study in DH patients finally showed that the hydroxylamine formation could be reduced, but not abolished, that methaemoglobin formation fell by nearly 30 per cent and the drug retained its clinical effects and improved patient tolerance. Subsequent studies underscored the possibilities of using cimetidine in patients who could only respond to high dapsone doses and would normally have had to endure considerable methaemoglobin formation. This method has reached clinical practice in some areas. Interestingly, it was clear that the rat was a poor model for man, in that cimetidine was far more effective as an inhibitor in the rat. It would probably have been undesirable, though, to use too potent an inhibitor long term, as endogenous CYP functions would have been severely affected. As a coda to this work, in 2003 the antioxidant dihydrolipoic acid (formed from lipoic acid in human erythrocytes *in vivo*) was found to partially block the reaction between the hydroxylamine and oxyhaemoglobin *in vitro*. Hence, a study could now be designed to use lipoic acid and cimetidine in combination to make an even larger reduction in methaemoglobin formation in patients on high-dosage dapsone, without completely blocking the CYPs.

Use of inhibition in alcoholism

The effects of alcoholism are covered in more detail in Chapter 7. Among the treatments for alcoholism is the use of the potent inhibitor of aldehyde dehydrogenase and CYP2E1, known as disulfiram (antabuse). This compound is taken by the alcoholic to help the abstinence process. In the alcoholic, ethanol is cleared by CYP2E1 and alcohol dehydrogenase to acetaldehyde, which is cleared by aldehyde dehydrogenase to acetic acid and water. If alcohol is imbibed during antabuse treatment, the clearance of ethanol to acetaldehyde occurs, but the process stops there and acetaldehyde accumulates causing a severe effect that includes flushing, nausea, vomiting and sweating. Even small amounts of alcohol will show this effect, even if the patient is genuinely abstinent. There are many medicinal and hygiene-based products, ranging from cough mixtures to mouthwashes, that can contain up to 30 per cent ethanol, so patient awareness is valuable in this context.

Summary

Inhibition of drug clearance has the greatest clinical impact on a patient's well-being, in terms of the rapidity of the effect and its severity. This is particularly important when the patient or health care professional is for a time unaware that a potent inhibitor has been consumed. Currently, in the light of the numbers of potent dietary and OTC inhibitors available to the patient, it is as important to educate the patient in the dangers of inhibition of narrow therapeutic index drugs as it is to educate the health care professional.

6 Conjugation and Transport Processes

6.1 Introduction

You might recall from Chapters 1 and 2 that drugs and many endogenous chemicals, such as steroids, are essentially oil-soluble (lipophilic) agents that exploit their lipophilicity and stability to carry out their biological function, crossing membranes, binding specific carrier molecules and finally entering cells to bind to the appropriate receptors. This lipophilicity and stability also means that they are very hard to control. In this context, control entails the termination of biological function and subsequent removal from the body. With steroid hormones, for example, the ability to modulate synthesis and destruction allows the exertion of exceedingly fine control over the structural and biochemical changes they induce. As radical chemistry was involved in their assembly, body clearance of such stable molecules means that radical chemistry must also be applied to change these oil-soluble agents to water solubility.

So the objectives of metabolizing systems could be summed up thus:

- To terminate the pharmacological effect of the molecule;

- Make the molecule so water-soluble that it cannot escape clearance, preferably by more than one route to absolutely guarantee its removal.

These objectives could be accomplished by:

- Changing the molecular shape so it no longer binds to its receptors;

- Changing the molecular lipophilicity to hydrophilicity to ensure high water solubility;

- Making the molecule larger and heavier, so it can be eliminated in bile as well as urine;

Human Drug Metabolism, Michael D. Coleman
© 2005 John Wiley & Sons, Ltd

- Efflux pump systems, which ensure that a highly water-soluble metabolite actually leaves the cell to enter the bloodstream, before it is excreted in bile and urine.

The CYP system ensures that virtually all lipophilic (and many hydrophilic) molecules can be oxidized and made at least slightly more water-soluble. However, many hydroxylated metabolites are not water-soluble enough to ensure that they remain in urine when filtered by the kidney and not be reabsorbed into the surrounding lipophilic tissue of the collecting tubes. So CYP-mediated metabolism can increase hydrophilicity, but it does not always increase it enough and it certainly does not make the molecule any bigger and heavier, indeed, sometimes the molecule becomes lighter as alkyl groups are removed during O, N and S dealkylations. CYP-mediated metabolism does not always alter the pharmacological effects of the drug either; in the case of the benzodiazepines and other drugs, metabolites do exert a great deal of pharmacological effect.

However, CYPs do perform two essential tasks: the initial destabilization of the molecule, creating a 'handle' on it. A crude analogy would be to liken a stable lipophilic molecule to a solid block of steel, and the CYP would be the high-speed drill that bores a hole in it, so that a hook or bolt could be attached. CYPs also 'unmask' groups that could be more reactive for further metabolism. The best examples of this would be the various dealkylation reactions. These reveal groups such as amines, hydroxyl and sulphides that can undergo more metabolism to make the molecule heavier, a different shape and more water-soluble.

This CYP-mediated preparation can make the molecule vulnerable to the attachment of a very water-soluble and plentiful agent to the drug or steroid, which accomplishes the objectives of metabolism. This is achieved through the attachment of a modified glucose molecule (glucuronidation), or a soluble salt such as a sulphate (sulphation) to the prepared site. Both adducts make the drug into a stable, heavier and water-soluble ex-drug.

Some oxidative metabolites are found in urine and some conjugated metabolites do not require 'Phase I' preparation prior to conjugation. However, with many drugs, their stability and lipophilicity mean that their clearance must take more than one metabolic operation to make them water-soluble.

A final problem is created by the formation of highly water-soluble metabolites, in that they can be too hydrophilic to easily leave the cell. The control of this process is sometimes termed Phase III of metabolism. In this case, a series of molecule pump systems have evolved, or efflux transporters, which provide a powered gradient to encourage the egress of these molecules into the interstitial cell fluid. Once out of the cell, there is no way back for such hydrophilic molecules and from the blood they are filtered by the kidneys into urine.

6.2 Glucuronidation

Introduction

This is the largest capacity Phase II clearance system in man and is accomplished by a set of enzymes known as UDP (uridine diphosphate) glucuronosyl transferases, or UGTs. These are found in many tissues, but the greatest concentration is in the liver. Once the UGT protein has been synthesized, its N-terminal signal sequence is clipped off and most of the rest of the enzyme is found inside the lumen of the endoplasmic reticulum attached to the membrane by a C-terminal transmembrane sequence and a multi-lysine stop transfer signal.

This places them in close proximity to the CYP isoforms and also ensures that they meet lipophilic agents directly themselves, so it is not always necessary for the CYPs to oxidize the drug prior to glucuronidation (Figure 6.1). These enzymes utilize and activate glucose and convert a huge number of chemicals to beta-D-glucopyranosiduronic acids, or glucuronides, by a nucleophilic substitution reaction. Interestingly, human UGTs do not function as rapidly as those of other animals, such as dogs.

In the majority of xenobiotics, glucuronidation appears to happen after some form of oxidative metabolism; however, there are a number of drugs

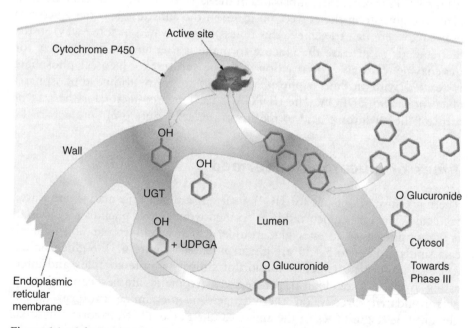

Figure 6.1 Scheme showing the approximate position of glucuronyl transferases (UGTs) in the smooth endoplasmic reticulum in relation to CYPs and Phase III efflux processes

that are cleared virtually entirely by direct glucuronidation, without any prior oxidative metabolism. These include lorazapam, oxazepam and morphine (Appendix B); the latter narcotic is cleared to a 3- and a 6-glucuronide. Glucuronidation is the major route of clearance for a vast array of chemicals: these include endogenous substances such as steroids, bilirubin, bile acids, fatty acids, retinoids and prostaglandins, as well as environmental pollutants, dietary constituents and of course drugs. Chemically, phenolics, carboxylic acids, hydroxylamines, amines, opiods and exogenous steroids can all be conjugated with glucuronic acid by these enzymes. The products are extremely water-soluble and provided that they are stable, ensure that the agent is cleared into urine or bile. In general, glucuronides are so radically different in shape and water solubility from their parent drugs that they do not exert any pharmacological effect. The most often quoted exception to this rule is morphine-6-glucuronide, which retains a potent opiate effect. UGTs have a seriously high capacity and are practically unsaturable; the first-generation anti-HIV agent AZT is a good example of this. This toxic compound was cleared entirely by UGTs and such is the capacity of these pathways that the drug had to be taken several times daily to remain in the therapeutic window.

Mode of operation

All the UGTs process their substrates in the same basic way. The enzyme must place the glucose in the correct position on the substrate and the glucose is not reactive enough to achieve this unless it is activated in some way. So the first stage is to prepare the glucose to make it thermodynamically easy for the enzyme to catalyse its reaction with the substrate. Glucose-1-phosphate is reacted with uridine triphosphate (UTP) to form uridine diphosphate-glucuronic acid UDPGA. The UDPGA is used as a co-factor for the attachment of the glucuronic acid to the substrate (see Figure 6.2).

Types of glucuronides formed

There are several options for UGTs to insert a glucuronic acid group into a molecule. The ether glucuronide as formed from simple phenols (Figure 6.2) is one option, as is an ester glucuronide, which would appear when chemicals similar to benzoic acid are glucuronidated (Figure 6.3). S-glucuronides can also be formed. Glucuronidation of amines is more complex and interesting from a toxicological perspective. Aromatic amines can either be glucuronidated directly on the nitrogen of the amine to form an N-glucuronide (Figure 6.4), or the amine can first be oxidized to form a hydroxylamine, where the glucuronide can be attached to either the nitrogen or the oxygen of the hydroxylamine to form an N-glucuronide or an O-glucuronide.

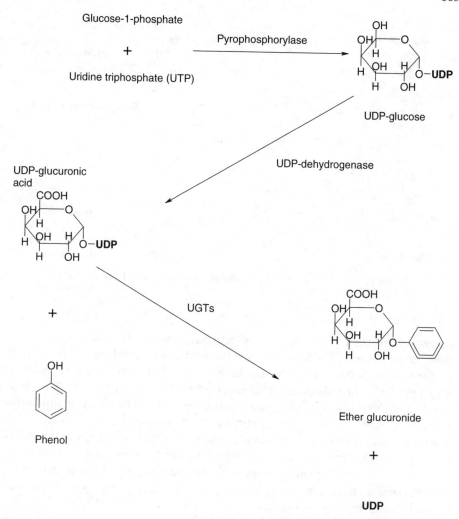

Figure 6.2 Process scheme for the preparation of glucose to UDP glucuronic acid, the co-factor for UGT-mediated formation of an ether glucuronide of phenol

With most aromatic amines, the N-glucuronide is formed directly from the amine and hydroxylation is unnecessary, although the N-hydroxy (hydroxylamine) Phase I metabolites can also be glucuronidated. The question is whether this would occur on the nitrogen (N-glucuronide) or the oxygen of the hydroxylamine (O-glucuronide).

The sulphone, dapsone, is an interesting example of the Phase II fate of an aromatic amine. In volunteers, the parent drug could be monoacetylated, which could then be N-hydroxylated along with the parent drug (CYP2C9) to form acetylated and non-acetylated hydroxylamines. These hydroxy-

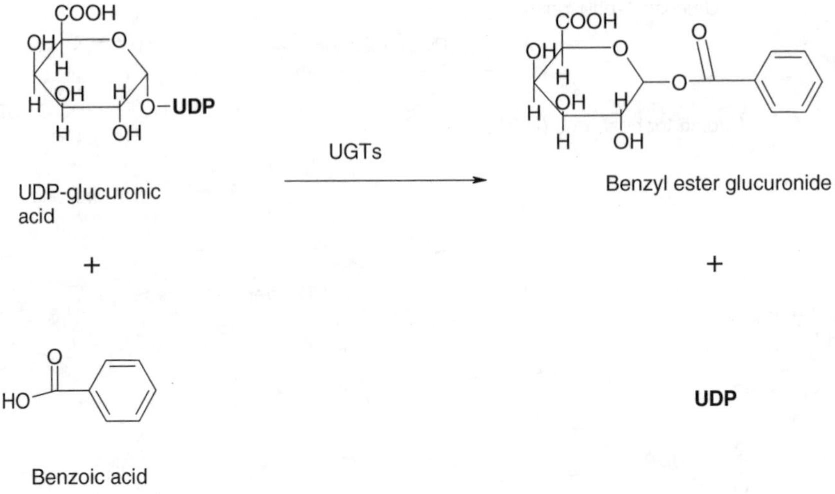

Figure 6.3   Formation of an ester glucuronide from benzoic acid

lamines were then predominantly glucuronidated, as around a third of the dose is recovered in 48 hours as glucuronides. Acid hydrolysis with β-glucuronidase (which splits the glucuronic acid off the drug or metabolite at acid pH) left intact dapsone hydroxylamine as the major metabolite. Irrespective of the position of the glucuronide, the hydroxylamine was just stable enough to survive after the glucuronic acid was hydrolysed away. With dapsone, oxidation to the hydroxylamine is so rapid that there is probably little opportunity for the parent amine to be directly conjugated to form an N-glucuronide. Subsequent studies with benzidine, a carcinogen that is N-hydroxylated and glucuronidated, suggest that the O-glucuronide formed from the hydroxylamine is less stable to hydrolysis than the N-glucuronides.

The stability and position of glucuronides on an amine are crucial issues with regard to the potential carcinogenicity. N-glucuronides in general are very susceptible to acid hydrolysis, which can occur in urine made acid by a diet rich in meat and dairy products. Human urine also contains β-glucuronidases, which operate most efficiently at acid pH. Those who have a predominantly vegetarian diet have more alkaline urine and little hydrolysis occurs. It appears that the acid hydrolysis of N-glucuronides of aromatic amines like benzidine leads to liberation of the parent amine and possibly the hydroxylamines in the urine. What occurs next is still under debate, but the released parent drug and other oxidative metabolites can lead to bladder cancer, which occurs in many workers exposed to benzidine in various dye industries, now sited in Third World countries. This is discussed in more detail in Chapter 8.

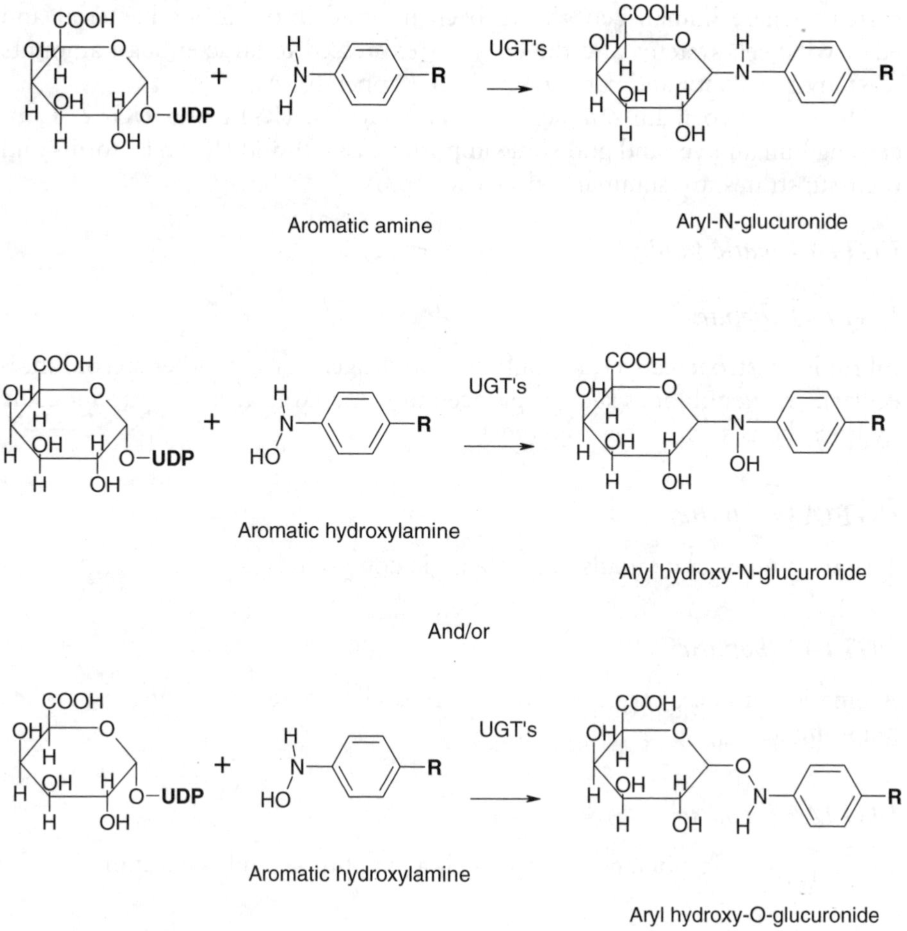

Figure 6.4   Scheme for glucuronidation of aromatic amines and hydroxylamines

UGT isoforms

Although these enzymes had been documented for many years, little detailed information about them was available until cDNA cloning technology allowed the expression of large quantities of the enzymes, so enabling the study of the different UGT isoforms. It emerged that in the same way different families of CYPs had evolved to metabolize broad groups of substrates, the same system applies to UGTs. More than 20 human UGT cDNAs have been cloned and sequenced and they are all structurally similar. The UGTs share a common 'backbone' with specific isoforms differing from each other in their N-amino termini. They have been extensively studied by expressing the human enzymes in various cellular heterologous systems. These are systems where human genes have been inserted into various bacterial and eukaryotic cell systems and the enzymes expressed in large enough amounts to study specificity and catalytic activity (Appendix A).

There are two main families of UGT enzymes: UGT1 and UGT2. Concerning human liver and gut, some important UGT1 and UGT2 isoforms and their substrates are summarized below.

UGT1A hepatic family

UGT1A1 (hepatic)

Bilirubin, oestrogenic steroids only (not androgens or any other steroid molecules), and xenobiotics such as paracetamol and large aromatic carcinogenic hydrocarbons such as benzopyrenes.

UGT1A3 (hepatic)

Tertiary amines, flavonoids, and phenolic compounds.

UGT1A4 (hepatic)

Aromatic amines, trifluoperazine, trycyclic antidepressants, such as imipramine.

UGT1A6 (hepatic)

Small, planar, phenolic chemicals, such as naphthols and paracetamol.

UGT1A9 (hepatic)

Both small and bulky phenolic chemicals, coumarins, flavones and amines.

UGT2B family

UGT2B4 (hepatic/extra-hepatic)

Xenobiotic and endobiotics.

UGT2B7 (hepatic)

Catechol oestrogens, morphine and naproxen.

UGT2B15 (hepatic)

Phenols and flavonoids and some sex steroids.

UGT2B17 (hepatic/extra-hepatic)

Xenobiotic and endobiotic compounds.

Gastro-intestinal tract UGTs

UGT1A10

Small and bulky aglycones.

UGT1A7

Endogenous ligands.

UGT1A8

Small and bulky phenolic chemicals.

Control of UGTs

Hopefully you will have read and understood the chapter on the induction of CYP isoforms, which outlined the sophisticated expression control system which has evolved to both coarse and fine-tune CYP isoform expression according to substrate 'load'. So it is entirely logical that there should be a similar system for the control of glucuronidation, given the capacity and importance of this Phase II system. Interestingly, it has been known for over 20 years that UGT1A1 glucuronidation is responsive to substrate 'load'. This effect was used beneficially in a study in pregnant women, who were asked to take phenobarbitone daily in the last few weeks of their pregnancies. The incidence and severity of neonatal hyperbilirubinaemia were greatly reduced. The women had to take at least ten 100mg doses to see the effect, showing that induction of the main route of bilirubin clearance, glucuronidation, had occurred. Since prolonged jaundice can affect neonatal hearing, phenobarbitone remains an effective method of stimulating the clearance of bilirubin in babies. However, due to its obvious sedating effect, which is detrimental for neonatal feeding, phenobarbitone treatment is not really a long-term practical approach and should be replaced with a non-sedating agonist. Rifampicin is also capable of inducing UGTs; however, this again is not a suitable agonist for this purpose due to the side effects of this agent, the least of which is to colour every bodily secretion orange.

That a barbiturate could induce glucuronidation expression demonstrated that this system was at least sensitive to known CYP inducers, and might be regulated in a similar way to CYP isoforms. 3-Methyl cholanthrene and oltipraz can also induce UGT1A1 in human hepatocytes. UGT1A6 and 1A9 are inducible through agonists of CYP1A1 (dioxins and betanaphthoflavone). Other information about UGT control came from clinical conditions that revealed that UGTs were polymorphic, but mainly in terms of their promoter systems. The most severe is Crigler–Najjar syndrome, classed as CN-1 and CN-2. CN-1 is fatal (without a liver transplant) due to non-expression of UGT1A1, because of a fault in the promoter system. CN-2 is a milder version with reduced UGT1A1 expression. A milder UGT1A1 syndrome is Gilbert's disease, which affects around 7 per cent of the population and this is another promoter defect that leads to poor expression of UGT1A1, particularly highlighted by an inability to clear major drug glucuronidation substrates like paracetamol. This is predominantly found in those of African ancestry, but it has been reported in Caucasians.

Research into the control of UGT expression is currently some way behind that of CYP isoforms, but it is emerging that UGTs are regulated by similar receptor systems to CYPs. Different receptor systems may induce specific UGTs, although nuclear receptors like the pregnane X receptor (PXR: Figure 6.5) and the constitutive androstane receptor (CAR; UGT1A1: Figure 6.6) are the most likely to be involved. The methods used to study UGT expression have centred on the UGT1A1, which glucuronidates bilirubin and animal models such as transgenic mice that express human nuclear receptors such as PXR and CAR. The transgenic mouse model allows an opportunity of watching the human receptors operate, although how close this actually is to the system in humans remains to be seen.

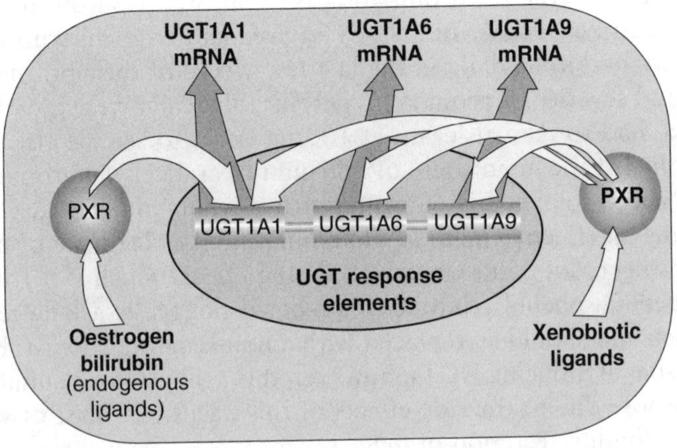

Figure 6.5 Control of UGT induction by PXR ligands, endogenous and xenobiotic

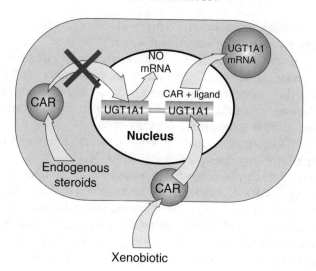

Figure 6.6 Proposed scheme of CAR-mediated control of UGT1A1: endogenous steroids can slow or stop UGT expression that may have occurred in response to other ligands, xenobiotic or endogenous

CAR and PXR-mediated regulation of glucuronidation

Obviously clinical experience with phenobarbitone has established it is a potent inducer of CYP isoforms and it is believed to exert its effect on the CYP genes through the CAR and to some extent the PXR nuclear receptors. So it is not unreasonable to assume that the phenobarbitone effect on UGT1A1 might also be mediated by CAR and possibly PXR as well (Figure 6.6). Using mice that expressed human CAR, it has been shown that inducers of CAR expression increase bilirubin clearance and that bilirubin itself stimulates CAR expression. In mice where the CAR gene has been removed (knockout mice) the responsiveness of UGT1A1 to the inducers and high bilirubin levels was lost. It is likely that CAR and PXR mediate UGT transcription in response to the presence of xenobiotics and endogenous substrates of UGT1A1.

It has been suggested that CAR does not become involved with the regulation of bilrubin glucuronidation until the rate of the process increases above a basal level. This is similar to the effect seen in Gilbert's disease, where some stimulus reveals the deficit in the system, which behaves like an idling car engine before the accelerator is pressed. CAR only begins to bind in quantity to the responsive elements in the UGT1A1 gene when bilirubin levels rise beyond a certain threshold. It is not clear whether bilirubin itself binds to CAR and it is also not clear whether other factors such as SRC-1, which is necessary for CAR-mediated CYP expression, are also necessary for human

UGT1A1 expression modulation. This will become clear once complete working human systems can be studied *in vitro*.

It has been proposed that neonates have, to varying degrees, a deficit in CAR expression that causes the poor bilirubin clearance. It has even been suggested that this may be an intended effect, on the grounds that bilirubin has antioxidant properties. However, in the light of the neurotoxic effects of this metabolite, this is a debatable point.

Concerning PXR, studies with the transgenic mice have shown that the PXR agonist rifampicin does increase UGT1A levels within a day or so of exposure. This effect can be reproduced using human cell lines such as HepG2 cells, which express PXR. Currently it is thought that PXR must bind with RXR (as with CYP isoform expression system control) prior to binding with the response elements (DR-3) on the UGT1A1 gene. It appears that transgenic mice with no PXR can still form glucuronides, so it is likely that CAR regulates basal levels of expression, while the PXR system responds and adapts to changes in levels of substrates.

Ultimately, it is likely that all the UGTs have similar control systems that are linked to CYP and efflux transporter expression. This makes sense, as both CYPs and the UGTs are meeting the same xenobiotic or endobiotic stimuli; this might be the gut wall, the liver or the kidney. Essentially, according to diet, chemical and drug exposure, each individual will possess a unique expression array of UGTs and CYPs which will be constantly fine-tuned throughout life. These enzyme systems are part of the same integrated multifunctional and highly adaptable response to lipophilic xenobiotic and endobiotic compounds.

Enterohepatic recirculation

This term usually refers to the recycling of bile salts during digestion, but can also be used to describe an apparent rise in blood drug levels hours after a single dose has been given. Since another dose has not been given, it is rather paradoxical to see a rise in blood levels just as the drug is gradually being eliminated from the system. This effect starts with Phase II clearance to a conjugate, usually a glucuronide, but it can also involve sulphates and amino acid. The conjugate is then excreted into bile and may be unstable when it reaches the gut. The conjugate could be chemically unstable, or is hydrolysed by gut bacteria; either way, free drug is then reabsorbed. This effect can extend the half-life of a drug and make its plasma levels variable and difficult to predict. In addition, it can expose the gut to levels of the parent drug which may be much more toxic than the conjugate (see Chapter 7, irinotecan). This effect is seen in NSAIDS and contributes to their gut toxicity. Opiates, antiparasitics such as ivermectin, many dietary antioxidant flavones and other phenolics are also enterohepatically recirculated. It can occur in steroids, although it is not thought to be clinically relevant in the cases of norethisterone and gestodene. Antibiotic administration can accelerate the clearance of enterohepatically recirculated drugs by killing the gut flora responsible for the hydrolysis of the conjugates.

6.3 Sulphation

Introduction

Sulphation is accomplished by a set of enzyme systems known as sulpho-transferases (SULTs) and they are found in most tissues to varying degrees of activity. The major sites of activity are the liver, small intestine, main intestine and colon. They are all cytosolic enzymes, i.e. they are never found in the endo-plastic reticulum or the more lipophilic areas of cells. Rather than directly attach the sulphate molecule to the xenobiotic, they require sulphurylase + APS phosphokinase to manipulate the sulphate into a form that is thermodynami-cally easiest for the enzyme to sulphate the xenobiotic (Figure 6.7).

The first step is to 'load' the sulphate into adenosine 5'phosphosulphate:

Sulphate	sulphurylase	Adenosine 5' phosphosulphate (APS)
+		+
ATP	$\longrightarrow$	P-Pi (Pyrophosphate)

APS	APS phosphokinase	PAPS
+		+
ATP	$\longrightarrow$	ADP

The co-factor known as PAPS (3'-phosphoadenosine-5'-phosphosulphate) acts as the final sulphate carrier.

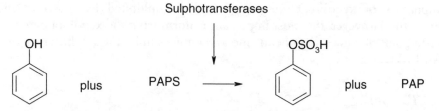

Figure 6.7   Basic reactions of sulphotransferases

The general aim of sulphation is to make the substrate more water-soluble and usually less active pharmacologically. Sulphated molecules are more readily eliminated in bile and urine. All the SULTs are virtually identical structurally in the area of the enzyme where they bind the co-factor, although there are obviously considerable differences in the substrate binding sites, which confer on the different enzymes the ability to bind groups of similar substrates in the same manner as CYP and UGT enzymes.

Although sulphotransferases do not have the vast capacity that the UGT systems possess, they are capable of forming large quantities of sulphate metabolites in a relatively short timescale. Again, our knowledge of this metabolizing system has benefited greatly from heterologous expression systems. However, the full range of the endogenous and xenobiotic-metabolizing roles of SULTs remains to be uncovered, as these enzymes are extremely important in many metabolic roles, particularly steroid metabolism in many different tissues, including the brain. They are especially active at the beginning of life as they are found in high levels during foetal development. Their roles regarding xenobiotic metabolism seem to be contradictory, with many SULTs involved in the activation of carcinogens, as well as the detoxication of other reactive species. All SULTs are believed to be subject to genetic polymorphisms, with a high degree of individual variation in their expression and catalytic activities; this is currently under investigation, particularly from the standpoint of individual risk factors for carcinogenesis.

Regarding classification of the superfamily of SULTs, it is assumed that 47 per cent amino acid sequence homology is indicative of same family members and 60 per cent homology for subfamily members. To date, there are 47 mammalian SULT isoforms so far discovered, which are derived from 10 human sulphotransferase gene families; SULTs1 and 2 appear to be the most important families.

SULT1 family

This is the major group of human sulphotransferases, which contains four subfamilies (1A, 1B, 1C and 1E) and a considerable number of isoforms, including 1A3, 1B1, 1C1, 1C2, and the oestrogen sulphotransferase 1E1. 1A3 (not found in the liver) as well as 1E1 are potent sulphators of xenobiotic oestrogens and are inhibited by oestrone and quercetin. However, the most important isoform from the xenobiotic metabolism point of view is the phenol and aryl amine sulphating sulphotransferase SULT1A1.

SULT2 family

These enzymes are hydroxysteroid sulphotransferases and there are only two subfamilies, SULT2A and SULT2B, with SULT2A1 and SULT2B1 being the best understood. There are a large number of individual enzymes which sulphonate a variety of sex hormones and hydroxysteroids. SULTB1 metabolizes sex steroids and predictably is found in the placenta, uterus and prostate and is thought to be heavily involved in the regulation of androgen levels.

SULT1A1

The genes which code for SULTs 1A1, 1A2 and 1A3 originate on chromosome 16; toxicologically and from the perspective of drug clearance, SULT1A1 has become more and more important as its role in the clearance and activation of xenobiotic molecules has been unravelled. The polymorphic variants of this isoform (designated SULT1A1*1/2) are found mainly in the liver and gut, but also the lung, skin and brain. SULT1A1 isoforms are capable of metabolizing a wide variety of hydrophobic molecules, and how they achieve this has become much clearer with the crystallization of the enzyme, showing its full structure.

This enzyme, being found in the aqueous cytosol, has been crystallized (SULT1A1*2). This is the main goal of any enzymologist, to be able to examine the detailed structure of an enzyme at leisure, essentially. This allows the exploration as to how the enzyme might accomplish its tasks. It is clear that the vaguely butterfly-shaped enzyme possesses a binding site for the cofactor PAPS as well as an L-shaped hydrophobic binding pocket which can accommodate two substrate molecules. To illustrate the subtle differences in these isoforms in terms of structure that lead to huge differences in function, SULT1A3 shares 7 out of 10 aromatic residues in its substrate binding site with SULT1A1, but it has much narrower specificity, only really metabolizing dopamine to its sulphate derivative. The 10 aromatic residues in SULT1A1's substrate binding pocket allows it to metabolize extremely hydrophobic substrates. The crystal structure does yield detailed knowledge of the enzyme's layout, but not always its function: SULT1A1 will process small entities such as paranitrophenol and much larger molecules such as thyroid hormones, although it is harder for the isoform to sulphate oestrogens. From the crystal structure, the oestrogens do not appear to fit the active site as well as the other molecules. However, the crystal structure is like a frozen image of the enzyme and it does not show how it actually operates; in the same way it is difficult to see today how King Charles II was such a successful womanizer from his later portraits. That the enzymes will sulphate such a variety of compounds, from phenols, to aromatic amines, polycyclic aromatics as well as sex steroids, shows that it can bind practically any shape molecule, from flexible ring structures and planar aromatics to what is termed 'extended fused ring systems', such as steroid-related molecules. It has been suggested that the active site alters its own conformation to process molecules such as steroids. This feature, which must involve the enzyme automatically sensing the structural characteristics of the potential substrate and then moulding itself around it, has been described as 'plasticity'. This confers tremendous flexibility on the enzyme and is likely to occur in many more enzymes that have very wide substrate specificity.

Control of SULT enzymes

The study of the control of SULT enzymes is very much in its infancy and much less is known about how their expression is controlled in comparison with CYPs. However, since we have seen that CYP isoforms and UGTs are modulated by PXR and CAR-type nuclear receptors, which also control other apparently disparate, but relevant systems, such as gut efflux transporter systems, it seems entirely logical that PXR and CAR also have some role in SULT expression. Indeed, for the liver and gut to coordinate a biochemical response to endogenous molecule regulation as well as the regulation of xenobiotics, some form of modulation of sulphation would appear to be essential. Some early indications from transgenic systems and human cell lines appear to support this. As SULT1A1 is part of the system for the clearance of thyroid hormones, which are closely controlled in concentration, it is most likely that CAR is involved in the regulation of this enzyme. Other work shows that the hydroxysteroid metabolizing SULTs, the SULT2 family, are inducible by dexamethasone through PXR effects in animal systems, so it is possible this might occur in man. As mentioned above, SULT isoforms vary greatly between individuals and differences in expression may have severe toxicological consequences, in terms of xenobiotic toxicity and carcinogenicity. There is also some evidence that diet is a strong influence on individual SULT profiles; SULT enzymes can also be inhibited by a number of different chemical agents, such as those that resemble substrates like chlorinated derivatives of dinitrophenol. However, antioxidants like quercetin and curcumin are also effective inhibitors. These agents exert protective effects against various cancers and a number of studies have revealed that SULT1A1 is capable of promoting the formation of reactive and highly unstable metabolites that are potentially carcinogenic.

6.4 The GSH system

Introduction

One of the main problems with the oxidation of various molecules by CYP enzymes is that they are often destabilized and sometimes form highly reactive products. The analogy used previously in this book was that of a child given a hammer and told to hit anything metallic hard. CYPs occasionally form metabolites so reactive that they immediately destroy the enzyme by reacting with it, changing its structure and, therefore, its function. Sometimes, this kind of damage can be self-limiting because the reactive species formed destroys the CYPs, so no more reactive species are formed until several days later, while more enzyme is assembled. Meanwhile, the chemical substrate itself is not a problem unless it is oxidized and it might well be cleared though other routes in the mean time.

The most dangerous forms of reactive species are those either evading UGTs and SULT enzymes, or inadvertently created by conjugation processes. These species escape into the cytosol and even into the nucleus, where potentially carcinogenic events may ensue. At the very least, such reactive species might react with cytosol and membrane protein structures, which eventually results in such high cellular damage that the cell necroses and disintegrates, or enters an apoptotic state (Chapter 8).

CYPs are not the only source of reactive species generated within cells. Around 80 per cent of our food intake is directed at maintaining our body temperature and a great deal of energy must be liberated from our food to accomplish this. Cells derive the vast majority of their energy through oxidative phosphorylation and this takes place in the 'engine rooms' of the cell, the mitochondria. With a car or any fuel-burning machine, aside from the achievment of the desired function, energy is also wasted in the form of heat and toxic exhaust gases. In cells almost all the oxygen we breathe is consumed in oxidative phosphorylation, forming ATP, heat and reactive oxidant species in the mitochondria that could cause severe damage to the structure and function of the cell if they were allowed to escape. So all cells, particularly hepatocytes, have evolved a separate system to accommodate such reactive toxic products and this is based on a three amino acid (cysteine, glycine and glutamate) thiol known as glutathione, or GSH. Thiols in general are extremely effective at reducing and thus 'quenching' highly reactive, electrophilic species. GSH has a very high redox potential of -0.33, and donates electrons to reactive species. During this process it loses its hydrogen ion and forms a glutathionyl radical (GS•), which is capable of causing oxidant damage itself, but more usually undergoes a complex series of reactions resulting in GSSG. This is now stable and is 'spent' and by itself it is useless in controlling reactive species.

To say that GSH can act as a cellular 'fire extinguisher' is an imperfect analogy, as it implies that GSH is only useful in emergencies. In fact, if cells are depleted of GSH by blocking its synthesis (by using buthionine sulphoxime), cell death ensues and the organism itself will die in a few days, due to uncontrolled activity of endogenous radicals. A better analogy for GSH would be the oil in a car engine. Without oil, the engine will essentially weld itself together and seize. To stretch the analogy somewhat, a combination of a good oil quality and pressure means that a well-designed car engine will last almost indefinitely. If GSH levels are not maintained in the cell over a long period of time, the cell wears out more quickly; for example, diabetic complications are linked with poor GSH maintenance. In fact, among its many functions, the GSH system acts like a cellular 'battery charger', recharging the oxidized spent versions of other antioxidants such as ascorbic acid and vitamin E.

GSH system maintenance

In the same way a central heating system maintains a set temperature, GSH levels are 'thermostatically' maintained in different subcellular 'pools' at preset levels. The ratio between GSH and GSSG will be very high in mitochondria, to ensure protection against reactive species, whilst the ratio is lower in other less radical-threatened areas of the cell such as the rough and smooth endoplasmic reticula. Overall, the hepatocyte maintains GSH at a very high (8–10 mM) intracellular level, whilst normal erythrocytes hold it at around 1–2 mM. Plasma levels are usually only in the micromolar range. Intracellular GSH concentrations are maintained by two methods: firstly, by a two-stage ATP-dependent direct synthesis (gamma glutamyl cysteinyl synthetase and glutathione synthetase), and secondly, by recycling the GSSG to GSH by the operation of GSSG reductase, which consumes cellular reducing power (NADPH; Figure 6.8). This system is so efficient that at any one time, 98 per cent is GSH and less than 2 per cent will be GSSG. The cell can completely restock its GSH level from nothing in less than 10 minutes. GSH levels are maintained through allosteric negative feedback mechanisms, where high GSH concentrations inhibit GSSG-reductase and the GSH synthetic enzymes. GSH maintenance can only be frustrated by a lack of raw materials (a sulphur containing amino acid, methionine or cysteine) or lack of reducing power. The cell will often succeed in maintaining high GSH levels even under severe attack by oxidative species. It is not usually necessary for GSH to leave a cell and it cannot cross membranes without a specific transporter such as MRP-1. Transporters actively pump GSSG out of cells in times of oxidative stress to prevent it reacting with other cellular thiols. GSSG egress is actually a good indicator of oxidative stress in a cell. When GSH quenches a reactive species it sometimes written as a GS-conjugate, which undergoes further processing to emerge as a mercapturate, which is excreted in urine (Figure 6.8).

Currently, over 30 essential cellular functions have been found for GSH, and the GSH system is so highly evolved that it does not solely rely on GSH spontaneously reacting with dangerous species. There are several enzymes that promote and catalyse the reaction of GSH with potential toxins to ensure that reactive species are actively dealt with, rather than just passive GSH-mediated reduction. Probably the most important from the standpoint of drug metabolism are the GSH-S-Transferases.

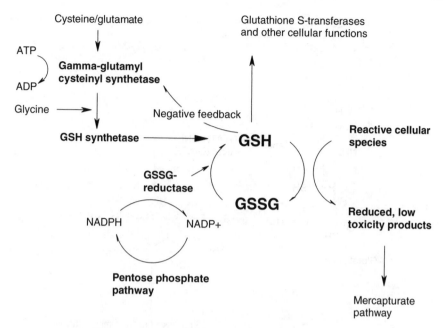

Figure 6.8   The GSH maintenance system in man

6.5   Glutathione S-transferases

Structure and function

The glutathione transferases, or S-transferases as they are sometimes known (GSTs), provide the essential active promotion of GSH reaction with electrophilic agents. This results in the formation of thioethers, which often are rearranged through further metabolism (mercapturate pathway) to form mercapturates, which are stable and non-toxic. These relatively small enzymes (around 25 000 Mwt) comprise about 5 per cent of total cellular protein and are all very similar in structure, with two subunits which strongly resemble a butterfly shape. The active site of a GST enzyme (found near the N-terminus of the enzyme) is obviously required to bind both a range of possible substrates as well as GSH. Thiols are also by their nature reactive and not very stable and to compensate for this, GSTs use hydrogen bonding at the GSH binding site to stabilize the thiol and prevent it from oxidizing before the substrate can be bound. A tyrosine residue in the GSH binding site is essential to carry out this thiol stabilizing process, where the pKa in the immediate environment of the GSH is lowered to 6–7, as thiols are stable in acidic environments.

Almost all the GSTs are found in the cytosol, although some are associated with the endoplasmic reticulum. The hydrophobic GSTs are structurally

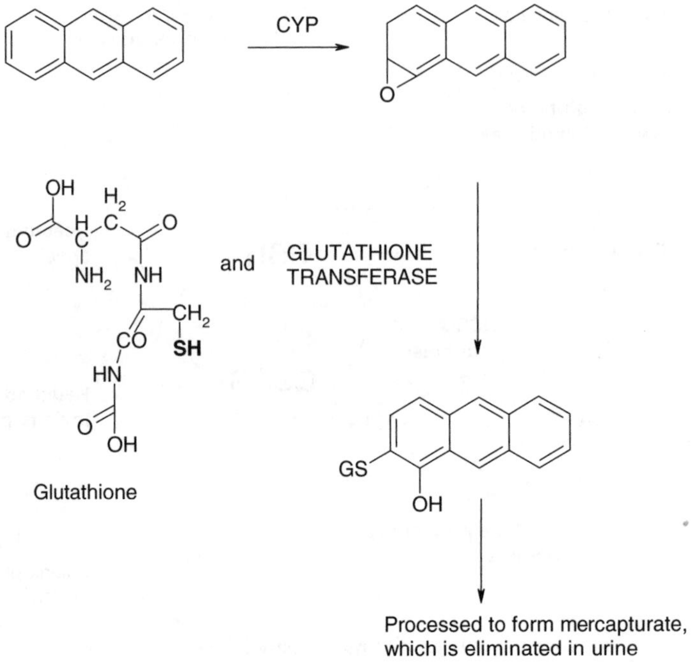

Figure 6.9 A typical GST catalysed reaction of GSH with a potentially reactive xenobiotic. The hydrophilic GSH molecule substantially increases the water solubility and molecular weight of the aromatic and will also detoxify it and ensure it will be transported out of the cell. It is unlikely anyone would make you learn the structure of GSH, but it is useful to look at it and appreciate that it is highly water-soluble

different from the cytosolic GSTs and they metabolize leukotrienes and prostaglandins. Aside from the detoxification roles of cytosolic GSTs, they can even repair damaged proteins, which have been S-thiolated. The major classes of mammalian enzymes are Alpha, Mu, Pi, Theta and Omega, although these enzymes are found right across the animal and plant kingdoms. In humans, the presence of mercapturates in urine (Figure 6.9) is usually a reasonably good indication of the formation of a reactive species somewhere in the hepatic handling of a xenobiotic agent.

GST classes

The GSTs are found in humans in several major classes. Generally, 60 per cent amino acid sequence homology is required for an isoform to be assigned to a particular class. The classes contain several subfamilies, with around 90 per cent common sequence homology. These enzymes are polymorphic and this is discussed in the next section.

GST Alpha class

GSTA1-1 is an important representative of the A class, which is found in only a few tissues of the body, including kidneys, intestine, lung, liver and testis. Finding GSTA1-1 in the blood is a clear sign of liver damage and is a more sensitive marker for the monitoring the progress of liver toxicity, as it is more closely associated with the liver than aspartate aminotransferase (AST) or alanine aminotransferase (ALT) and is more rapidly eliminated, so a more up-to-date picture of liver pathology is available. The substrate-binding site of the Alpha GSTs is most efficient at processing small hydrophobic molecules. There are three other human GST A isoforms, including GSTA2, 3 and 4. The catalytic action of GSTA4 is inhibited by ethacrynic acid, lipid hydroperoxides and 4-hydroxyalkenals (products of lipid breakdown). These enzymes are also capable of carrying out GSH peroxidase activities.

GST Mu class

The representative Mu class GSTM1-1 has a larger more open active site than the alpha GSTs and it contains a deeper binding cleft than the GST P variants. GST M1's are found in the liver, brain, testis, kidney and lung and will oxidize many bulkier electrophilic agents, such as 1-chloro-2,4-dinitrobenzene (CDNB); aflatoxin B1-epoxide; and trans-4-phenyl-3 buten-2-one and benzpyrene diols.

GST Pi class

GSTP1-1 is widespread, except for the liver, but is especially common in tumour cells. It will process a variety of toxicologically dangerous agents as well as endogenous species; these include CDNB, acrolein, adenine, propenal, benzyl isothiocyanante and 4-vinylpyridine. Aside from their functions in xenobiotic metabolism, GST Pi's and the Mu class GSTs appear to regulate a mitogen-activated protein (MAP) kinase pathway that is part of the apoptosis control system. The role of GSTP1 is especially troublesome in the induction of resistance to alkylating agents in cancer chemotherapy. Part of this process is the upregulation of GSH formation, but it also appears that GSTP1 and other isoforms in the series defend the tumour cells by direct detoxification as well as by blocking apoptosis through their effects on MAP kinase. Indeed, GSTP1 is such a problem within cancer therapeutics, that current research is directed at inhibitors of these isoforms to prevent the development of resistance to anti-neoplastic agents. These include ethacrynic acid and TER 199, which is a GSH analogue. It is also apparent that many flavonoids are also potent GSTP1 inhibitors.

GST Theta class

Enzymes differ from the other GSTs as they do not use the tyrosine residue to catalyse the reaction between the substrate and GSH. Serine accomplishes this activity in the GST-T isoform and it is likely that the site is capable of some structural rearrangement that assists in the catalytic process. This GST is associated with the metabolism of environmental and industrial carcinogens, including planar polycyclic aromatic hydrocarbons, halomethanes, dihalomethanes and ethylene oxide. Interestingly, GST-T in erythrocytes is identical to the hepatic version, so methyl bromide or ethylene oxide turnover by the enzyme in sampled erythrocytes is used to determine if an individual expresses this isoform.

GST Omega class

Enzymes process CDNB, 7-chloro-4-nitrobenzo-2-oxa-1,3-diazole, *p*-nitrophenyl acetate particularly effectively and are found in most tissues. These isoforms are thought to be responsible for protein repair, where thiol adducts are trimmed off cytosolic structures as the enzyme acts as a thiol transferase. It has a very large and open hydrophobic binding site, which allows it to bind polypeptide chains. This isoform is also involved in preventing cellular apoptosis by blocking calcium ion mobilization from intracellular stores.

Control of GSTs

As GSTs can be induced by the presence of alkylating agents and various other reactive species, it is thought that these vital cellular defence enzymes are tightly controlled through similar nuclear receptor systems as the CYPs, UGTs and the SULT enzymes. It certainly would be logical for a system that could detect potentially threatening lipophilic molecules, also to detect the unstable products of their oxidation. To a great extent, the risks run by the oxidation of potentially reactive molecules by CYP oxidation are nullified by the GST system. It is likely that the reactive species bind to the RXR nuclear receptor system and increased expression of the GST results from an RXR/xenobiotic complex binding to DNA response elements on the GST genes. Certainly, some analogs of retinoic acid, as well as the thiazolidinediones (troglitazone, rosiglitazone, pioglitazone), which bind other receptor systems, can cause RXR to induce GSTA2 in human cell systems.

It would also be logical if this system reacted more swiftly than, say, the induction effects of barbiturates and other lipophilic molecules. It may be that the very reactivity of such molecules as aromatic epoxides is exploited to mount a response to detoxify them. GSTs appear to interact with a number of cellular regulatory systems as mentioned already, so these enzymes can respond to 'homegrown' as well as xenobiotically generated reactive species. It would be expected from an evolutionary standpoint that organisms which possess an unusually high capacity to respond to a xenobiotic toxic threat which is far in excess of endogenous molecules will thrive at the expense of organisms which cannot neutralize the reactive species and clear them from their cells. This appears to be the case in humans, as there is considerable variation in the phenotype of these enzymes, conferring a wide defence for our species from environmental toxicity at the expense of the individual.

6.6 Epoxide hydrolases

Types of epoxide hydrolases (EHs)

Epoxide hydrolases are important multifunctional enzymes for both the deactivation and activation of reactive species; in addition, they have a number of equally important endogenous functions. In the same way as CYPs, higher organisms have 'appropriated' epoxide hydrolases from bacteria, with little real change in structure and function. From the drug/toxin metabolism standpoint, their main function is to convert any potentially reactive epoxide, formed by CYPs, to a diol (also known as dihydrodiols), which is usually less reactive, more water-soluble and more likely to be cleared by GSTs. There are two main variants of epoxide hydrolases:

- Microsomal epoxide hydrolase (mEH, or EPHX1) exists as two 'Types'. *Type I* is ideally positioned in the hepatic endoplasmic reticulum to 'intercept' epoxides of polycyclic aromatics (like styrene 7,8 epoxide), or drugs (carbamazepine 10,11 epoxide; Figure 6.10) formed by CYPs

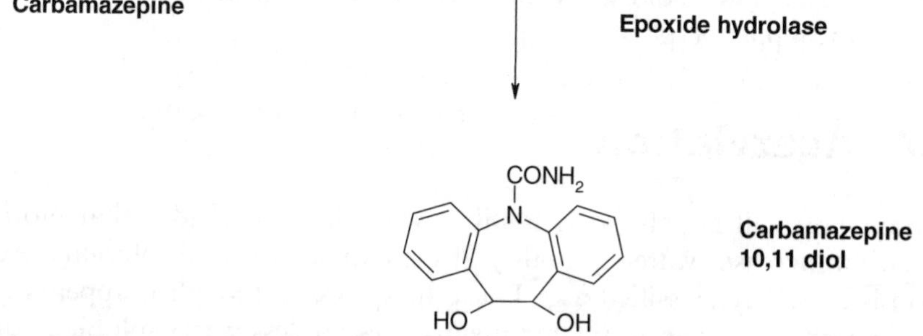

Figure 6.10 A typical microsomal epoxide hydrolase reaction: formation of carbamazepine 10,11 diol, which is thought to have anticonvulsant activity

and make them into diols. *Type II* mEH is found in the hepatocyte plasma membrane, where it controls the uptake of bile acids in the liver in association with a taurocholate binding protein; this system is involved in a number of endogenous processes, such as the control of cholesterol metabolism.

- Soluble epoxide hydrolase (sEH) also forms diols from many endogenous and exogenous epoxides. Unlike mEH, it has been found in most tissues as well as the liver, lung and kidney, as it is often closely associated with CYP enzymes such as CYP2C8 and 9. This enzyme appears to regulate many pathways related to endogenous systems such as fatty acid and leukotriene epoxide metabolism and is involved in blood pressure regulation and inflammatory responses. It appears that epoxide hydrolases are controlled by a number of DNA transcriptional factors and, in common with other Phase I and II enzyme systems, are likely to respond to increased substrate load through nuclear receptor regulation.

EH mechanisms of action

The mechanisms of action of these enzymes have been described (Figure 6.11), partly on an experimental basis and partly on the crystallization of sEH. It appears that although the enzyme has a low turnover number, it manages to catalyse the formation of diols extremely quickly, using tyrosine residues as proton donors and the carboxy group of an aspartate residue, which forms an intermediate enzyme–substrate ester, which then slowly hydrolyses to give the diol. This latter step is rate-limiting, although it is likely the enzyme accelerates the process of hydrolysis, as ester bonds are usually stable.

Epoxide hydrolases are thought to be responsible for the formation of diolepoxides of polycyclic aromatics, which are potent carcinogens. There are slow and fast versions of these enzymes and there is considerable human variation in their phenotypes.

6.7 Acetylation

By now, you will hopefully be familiar with the central idea that biotransformation increases water solubility at the expense of lipid solubility. Acetylation is generally classified as a Phase II process, although it appears to be rather contradictory as acetylated metabolites are less water-soluble than the parent drug; indeed, this often makes acetylated metabolites difficult to eliminate in urine. *In extremis*, acetylated metabolites of some old sulphonamides

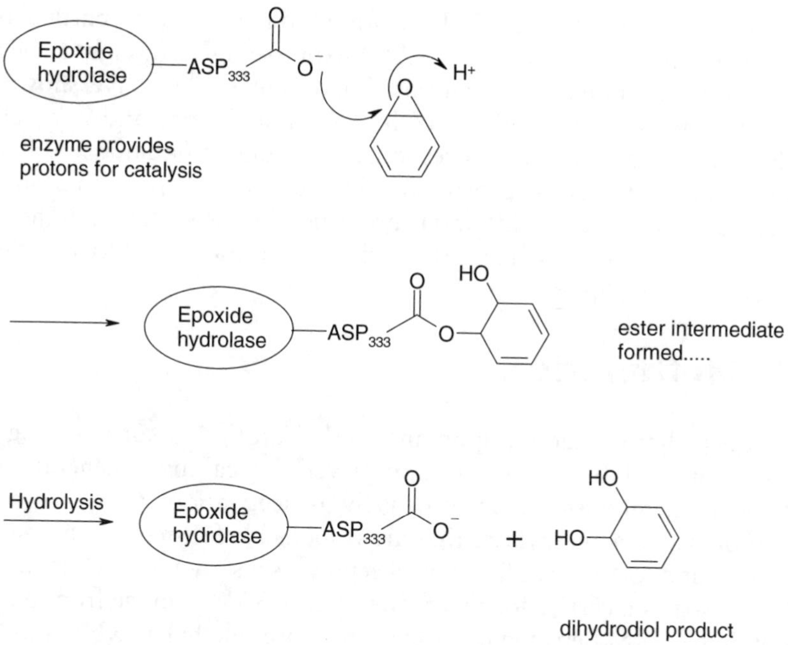

Figure 6.11 Mechanism of action of epoxide hydrolase in the conversion of a typical CYP-formed epoxide to a dihydrodiol

were so poorly water-soluble that they crystallized (painfully) in the patient's kidneys. You may be wondering what acetyltransferases are actually for, since they do not at first appear to contribute positively to the clearance of their substrates. There are a number of acetyltransferase gene families found in most cells and they have a large number of functions connected with cell homeostasis; for example, histone acetyl transferases (HATs) regulate DNA transcription through activating histone proteins by acetylating them, whilst some hormones such as melatonin are regulated through acetyltransferases. Although most metabolic reactions are to some extent reversible, acetylation is much more reversible than most. Indeed, there are many of these enzymes that are predominantly deacetylases, as well as acetylases. Many acetylated molecules can act as 'on' and 'off' switches in the regulation of the functions of nuclear receptor systems. The acetyl transferases relevant to human drug metabolism include two families of genes which are expressed, N-acetyl trans-ferase 1 (NAT-1) and N-acetyltransferase 2 (NAT-2). These enzymes use acetyl Co enzyme A as a co-factor to acetylate their substrates by using what is known as a double displacement (ping-pong) mechanism. There are two sequential steps to the reaction: firstly, the acetyl group is moved from acetyl CoA to form an acetylated enzyme intermediate, then the substrate is acety-lated and CoA is released. Iodacetate and N-ethylmaleide are irreversible inhibitors of the process, whilst reversible inhibitors (salicylamide) are similar in structure to the substrates. NAT-1 is found in many tissues, particularly in the colon, but also in erythrocytes. NAT-1 expression was thought to be fairly constant through human populations, but recent studies have shown that there is at least a twofold difference in some populations and it is believed that NAT-1 may be inducible in response to certain xenobiotic and endogenous substrates. It prefers to process substrates such as para-aminobenzoic and para-aminosalicyclic acids and is not generally associated with the acetylation of drugs. The consequences of genetic variation in acetyltransferases are discussed in Chapter 7.

6.8 Methylation

As with acetylation, adding lipophilic methyl groups to various drugs that decrease water solubility does not appear very logical in the general context of Phase II metabolism. However, as with acetylation, there are a huge number of cytosolic methylases that are responsible for many stages in DNA regulation and other cellular housekeeping tasks. S-adenosyl methionine (SAM) is used as a carrier for the methyl group. SAM is made from ATP and L-methionine. SAM-dependent methyltransferases methylate RNA and DNA, many proteins, polysaccharides, lipids and many other molecules. N, O and S-methyltransferases can be found in human systems.

N-methyltransferases can methylate various histamine-related compounds and amines. In the brain and the liver, catechol-O-methyl transferase (COMT) O-methylates the phenolic groups of a number of catecholamine neurotransmitters, including adrenaline and noradrenaline, although it also methylates dopamine; tolcapone (unfortunately a hepatoxin) was developed to inhibit the enzyme to increase dopamine levels in the brain in Parkinsonism. This drug was withdrawn in 1998 but re-introduced on a restricted basis in 2004. Methyl transferases can also methylate adrenaline, thiouracil, histamine and pyridine derivatives.

6.9 Esterases/amidases

There are a number of drugs that possess ester or amide linkages and these are vulnerable to the activity of esterases and amidases. Esterases are sometimes known as carboxylesterases and can overlap in activity with amidases (Fig. 6.12). These enzymes clear procaine, acetyl salicylate and chloramphenicol, although genetic polymorphisms can prolong the clinical effects of a number of neuromuscular blocking drugs (succinylcholine, atracurium mivacurium) which are also hydrolysed by esterases. There are many esterase enzymes in various tissues and the plasma, but the liver and kidney enzymes can hydrolyse the drugs listed above as well as several organophosphate and carbamate insecticides and herbicides. All the esterases, which include neural

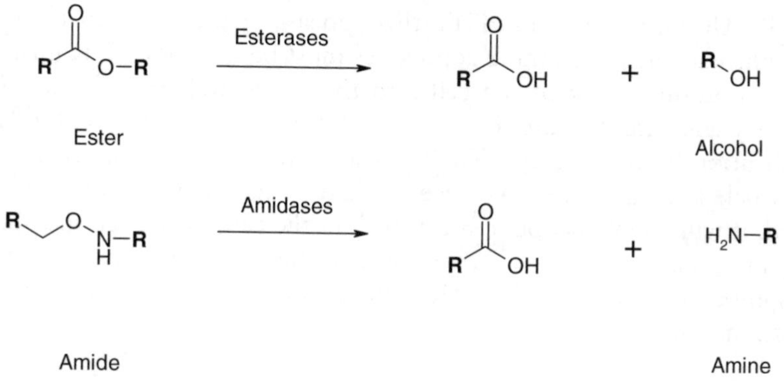

Figure 6.12 Esterase and amidase reaction sequences

acetylcholinesterase and butylcholinesterases, operate in a fairly similar manner, using an anionic and esteratic site to bind the substrate and a serine hydroxyl group to catalyse the hydrolysis of the ester linkage. Once an amidase has hydrolysed an amide, if an aromatic amine is released, the subsequent Phase I N-hydroxylation of the amine can cause systemic toxicity.

6.10 Amino acid conjugation (glycine or glutamate)

This is a comparatively minor but specialized route of Phase II clearance. Conjugation with amino acids generally involves glycine and occasionally glutamate. Glycine conjugation is the main route of clearance of salicylate, and a number of small aromatic alcohols and carboxylic acids can also act as substrates for the enzymes that catalyse the process, acyl-CoA synthetase and N-acyltransferase. The enzymes are found in the liver and kidney, but it appears that in the case of salicylate glycine conjugation the kidney is the main clearance organ. The amino acid is attached to the drug through an amide bond and can depend on cellular glycine supplies. Small organic acids like benzoic acid, a food preservative, are also cleared to hippuric acid derivatives though glycine conjugation.

6.11 Phase III transport processes

Introduction

Obviously once xenobiotics have been converted into low-toxicity, higher-molecular-weight and high-water-solubility metabolites by the combination of CYPs, UGTs, SULTs and GSTs, this appears at first sight to be 'mission accomplished'. However, these conjugates must be transported against a concentration gradient out of the cell into the interstitial space between cells. Then they will enter the capillary system and thence to the main bloodstream and filtration by the kidneys. The biggest hurdle is the transport out of the cell, which is a tall order, as once a highly water-soluble entity has been created, it will effectively be 'ion-trapped' in the cell, as the cell membrane is highly lipophilic and is an effective barrier to the exit as well as entry of most hydrophilic molecules. In addition, failure to remove the products of Phase II reactions can lead to:

- Toxicity of conjugates to various cell components;

- Hydrolysis of conjugates back to the original reactive species;

- Inhibition of Phase II enzymes.

If the cell can manage to transport them out, then they should be excreted in urine or bile and Phase II detoxification can proceed at a maximal rate. This situation is complicated by processes such as enterohepatic recirculation, where conjugates are hydrolysed and parent drug appears in the gut for reabsorption and transport by the efflux pump systems.

Consequently, an impressive array of multi-purpose membrane bound transport carrier systems has evolved which can actively remove hydrophilic metabolites and many other low-molecular-weight drugs and toxins from cells. The relatively recent (1990s) term of Phase III metabolism has been applied to the study of this essential arm of the detoxification process.

Efflux transporters

The main thrust of research into efflux transporters has been directed at the ABC-type transporters P-glycoprotein (chapter 5) and multi-drug resistance associated proteins (MRP1 and 2, also known as MDRs). This is because these ATP-consuming transporters are partly responsible for the resistance of cancer cells to chemotherapy and indeed, generic MDRs, or multi-drug resistance transporter proteins, are also used throughout the bacterial world to evade the effects of antibiotics. P-glycoprotein is intended to pump out relatively bulky lipophilic agents (orally administered drugs especially) and is sited in places where it will encounter them, such as the small intestine. It can pump out some hydrophilic molecules, although it has less of a role in the clearance of conjugated water-soluble metabolites than other transport systems, such as MRPs 1–3.

MRP1–3 (GS-X pumps)

So far, six MRP genes have been identified and their enzyme products have been known by a number of names, including GS-X and MOAT (multi-specific canalicular organic anion transporter) pumps. They have approximate molecular weights of around 190 000 and usually pump out molecules of toxicological significance, like GSH conjugates, steroid glucuronides and sulphated metabolites. They are found in most tissues, such as the liver, lung, testis and skin, and they are thought to act in a coordinated manner with GST enzymes. MRP1 may have evolved to remove GSH-related and other conjugates from cells (and is particularly important in the lung), whilst MRP2 is responsible for pumping bilirubin glucuronides into the bile in humans. A condition known as Dubin Johnson syndrome is associated with non-expression of MRP2 and patients cannot clear bilirubin conjugates efficiently. MRP1 and MRP 2 can both apparently use GSH in a co-transport capacity to clear non-conjugated and conjugated agents like methotrexate and vincristine and conjugated nitrosamines.

MRP1 is usually associated with substrates like GSH-related conjugated products, such as the GS conjugates of etoposide and melphalan, as well as aflatoxin B1 metabolites and several tobacco-related nitrosamine glucuronides. It is thought that MRP1 and 2 have multi-point binding pockets which enable them to bind the hydrophobic and polar areas of conjugated metabolites simultaneously at several points on the substrate. There is some evidence that the MRP proteins are controlled by nuclear receptor systems; MRP3 which is also known as D-MOAT, is known to be induced by phenobarbitone and the carcinogen 2-acetylaminofluorene. MRP 5 (was MOAT-C) is known to export various pyrimidine bases and is linked to resistance to the anti-cancer agent 6-mercaptopurine.

DNP-SG ATPase

This pump system was one of the earlier ones to be identified and this was named as it was shown first to use to be stimulated by S-(2,4-dinitrophenyl)glutathione (DNP-SG) and ATP was consumed. This broad specificity pump system is found in most tissues and it is unusual in that it will transport both anionic (e.g. glutathione-related conjugated metabolites) and cationic (doxorubicin) substrates. Patients who cannot express MRP2 have a residual anionic efflux ability and this is thought to occur through the operation of DNP-SG ATPase.

Other pump systems

There are a number of other non-ATP dependent pump systems which work in concert with the MRP series of efflux pumps, such as RLIP76, a non-ABC,

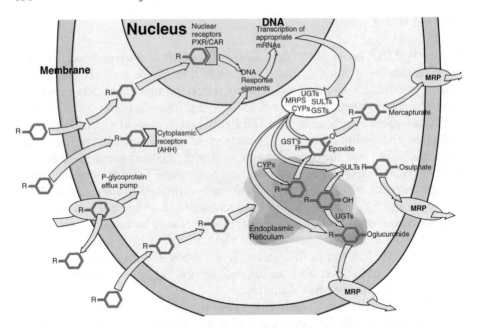

Figure 6.13   A scheme showing Phase I, II and III systems operating in concert for the detection and elimination of xenobiotic molecules such as aromatic hydrocarbons

GTPase-activating protein which transports GSH-related and other Phase II products. It is clear that detoxification enzyme and MRP activities are linked together, so the clearance of Phase II conjugates is exquisitely responsive to load. Figure 6.13 shows a scheme that tries to sum up the whole Phase I–III system, which operates predominantly in the liver, gut, lung and kidney, as well as to a lesser extent in other organs such as the brain and skin.

7 Factors Affecting Drug Metabolism

7.1 Introduction

As you are may be aware, drugs are initially tested at the preclinical stage in animal populations which are usually inbred and display little variation from animal to animal. Data from animal studies in one country are usually comparable with that of another, provided the animal species and strain are the same. This provides a consistent picture of the basic pharmacological and toxicological actions of a candidate drug in a living organism, although controversy rages over the value of this picture. Currently, animal data, combined with human tissue studies, are intended to give some approximation as to how the drug might affect humans. Unfortunately, you might also be aware that some drugs reach the clinic only to be withdrawn or have severe strictures placed on their usage, based on some form of toxicity or unintended pharmacological effect. Although it has been obvious since animal testing began that there would be large differences in the way a drug might perform in man compared with animal species, perhaps in the last 15–20 years it is clear just how vast these differences can be. Unfortunately, there is no experimental model yet designed that can not only consider human biochemistry and physiology, but also the effects of age, smoking, legal and illegal drug usage, gender, diet, environment, disease and finally genetic variation. Indeed, many clinical studies have revealed enormous differences in drug clearance and pharmacological effect even in age, sex and ethnically matched individuals. In effect, this means that the first year or so of a drug's clinical life is a vast, but monitored experiment, involving hundreds of thousands of patients and there is no guarantee of success. This chapter discusses some of the factors that can influence drug metabolism and their impact on the achievement of our goal of maintaining drug levels within the patient's therapeutic window.

Human Drug Metabolism, Michael D. Coleman
© 2005 John Wiley & Sons, Ltd

7.2 Genetic polymorphisms

Introduction

Apparently, cheetahs are all genetically identical and can receive skin grafts from any other cheetah like an identical twin could in humans. The same goes for elephant seals. Environmental and hunting pressures shrank the species to such small numbers that only one genetic variant now exists. The long-term survival of this type of population is unlikely, as genetic diversity is vital to ensure that no one toxin, bacteria or virus can eliminate all the population. In practice, genetic diversity is manifested in differences in single DNA nucleotides and/or whole genes that code for particular proteins. This results in a proportion of a population which expresses a protein that is different in structure and function to the majority. These differences may manifest as a substitution of a single amino acid with another, or a whole amino acid sequence may be different. These are termed 'polymorphisms' and their study is termed 'pharmacogenetics' or 'pharmacogenomics'. A polymorphism is a genetic variant that appears in at least 1 per cent or more of a population. The range of effect is wide: the polymorphic protein may simply not be as efficient as the majority, or it may be completely non-functional. If you recall earlier chapters where enzyme structures have been described, you might remember (hopefully) that a single amino acid in a precise position is often vital for the enzyme to function. The most common polymorphisms seem to be due to a change in one nucleotide, which means that the gene now specifies the wrong amino acid in a critical position, so reducing catalytic activity or it means a full stop occurs too early on the gene and incomplete mRNA is made which causes translation of an incomplete protein that is also ineffective and/or unstable. These are called SNPs or single nucleotide polymorphisms and can occur anywhere in the regulatory regions of genes in addition to the genes themselves. They can either be catalytically incompetent, or unstable, which leads also to incompetence. From basic genetics, you might recall that an individual who is heterozygous for a particular defective gene may either partly express the faulty protein or not at all, but a homozygote certainly will.

Polymorphisms arise due to mutations, but persist in human populations due to factors that may involve some advantage of the milder forms of the polymorphism (heterozygotes). If a faulty enzyme's endogenous function can be shouldered by other systems, then even homozygotes for the polymorphism may never be aware of their genetic make-up, as they suffer no symptoms. Glucose-6-phosphate dehydrogenase deficiency (G-6-PD) in Afro-Caribbeans is only a problem if the individual takes antimalarials such as primaquine or dapsone (Chapter 8), which generate toxic species that overwhelm the G-6-PD individual's compromised oxidant defence mechanisms. Similarly, if some xenobiotic agent can only be cleared, or detoxified, by a particular enzyme that is subject to a polymorphism, then the extremes may occur of either drug failure or drug toxicity. Any given drug response is based partly on the sensitivity of the appropriate receptor and the amount of drug in the system. Both these factors are subject to polymorphisms and the following sections concentrate on polymorphic effects on the mechanisms that govern drug clearance. Most polymorphisms are a problem clinically due to an inability of the poor metabolizers to remove the drug from the system. Drug failure can occur if the agent is administered as a pro-drug and requires some metabolic conversion to an active metabolite. Drug accumulation can lead to unpleasant side effects and loss of patient tolerance for the agent.

Genetic polymorphisms in CYP systems

CYP1A1

CYP1A1 is of greatest significance as the inducible producer of potentially carcinogenic species from PAHs. The presence of high levels of this isoform has often been seen in tissues affected by cancers, such as the lung and breast. The enzyme has evolved as a protection against PAH-like molecules, activating them into epoxides or other reactive species, which are then conjugated by adjacent conjugative systems to non-reactive excretable products. Why this system is linked to many cancers may be due to a variety of reasons, such as the large inter-individual variation in the degree of induction (Chapter 4) of CYP1A1, as well as polymorphisms in the isoform itself. From Chapter 4, it can be recalled that there are several steps in the induction of this CYP, such as the Ah receptor, and the proteins used in these steps are all vulnerable to genetic mutations. There are four currently described polymorphic forms of CYP1A1, of which CYP1A1*2 and CYP1A1*3 are the most studied. These differ only in one amino acid from the other forms and it has been suggested that this makes them easier to induce so forming more reactive species, which in turn increases cancer risk. This is very difficult to prove experimentally and many more studies need to be done to substantiate this.

CYP2A6

This CYP has toxicological and endogenous roles in the clearance of a number of substrates (Chapter 3), such as nicotine. There are some polymorphisms associated with the isoform, with about four mutant types of the non-functional enzyme expressed. Some non-functional mutants exist in low proportions (<3 per cent) of Caucasians, although one particular mutant is found in up to 20 per cent of Chinese and 5 per cent of Japanese individuals. The clinical relevance of the polymorphism may become important if the

PAF (platelet-activating factor) antagonist SM-12502 becomes widely used, as this agent is solely oxidized by 2A6.

CYP2D6

This CYP, whose gene is found on chromosome 22, does not appear to have a vital endogenous function. It is non-inducible, but it was noticed in the 1970s that the clearance of some (now obsolete) drugs (sparteine and debrisoquine), was greatly retarded in a small proportion of Caucasian populations. The enzyme is still sometimes termed 'debrisoquine hydroxylase', or 'spartein/debrisoquine hydroxylase'. Subsequent research has shown that 2D6 is subject to a variety of defects that include one-nucleotide deletions as in SNPs or two nucleotide deletions, or even the complete deletion of the gene, so the 2D6 protein does not appear at all. If a patient is homozygous for any of these deletions, then they are poor metabolizers of CYP2D6 substrates. The frequency of homozygotes or poor metabolizers varies according to race – around 3–10 per cent of Caucasians, 4 per cent of Afro-Caribbeans and less than 1 per cent of Orientals exhibit this effect. Potentially, in Europe, there could be more than 30 million poor metabolizers of 2D6-cleared drugs and maybe 10–15 million in the USA. Normal, or 'wild type' individuals for this gene are sometimes called extensive metabolizers. The manifestation of this polymorphism can lead to plasma levels in poor metabolizers that are up to *10 times* those of the extensive metabolizers. There is also evidence that heterozygotes show some degree of impairment in the enzyme. There is even a condition where multiple forms of the 2D6 gene are encoded in the subject's DNA, which can lead to up to 13 versions of the enzyme appearing instead of one. These individuals are known as ultra-rapid metabolizers and have to take drug doses that can be several times more than the normal 'wild type' individual and perhaps 20 times more than a poor metabolizer. These ultra rapid metabolizers are found in some Arabic populations and in north-eastern Africa, where the multiple copies of the gene are believed to be a form of 'induction' for an enzyme that cannot be induced. This may be in response to dietary pressure of certain toxins found in that area. Clearly in poor metabolizers, there is a risk of a variety of clinical problems that centre, as you might expect, on both drug toxicity as well as drug failure.

CYP2D6 and antipsychotics

As if the problems of schizophrenics were not enough, the drugs available to control the symptoms are well known for their extensive and unpleasant side effects. Among the most difficult to control and distressing effects are tardive dyskinesias (TDs) which are involuntary movements of the lips, tongue, face, arms and legs, which begin to occur during the first year or so of treatment with some of these drugs. TDs are part of a series of involuntary disorders known as 'extra-pyramidal effects'. After around 10 years or so on antipsychotic drugs, more than half the patients will have developed permanent TDs. The causes of TDs and related dyskinesias could be related to neurological damage caused by the drugs and/or their metabolites. TDs can be present without the drugs, although the drugs do make them significantly worse. Patients with CYP2D6 polymorphisms are much more prone to TD symptoms to the point that the drugs cannot be tolerated, and interestingly, patients who are heterozygous for the polymorphism also are more likely to develop TDs. The use of risperidone, (a CYP3A4 as well as 2D6 substrate) and the 'Amplichip' CYP DNA microarray test system, which uses patient blood samples to determine CYP2D6 and 2C19 status in advance of drug administration, will hopefully prevent antipsychotic toxicity, as well as sudden deaths in schizophrenics due to torsades des pointes-induced heart failure.

Tricyclic antidepressants (TCAs)

These drugs were the mainstay of treatment for depression until the advent of the SSRIs and newer mixed-function agents such as mirtazapine. They are seen as essentially superseded drugs, although they are still used in a number of complaints aside from depression, such as intractable pain. They were difficult to use and dangerous from a number of perspectives, not least because they took so long to show any clinical benefit (six weeks or more) and their atropine-like side effects (dry mouth, constipation, etc.). If the patient did not respond to these drugs, then the patient might choose to overdose. This combined with a narrow therapeutic index led to many TCA fatalities. Inability to clear these drugs due to a patient's status as a 'poor metabolizer' would provide the twin problem of a high level of the atropinic side effects, combined with an even narrower therapeutic index in that patient and a risk of death from a modest overdose.

Beta-blockers

Failure to clear beta-blockers such as timolol, propanolol, pindolol and metoprolol can accentuate considerably their side effects, which include bronchospasm, heart problems, headaches, sexual dysfunction, nightmares, depression, problems with glucose metabolism and general tiredness.

SSRIs

The metabolism of SSRIs is complex, as they are both extensively oxidatively (often demethylated) metabolized by, as well as actively inhibiting, CYP2D6, as well as other isoforms. Citalopram is metabolized by 2D6 to several demethylated derivatives and undergoes some 2C19 clearance also. Fluoxetine is N-demethylated by 2D6 to the irreversible inhibitor norfluoxetine, although other CYPs are involved. Polymorphisms in 2D6 are likely to affect citalopram and fluoxetine much more than paroxetine, which is cleared by 2D6 at low concentrations only, but inhibits it at higher concentrations. Fluvoxamine and sertraline are not dependent on 2D6 for clearance, although sertraline can inhibit the enzyme *in vivo*. Combinations of SSRIs and TCAs can cause severe drug accumulation in 'wild type' individuals, so the effects would be even worse in those subject to polymorphisms.

Antiarrhythmics

Flecainide, mexiletine and encainide have potent effects on cardiac electrophysiology and these are sensitive to dosage, so 2D6 poor metabolizers run the risk of high concentrations of these agents increasing arrhythmias rather than reducing them.

Opiate analgesics

These include codeine, fentanyl, meperidine, propoxyphene and pethidine. Codeine is a pro-drug, as it is a methylated version of morphine and must be O-demethylated by 2D6 before the liberated morphine can act analgesically. In poor metabolizers, codeine will therefore have little efficacy. Oxycodone is normally converted to oxymorphone partly by 2D6 and this drug's efficacy is also impaired in poor metabolizers. Tramadol is much less toxic than morphine, and is O-demethylated to an active metabolite that has opioid effects. In poor metabolizers, less of the O-demethylated metabolite is formed, but parent drug levels are not that much higher than wild-type individuals, so it appears to be less subject to 2D6 polymorphism problems than codeine and other substrates of this isoform. Fentanyl is a highly potent opiate that is predominantly cleared by N-dealkylation by 3A4 and by 2D6 to norfentanyl and other metabolites. Poor metabolizers will be in danger of an intensification of the opiate effects from a relatively low dose.

Other drugs

Venlafaxine is a noradenaline and serotonin reuptake inhibitor and is often a second-line treatment in depression after SSRIs have failed to help. It is much safer than the TCAs as it is not toxic, nor does it cause all the anticholinergic effects seen with the TCAs. Unfortunately when it was first used efficacy was not impressive and side effects were high (restlessness and nausea). This may be because it was usually tried after SSRIs had failed and fluoxetine is a potent 2D6 inhibitor through its norfluoxetine metabolite. This effect can last for weeks and it appears that venlafaxine is oxidized to two major active metabolites, O-desmethyl venlafaxine (ODV) and N-desmethyl venlafaxine (NDV). The SSRI effect may have impacted on the efficacy of venlafaxine, while retarding its clearance and increasing the side effects. This suggests that a longer 'washout' period is required before venlafaxine is started after SSRIs have been abandoned. Trazodone, another non-TCA or SSRI alternative antidepressant, is also cleared by 2D6, although it is not clear to what extent poor metabolizers are disadvantaged in efficacy by the polymorphism.

CYP2C8

The significance of polymorphisms in CYP2C8 is still emerging, mainly in relation to the metabolism of the anti-cancer agent taxol. It is thought that 20 per cent of Caucasians are heterzygotes for SNPs for this isoform. So far, five polymorphic forms have been identified, CYP2C8*1–5. CYP2C8*3 and possibly *4, found in Caucasians, has been suggested to be defective compared with the wild type in the clearance of taxol and arachidonic acid, although later studies suggest that this polymorphism may not be clinically significant. It has also been suggested that the regulation of CYP2C8 expression is subject to polymorphism.

CYP2C9

This enzyme has been intensively studied and emerged as a major factor in the clearance of a number of drugs, such as non-steroidal anti-inflammatories (diclofenac, ibuprofen, naproxen), the hypoglycaemic sulphonyl ureas such as tolbutamide and glipizide, as well as the angiotensin II blockers losartan and irbesartan and a number of other drugs such as dapsone, some sulphonamides, amitryptyline, SSRIs, phenytoin, tamoxifen and S-warfarin. It is found on chromosome 10 and is subject to a polymorphism that is relatively low in frequency in Caucasians, at around 1–3 per cent. The levels in Orientals are much lower, at around 0.5 per cent, although in Hong Kong Chinese the frequency is slightly higher. Warfarin is cleared by 2C9 to an inactive 7-hydroxy derivative and in poor metabolizers the drug could potentially accumulate on the 'normal' dose and lead to excessive anticoagulation. However, clinically, patients are monitored by the ability of their blood to coagulate in a set time (INR, as mentioned in Chapter 5: – usually set in the range 1.5–3), so drug levels are carefully titrated against the pharmacodynamic effects of the drug, rather than just a set dosage. Some can be fully anticoagulated on half a milligram of warfarin, less than a tenth of the dose required for others. Problems might arise in the initial stages of therapy, where disproportionate anticoagulation may occur from a modest loading dose, which should appear unusual to the experienced physician. The clinical impact of a 2C9 polymorphism may be a problem on the basis of its relative rarity; there is less awareness of 2C9 polymorphisms, compared with those of 2D6. Even so, low 2C9 activity may potentially affect more than half a million individuals in the UK alone.

CYP2C19

This CYP (chromosome 10) was discovered to be polymorphic in the mid 1990s, and it is involved in the clearance of a considerable number of drugs, which include phenytoin and the usual probe drug S-mephenytoin as well as phenobarbitone and several other barbiturates, plus benzodiazepines, citalopram, cyclophosphamide, indomethicin, lansoprazole, omeprazole, primidone, R-warfarin, proguanil, propranolol, nelfinvir and clomipramine. The frequency of the polymorphism is low in Caucasians, 3–5 per cent, about the same in Afro-Caribbeans (2–5 per cent) but much higher in Orientals (15–20 per cent). Two mutations account for 99 per cent of the Oriental poor metabolizer phenotypes, but less than 90 per cent of the Caucasian phenotypes, so other genetic defects account for the polymorphisms in this group. Again, the mutations are SNPs.

CYP3A

Since the CYP3A group (chromosome 7) metabolize around half of all drugs, intensive efforts have been made to account for variation in the metabolism of CYP3A substrates, which can be up to tenfold in terms of drug clearances and up to 90-fold in liver protein expression. This is partly due to the responsiveness of the CYP to all the inducers and inhibitors that enter human systems. It appears that CYP3A drug clearance can be resolved mostly in terms of the sum of CYP3A4 and 3A5 isoforms, although a CYP3A7 and a CYP3A43 (very low levels of expression) have also been found. In wild-type individuals, the ratio between the two major CYPs can be about 50:50.

Regarding CYP3A4, it does appear to be remarkably well conserved across humanity and no major variants in its structure have been found in levels high enough (>1 per cent) to be classed as a significant polymorphic. The PXR binding elements in the regulatory area of the gene do not appear to vary much either, although there is a fault in the promoter of CYP3A4 in some individuals, who possess a CYP3A4*1B, which has been suggested to lead to reduced CYP output in response to hormone stimulus. This is said to lead to greater hormone levels that might promote neoplasms, such as in prostate cancer. This is so far unproved. Other rarer varials of CYP3A4 include CYP3A4*2 and *3, as well as *4–6, found in Chinese individuals. It is likely that the full extent of the variation in CYP3A4 is still to be discovered in other aspects of its regulation.

While it is thought that 3A4 is not subject to an obvious major polymorphism, CYP3A5 definitely is. CYP3A5*1 is the functional version, whilst a single nucleotide polymorphism causes the misreading of the CYP3A5 gene leading to the formation of shortened and catalytically inadequate CYP3A5*3. CYP3A5 is absent or non-functional in nearly 70 per cent of Caucasians, but only in 40 per cent of Afro-Caribbeans. Although this looks radical, the net effect has not been fully assessed and may not be so great since CYP3A4 and 3A5 appear to be very similar in their activities. Certainly with antipsychotics like haloperidol, there is little difference in the way CYP3A4 and 3A5 handle the drug or behave in the presence of inhibitors. Predisposition to neoplasms linked with hormone metabolism are thought to be most likely associated with polymorphisms in CYP3A5, such as the *3 variant, rather than CYP3A4.

Other CYP polymorphisms

There is evidence that CYP2B6 (chromosome 19) is polymorphic: it affects around 3–4 per cent of Caucasians. This CYP is known to metabolize a relatively small group of drugs, which includes phenobarbitone, bupropion, cyclophosphamide, methadone and ifosfamide.

Other polymorphic enzymes relevant to drug disposition

The enzyme dihydropyrimidine dehydrogenase is subject to a polymorphism and since it is responsible for the clearance of the nucleotide antimetabolite, 5-fluorouracil, this leads to neurotoxicity due to accumulation of this drug. Drug efflux transporters such as P-glycoprotein are subject to polymorphisms and are implicated in therapeutic resistance to epilepsy drugs. It is not clear to whether other drug efflux transporters are subject to these polymorphisms, such as MRP1–3 families, although it is highly likely that they are. The ability to remove a potential toxin that cannot be cleared by any other means would confer advantage to certain individuals, although in the case of drug therapy, this can be a positive disadvantage.

Conjugative polymorphisms: acetylation

Acetylation was the first polymorphism to be investigated and was based on the observation that the antitubercular drug isoniazid caused a different level of neural toxicity in Japanese compared with US patients. Although there are two N-acetyltransferase isoforms, NAT-1 and 2, NAT-2 (found mostly in the liver) is relevant to drug polymorphisms. It acetylates drugs such as isoniazid, dapsone and the sulphonamides. There are three distinct groups: fast, intermediate and slow acetylators. The highest frequencies of fast acetylators are in Asian countries, particularly Japan, with over 90 per cent of the population. Frequencies in the Indian subcontinent are much lower, at around 30 per cent; with European populations around 40 per cent are fast/intermediate acetylators.

This polymorphism has dramatic effects on the plasma levels of the parent form of acetylated drugs. With fast acetylators, perhaps only 20 per cent of drug-related material in the plasma will be parent drug and therefore clinically effective (assuming metabolites are not active). This situation could lead to potential treatment failure. In contrast, in the slow acetylators, more than 80 per cent of drug-related material in the blood will be parent drug and these levels may be so high as to approach toxic levels in some individuals. Obviously in drug therapy, most people will be prescribed a standard dosage of any given drug, so it is clear that the difference in plasma levels across even a small group of patients of differing phenotypes will be potentially huge, leading to a risk of toxicity in one group and possibly drug failure in another.

Acetylation and sulphonamides

In a study in patients taking sulphasalazine (sulphapyridine and 5-aminosalicylate linked by an azo bond) for ulcerative colitis, parent drug (sulphapyridine) plasma levels were between three- and fourfold higher in the slow acetylators compared with the fast acetylators, whilst the acetylated drug was found in approximately threefold higher levels in the fast acetylators compared with the slow.

Despite the potential problems caused by wide disparities in plasma concentrations between populations and individuals, sulphonamides were cheap, effective and were used in vast amounts as broad-spectrum antibacterials for over 50 years. In fast acetylators, providing there was enough drug in the plasma to suppress bacterial growth or exert an anti-inflammatory effect, efficacy would be adequate. However, in some individuals, it is likely that sustained low plasma levels of the drug contributed to the selection of resistant bacterial populations that reduced drug effectiveness. Resistance was offset by the use of sulphonamides in combination with 2,4 diamino-pyrimidines (pyrimethamine and trimethoprim) which are synergistic in effect, as the drugs attack the bacterial/protozoan DNA synthesis process in two places, thus requiring much lower plasma concentrations to be effective. Currently, a combination of sulphamethoxazole with trimethoprim (SMX and TMP) is highly effective in treating *Pneumocystis jaroveci*-induced pneumonia in HIV-positive individuals who have T-cell counts below 200.

Sulphonamides and their combinations also fell out of favour for broad-spectrum antibacterial usage, because of a relatively high rate of adverse reactions, which included some gruesome conditions such as Stevens–Johnson syndrome (Chapter 8). Indeed, more than half of HIV patients taking the

SMX/TMP combination suffer from milder adverse reactions such as various rashes, which can abolish patient tolerance of the drugs. These reactions are not connected with the parent drug or the acetylated metabolites, which are not cytotoxic on their own. Unfortunately, all aromatic amine-based drugs such as sulphonamides and sulphones and other substrates of NAT-2 are also subject to extensive CYP-mediated (usually CYP2C9) oxidative metabolism. These metabolites are the main route of clearance of these agents and they are mostly hydroxylamines, which are usually eliminated as Phase II sulphates or glucuronides. However, enough of the cytotoxic hydroxylamines escape Phase II to be the cause of the adverse reactions associated with these drugs.

So you can see that NAT enzymes could be seen as detoxification pathways for aromatic amine-related drugs; this is because once an amine has been N-acetylated, then there should be less opportunity for it to be oxidized by the CYPs to hydroxylamines (Figure 7.1). This would only apply if the

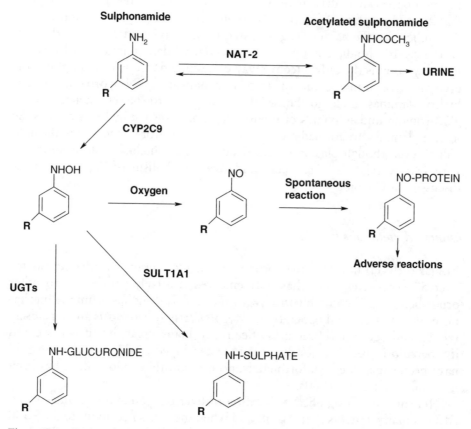

Figure 7.1 Basic scheme for sulphonamide metabolism and how adverse reactions are related to metabolism

acetylated derivative was excreted into urine and did not undergo further oxidative metabolism. With sulphapyridine, a modest amount (approximately 20 per cent) of the dose was found in urine as the acetylated derivative, so providing some support for other studies which suggested that in drugs which only possess one aromatic amine (sulphonamides), the frequencies of adverse reactions related to the oxidative metabolites were lower in fast acetylators and correspondingly higher in slow acetylators. So it appears that the slow acetylators are more vulnerable than fast acetylators to toxicity from the oxidative route of metabolism.

Sulphones

However, in drugs with two aromatic amine moieties, such as dapsone, this protective effect does not apply, as diacetylation is a minor pathway in dapsone metabolism and only a few per cent of the dose is found in urine as the monoacetylated derivative and trace amounts of the highly lipophilic diacetylated sulphone (Figure 7.2). Monoacetylated dapsone is much more lipophilic than the parent drug, so essentially, acetylation can delay dapsone clearance, by 'holding it up' in the acetylation/deacetylation pathway. N-hydroxylation is the only effective way of making dapsone less lipophilic and even the free amine group of acetylated dapsone is N-hydroxylated. The hydroxylamines undergo Phase II metabolism to be eliminated as N-glucuronides and sulphates of monoacetyl and dapsone hydroxylamines. So hydroxylamines are formed regardless of the acetylator phenotype of the individual, even though plasma parent drug levels are higher in slow compared with fast acetylators. The toxic oxidative metabolism of dapsone will be discussed in Chapter 8.

Isoniazid metabolism

Isoniazid (INH) has been the cornerstone of the therapy of tuberculosis for over 50 years. Resistance has only emerged relatively slowly due to other drugs being used in combination with INH. This drug has a unique mechanism of action that only operates in *Mycobacteria tuberculosis* and its closely related pathogens. INH remains effective in many areas, but it is toxic and if tuberculosis were a major disease of the developed world, it certainly would have been superseded. Unfortunately, no new antituberculosis drug has been introduced since the 1960s.

INH can lead to significant elevation of liver transaminase enzymes (AST, ALT) in many patients that take it, and when the levels rise about to 300–500 (around 10-fold normal) mild hepatotoxicity may be occurring. Hepatotoxicity can be serious in round 1–2 per cent of patients and lead to liver

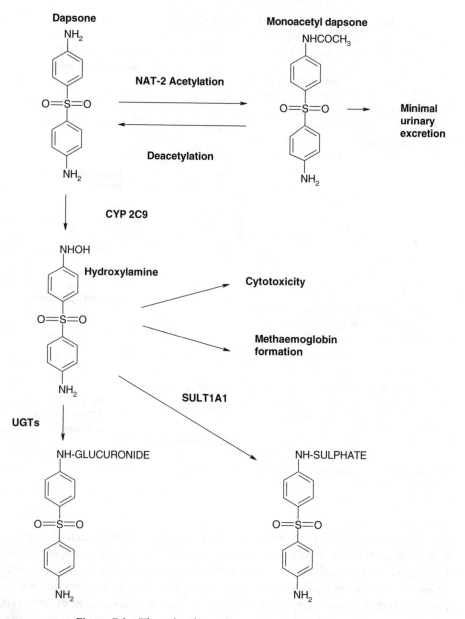

Figure 7.2 The role of acetylation in dapsone metabolism

failure if the drug is not stopped immediately. It is a substrate for NAT-2 and it is believed that slow acetylators are most at risk from INH hepatotoxicity; it has been suggested that CYP-mediated metabolism is linked with the toxicity. NAT-2 forms N-acetyl isoniazid that can hydrolyse to form the acetyl hydrazine, which is a potent nucleophile in its own right and does not need

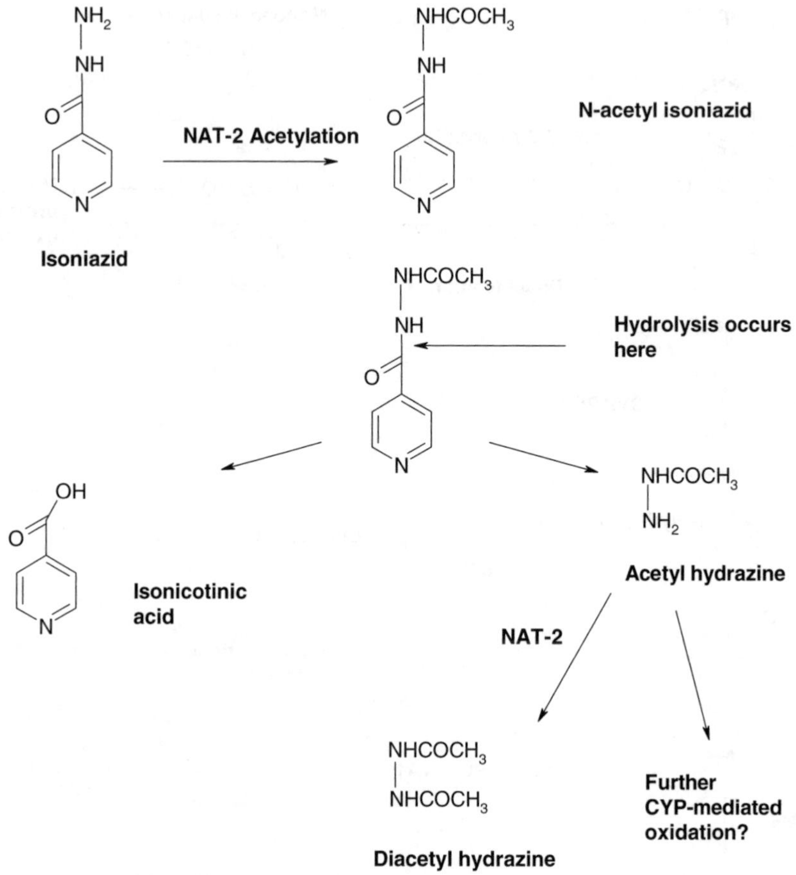

Figure 7.3 Acetylation and isoniazid metabolism

any more metabolism to be cytotoxic. It is not clear with isoniazid metabolism how acetylation is protective; from Figure 7.3, it might be expected that fast acetylators would form more acetylhydrazine and then be more susceptible to toxicity, than the slow acetylators, but this is not borne out by clinical studies. Slow acetylation appears to be associated with greater risk of liver toxicity and any concurrent therapy (or heavy alcohol use) that induces CYP2E1 increases the risk of liver damage. It is more likely that acetyl isoniazid is accommodated by Phase II detoxification and that CYP2E1 forms a much more toxic metabolite, perhaps directly from isoniazid itself, without acetylation being necessary. This would account for the protective effect of acetylation, which essentially promotes the formation of a relatively reactive but containable metabolite (acetyl hydrazine), so restricting entry of the parent drug or even acetyl hydrazine itself into oxidative metabolism.

Toxicological significance of acetylation

To complicate this situation further, some acetylated metabolites can undergo further oxidation themselves to form highly reactive cytotoxic and carcinogenic species. Indeed, in recent years, acetylation has become intensively studied almost entirely due to its role in the carcinogenic activation of aromatic amines and this is discussed briefly in Chapter 8. Perhaps the best context to see acetylation is a homeostatic process that unfortunately xenobiotics do enter and undergo metabolism, often leading to outcomes that are at best rather equivocal.

Conjugative polymorphisms: methylation

A particularly dangerous polymorphism clinically was identified in the 1980s for one of the Phase II methyltransferases. *S*-methylating thiopurine *S*-methyltransferase (TPMT) is capable of *S*-methylating thiopurine derivatives. There are other enzymes which can accomplish its activities, and it does not seem to have an absolutely vital endogenous task to perform. However, mercaptopurine and azothioprine are antimetabolites that mimic purine to disorder DNA metabolism in malignant cells. These drugs are effective in some childhood leukaemias, and are activated to 6-thioguanine nucleotides by an enzyme called HGPRT. TPMT is the main route of clearance of these toxic 6-thioguanines and this polymorphism can greatly distort the clinical behaviour of this drug in the patients. Those who are poor metabolizers and have low TPMT expression can suffer from lethal myelosuppression and abnormally high levels of the active 6-thioguanine nucleotides. The polymorphism is due to a single nucleotide change that leads to two alterations in the amino acid sequence of the enzyme. The frequency has been estimated worldwide to around $1:300$, although about 4 per cent of Caucasians express the TPMT poor metabolizer polymorphism, whilst it is virtually absent in Chinese/Japanese. The faster metabolizers clear the thiopurines too quickly and reduce their cytotoxic efficacy, leading effectively to drug failure. Drug failure in the context of a progressive and life-threatening disease is obviously extremely serious. A test was developed for TPMT expression based on the fortunate fact (in common with GST-theta and NAT-1) that enzyme expression in red cells is the same as systemic expression. This means that the patients are tested for TPMT expression prior to therapy and the drug's toxicity is not now life-threatening, although as you may know if you have seen any antineoplastic drugs used, they all exert fairly horrendous side effects anyway.

Conjugative polymorphisms: glucuronidation

It is believed that polymorphisms in UGTs are found in the promoters, or the controlling systems, of these isoforms. One of the main UGTs, UGT1A1, is subject to polymorphisms as described in Chapter 6. The most severe, Crigler-Najjar syndrome-1 is fatal, but CN-2 is survivable and Gilbert's syndrome is also relatively mild and is the commonest UGT polymorphism, with up to 19 per cent of some ethnic groups affected. It is apparent that susceptibility to some cancers linked with exposure to environmental toxins such as PAHs as well as hormone-dependent cancers, may be influenced by UGT status. Genetic variation in human UGTs has been reported to be as high as 100-fold. More immediatedly, if a drug relies on the clearance of a reactive toxic metabolite to a glucuronide, then the various UGT1A1 polymorphisms strongly predispose the individual to toxicity. This is most clearly shown in the use of the anticolorectal cancer drug irinotecan. This drug is a topoisomerase-I inhibitor and is a pro-drug which is metabolized to the active species SN-38. This species is associated with severe diarrhoea in some individuals as it is directly toxic to the gut. Glucuronidation normally protects the gut as the conjugate is not toxic and UGT1A1 polymorphisms abolish this protective pathway, thus precluding these patients from the benefits of the drug. It is likely that other UGTs are also subject to polymorphisms.

Conjugative polymorphisms: sulphation

Understanding of sulphation and its roles in endogenous as well as xenobiotic metabolism is not as advanced compared with that of CYPs; however, the role of SULTs in the activation of carcinogens is becoming more apparent. One of the major influences on SULT activity is their polymorphic nature; in the case of one of the most important toxicologically relevant SULTs, SULT1A1, this isoform exists as two variants, SULT1A1*1 and SULT1A1*2. The *2 variant differs only in the exchange of one amino acid for another. This single amino acid change has profound effects on the stability and catalytic activity of the isoform. The *2 variant is found in approximately 32 per cent of Caucasians and is unstable and so has a shorter half-life than the *1 variant (wild type) and consequently its general activity is lower than the *1 variant. The *2 variant is also less subject to substrate inhibition, which may have consequences regarding the general feedback metabolic control of the *2 variant. Although susceptibility to carcinogenesis depends on myriad factors, SULT activity regarding some specific carcinogens such as acetylfluorene may be an important determinate of exposure to DNA-damaging reactive species.

Other Conjugative polymorphisms

GSTs are polymorphic and much research has been directed at linking increased predisposition to cytotoxicity and carcinogenicity with defective

GST phenotypes. Active wild-type GSTMu-1 is found in around 60 per cent of Caucasians, but a non-functional version of the isoform is found in the remainder. This is caused by a gene deletion that also occurs in GST-Theta isoforms. It is difficult to link a lack of expression of GST isoforms and increased DNA damage, partly because other detoxifying enzymes such as epoxide hydrolase (mEH) might be operating and masking the effects on the test cell system. mEH itself is subject to a polymorphism, with a fast and slow variant of the enzyme. Carcinogenesis may be due to a complex mix of factors, where different enzyme expression and activities may combine with particular reactive species from specific parent xenobiotics which lead to DNA damage only in certain individuals. Resolving specific risk factors may be extremely difficult in such circumstances.

Polymorphism detection: clinical issues

If a drug company could afford to choose not to develop a drug that is a 2D6 substrate it probably would not proceed with the agent, due to the inevitable problems that would arise from its clinical usage. Drugs are, of course, some way down the line of evaluation before their hepatic metabolism is fully elucidated and the primary driving force has tended to be efficacy, rather than eventual route of clearance, or non-clearance, for that matter. Until recently it has been assumed that medical staff will be made aware that the drug's clearance is subject to a polymorphism and everyone hoped for the best. The potentially terminal blow to a drug company's finances when a drug is withdrawn before they have recouped their investment can be averted if pharmacogenetic testing procedures take place as early as possible in the development of the drug. The most successful companies have been doing this for a number of years and are well aware that a new drug has a considerable chance of clearance via some sort of polymorphic route. From the clinical perspective, the point has been raised that in the future, it might be considered unethical to prescribe a drug which is subject to a polymorphism to an individual without first determining whether they are a poor metabolizer or not. Currently, DNA testing using gene amplification techniques can provide an accurate pharmacogenetic profile of an individual's possible polymorphism for CYP2D6, 2C9 and 2C19. This technology has now reached the clinic, and should benefit patients such as those prescribed antipsychotic drugs. As has been outlined already, most of those using antipsychotics that are also 2D6 poor metabolizers suffer high levels of side effects of these drugs. At the moment, it is generally agreed that medical staff do have access to information on the radical effects of polymorphisms in certain drugs and current awareness is increasing. Some advances in the prevention of adverse reactions have been enthusiastically adopted and been highly successful; for example, the agranulcytosis-inducing tendencies of the antipsychotic clozapine (Chapter 8) have been abolished by restricting its usage to those with a normal white cell count. This has retained a drug that has a vitally important niche in patients who do not respond to other antipsychotics. The introduction of the TPMT genotyping discussed earlier is another good example. However, other potential beneficial drugs, such as the use of radioprotective thiols to attenuate toxicity in cancer chemotherapy, have never really reached clinics, even though they would reduce morbidity and mortality. It is to be hoped that 2D6 genotyping will eventually be successful in groups of vulnerable patients who have little therapeutic alternative to a 2D6-cleared drug and are poor metabolizers.

7.3   Effects of age on drug metabolism

The effects of age on drug clearance and metabolism have been known since the 1950s, but they have been extensively investigated in the last 20 or so years. It is now generally accepted that at the extremes of life, neonatal and geriatric, drug clearance can be significantly different from the rest of humanity. In general, neonates, i.e. those less than four weeks old, cannot clear certain agents due to immaturity of drug metabolizing systems. Those over retirement age cannot clear the drugs due to loss of efficiency in their metabolizing systems. Either way, the net result can be toxicity due to drug accumulation.

The elderly

As every aspect of the body declines fairly precipitously beyond the age of around 70, the ability to clear drugs is no exception. Unfortunately, most elderly people are taking not just one, but sometimes rather complex combinations of drugs, which is termed 'polypharmacy'. Some have estimated that the average 70-year-old could be taking eight drugs or medications daily. It seems that the inability of older people to clear drugs is not necessarily related to the efficacy of their CYP-mediated oxidations, which are often not much different from that of younger individuals. Studies with the major CYPs 1A2, 2E1, 3A4/3A5, 2C8 and 2C9 have shown that these enzymes function catalytically as well in elderly livers *in vitro* as younger livers do. However, functioning in a laboratory with enough oxygen and NADPH may not necessarily be an accurate picture of whether the CYPs are operating efficiently in elderly livers *in vivo*. It has been suggested that elderly livers do not supply enough oxygen to the CYPs *in vivo*, which is known as the 'oxygen limitation theory'. This, however, is rather academic, as the major limitations on drug clearance in the elderly are due to other more pressing physiological factors. There are significant changes in the liver itself, as it decreases in mass and its blood flow is reduced as we age. This occurs at the rate of around 0.5–1.5 per cent per year, so by the time we hit 60–70, we may have up to a 40 per cent decline in liver blood flow compared with a 30-year-old.

Other factors include gradual decline in renal function, increased fat deposits and reduction in gut blood flow, which affects absorption. This is most noticeable in drugs that have a high 'intrinsic clearance' (Chapter 1), in that their clearance is directly related to blood flow; propranolol is a good example, while phenytoin is a low intrinsic clearance drug and is less affected by age. The problem arises that the drug's bioavailability increases due to lack of first-pass clearance; this means that from a standard dose, blood levels can be considerably higher than would be expected in a 40-year-old. This can be a serious problem in drugs with a narrow therapeutic index, such as anti-arrhythmics. In addition, average doses of warfarin required to provide therapeutic anticoagulation in the elderly are less than half those required for younger people. The person's lifelong smoking and drinking habits also complicate this situation. Among the drugs known to be cleared more slowly in older people are antipsychotics, paracetamol, antidepressants, benzodiazepines, warfarin, beta-blockers and indomethicin.

Nearly 20 per cent of elderly people are believed to be clinically depressed and SSRIs are now the first-line treatment for this condition. It is recommended that the dosages for several of these drugs should be reduced in older patients (paroxetine and nefazodone), while fluoxetine is such a potent inhibitor of CYP2D6 and other CYPs, it is highly likely to interfere with the clearance of co-administered agents for a considerable time span, probably more than 10 days in the elderly. Obviously, the inhibitory effects of SSRIs on 2D6 and to a lesser extent on the 3A series suggest that extreme caution should be exercised when prescribing these drugs to the 'polypharmaceutical' elderly.

Neonates

Babies are classed as neonates when they are less than four weeks old, although in some reports, older babies are sometimes included as neonates. What research that has been done in neonates has revealed that CYP activities are less than half and perhaps as little as one-third of adult activity. This is reflected in the inability of neonates (full term and premature) to clear many drugs that rely on the major CYPs for their clearance. Often, drug half-lives can be up to 10 times longer than those of adults. There is even a marked difference between premature neonates and full-term babies; on average, the premature neonates clear drugs less than half as quickly as full-term neonates. This is a combination of poor renal clearance and poor CYP oxidative performance. Predominantly renally cleared drugs such as cimetidine, vancomycin and ampicillin are cleared at less than one-third the rate of adults.

This is partly a function of immaturity of kidney function and may also be related to fluid intake that can be variable if the babies are not parentally fed. Interestingly, there is little difference between renal drug clearance of premature and full-term neonates.

Oxidative metabolism in neonates

Regarding CYP-mediated oxidative drug clearance, foetal liver contains a number of unique CYP enzymes, such as 3A7; however, this CYP clears 'standard' 3A4 substrates such as carbamazepine much more slowly than mature 3A4 and it is likely that foetal CYP enzymes are sufficient for the clearance of endogenous substances such as steroids but are not really capable of clearing many xenobiotics. Premature neonates clear CYP1A2 (caffeine) 3A (midazolam, nifedipine) substrates less than half as efficiently as full-term babies. Caffeine is cleared about nine times less quickly in premature neonates than adults. However, the difference between adult and neonate drug clearance virtually disappears by 2–6 months in age. In the first few months of life CYP activities increase at an extremely rapid rate, to the point that drug clearance can be quicker in toddlers than adults, as children have the matured CYPs and renal sufficiency as well as higher hepatic blood flow. The use of midazolam in the sedation of neonates in intensive care units illustrates the difficulties in balancing dose and effect. Although this drug is preferred as its half-life is short and so can provide brief periods of sedation, doses used are often too high, leading to excessive sedation. There is wide variability between neonates of similar ages in the clearance of the drug – indeed half-life determinations vary from 5 to more than 12 hours. Doses used for neonates must be considerably lower than those used for older babies.

Conjugative metabolism in neonates

It has long been known that with glucuronidation, neonates and term babies have less than adequate activity in their UGT expression systems. This is clear in the relatively high incidence of jaundice in newborns, which is due to immaturity of UGT-mediated bilirubin clearance. Indeed, in babies who are not jaundiced, their low UGT capability can be revealed by drug administration; in the 1950s, the use of chloramphenicol for infections in babies led to 'grey baby syndrome' where the drug was cleared to a hydroxylamine (probably by 2C9) which would be glucuronidated in adults, but in children the poor UGT capability led to the metabolite escaping the liver and causing methaemoglobin formation. Chloral hydrate used to be used as a sedative in neonates; however, it is cleared to trichloroethanol, which is not only poorly glucuronidated by neonates but also competes with bilirubin for this pathway and jaundice can be exacerbated.

Premature neonates' ability to clear drugs that are almost entirely glucuronidated (lorazepam, morphine, AZT) is more than fourfold slower than that of adults. In general, glucuronidation systems mature more slowly than other Phase I and II systems according to current knowledge. In studies in human foetuses at 20 weeks' gestation, there was no evidence of any expression of UGTs. At 6 months, UGT1A1, 3, 4, 6 and 9, as well as 2B4, 7, 10 and 15 were expressed, although activities were much lower than adults. Indeed, in children around toddling age (1–2 years), their clearance of ibuprofen, amitryptiline and oestrone was more than tenfold lower than that of adults. This is particularly significant for the use of morphine in neonates and young children as this agent is cleared by glucuronidation. With paracetamol, clearance in neonates and babies is just over half that of older children. Although the drug is cleared mostly by glucuronidation in adults, in neonates it is eliminated mostly as a sulphate. Interestingly, paracetamol is not as toxic to neonates and children as it is to adults, mainly because their CYP2E1 is of lower activity and only very low levels of the hepatotoxic quinoneimines are formed. Those that do appear are detoxified by the glutathione system, which is more active in neonates than adults. Some reports have gone as far as to suggest that neonatal paracetamol overdose is virtually harmless.

Overall, drug clearance in premature neonates can be 10 times less than adults and they possess little ability to glucuronidate drugs. Term neonates also have immature Phase I and II systems, but by 2–3 years old the system is virtually adult, as CYP systems and Phase II systems are more or less mature.

7.4   Effects of diet on drug metabolism

The old saying 'you are what you eat' still has resonance and diet can influence the clearance of drugs. Some of the possible diets that are available in Western countries can be more toxic than many drugs; in 2004, a man in the US decided to eat only super-size portions from a well-known purveyor of fast food. After three weeks or so of this, his doctor instructed him that if he did not stop he would die imminently. Food contains a vast array of chemicals, such as antioxidants, plant toxins, preservatives, polyphenols, polycyclic aromatics and various other environmental pollutants. It is clear from the preceding chapters that the profile of our Phase I and II systems has been designed to respond to the pattern of our xenobiotic intake and since most of our dietary habits vary relatively little over our lives, our metabolizing systems adapt to the xenobiotic stimuli in our food intake also. Many of the compounds absorbed from our diet are as potent as drugs in terms of induction or inhibition of CYPs.

Polyphenols

Thousands of polyphenols are found in plants, vegetables, fruit, as well as tea, coffee, wine and fruit juices. These molecules have specific uses in the plants, either as antioxidants to extend the 'shelf-life' of fruit on the plant to maximize the attraction to insects and birds to spread seeds, or as toxins to ensure a hideous lingering death for any animal that has the nerve to eat the plant. These compounds are a broad classification and can include phenolic acids, stilbenes, flavonoids and lignans. Each subclass, such as the flavonoids, have a wide array of related agents (flavonols, isoflavones, etc.). The drastic effects of the polyphenols such as naringenin and bergamottin from grapefruit juice on CYP3A activity have already been discussed in Chapter 4. These agents can have profound effects on endogenous metabolizing systems. Flavonoids such as quercetin and fisetin are excellent substrates for COMT, so competitively inhibiting the metabolism of endogenous catecholamine and catechol oestrogens. Quercetin and other polyphenols are found in various foods such as soy (genestein) and they are potent inhibitors of SULT1A1 which sulphate endogenous oestrogens, so potentiating the effects of oestrogens in the body. Many of these flavonoids and isoflavonoids are manufactured and sold as cancer preventative agents; however, it is more likely that their elevation of oestrogen levels may have the opposite effect.

It is also likely that various polyphenols influence other endogenous substrates of sulphotransferases, such as thyroid hormones and various catecholamines. It is gradually becoming apparent that polyphenols can induce UGTs, indeed; it would be surprising if they did not. Certainly drug-efflux transporters are modulated by polyphenolic isoflavones. This effect has been seen with P-glycoprotein and MRP1–3. The flavonoid chrysin, found in honey, is a potent inducer of UGT1A1. Overall, it is likely that there are a large number of polyphenols that are potent modulators of CYPs and Phase II enzymes.

Barbecued meat

In the UK, the weather effectively prevents the excessive consumption of so-called charbroiled, or barbecued meat. However, many fast-food outlets claim that their burgers are 'flame-broiled', so it is possible through some modest effort to maintain a high consumption of barbecued meat in the UK. However, this exposes the consumer to a combination of polycyclic aromatics, nitrosoamines and hetercyclic aromatic amines which all induce CYP1A2 and CYP1A1. If consumption is heavy enough, the clearance of drugs such as amitryptiline, clozapine, fluvoxamine, mexiletine, haloperidol, naproxen, olanzapine and paracetamol will be increased significantly. GSTs and UGTs can also be induced, so that the carcinogenic effects of the induction of these CYPs can be offset to some extent. An even more effective way to offset the effects of induction is to consume considerable amounts of vegetables with cooked meats. These contain a variety of inhibitors of these CYPs, so reducing the risk of activating the polycyclics and ameliorating the inducing effect on any prescription drugs that might be washed down with the barbecue.

Cruciferous vegetables (sprouts, cabbage, broccoli, cauliflower)

It is often quoted in lectures in drug metabolism that Brussels sprouts are potent modulators of drug-metabolizing enzymes. It is clear that sprouts and other cruciferous vegetables are a less than popular choice in student cuisine. Indeed, a former US President (George H.W. Bush) was once heard to refuse to eat broccoli. However, this type of vegetable can be highly beneficial; it contains polyphenols, glucosinolates and isothiocyanates; one of which (sulfuraphane) has therapeutic promise. These compounds markedly induce glutathione S-transferases (GSTs) in the gut and liver, particularly GST Alpha. To get the effects, it takes around 1–2 weeks and you have to eat around 200–300 g/day. These vegetables also induce CYP1A2, but you need to eat about 500 g/day to get that effect. It appears unlikely that many would consume nearly 0.5 kg of cruciferous vegetables per day, but it is technically possible. Drugs cleared by 1A2 include clozepine, caffeine and theophylline. If an individual does consume a high quantity of cruciferous vegetables on a daily basis, then they are likely to show significant accelerated clearance of these drugs.

As with CYP induction, the response time for GST induction is fairly rapid and if the vegetables are removed from the diet, the effect disappears equally quickly. This illustrates the problem of deciding whether these effects are actually beneficial. Most authorities recommend cruciferous vegetables as they increase detoxification enzymes such as the GSTs in many tissues and can reduce the risks of various gut cancers. However, CYP1A2 is highly effective in activating aromatic amines to carcinogens. However, this should not be a problem, as GSTs are highly efficient at detoxifying reactive species such as hydroxylamines. It is likely that a balanced diet where these vegetables are a relatively modest component (around 200 g/day) is likely to lead to beneficial increases in GSTs while minimizing the CYP induction effect. Certainly the smell of boiled cauliflower in your house could well erode your popularity amongst your friends. In addition, the prospect of consuming these vegetables may seem less than appealing, but it is significantly better than dying of cancer. It is worth remembering that if you put enough cheese (particularly stilton) on them, you can hardly taste them at all.

Other vegetable effects on metabolism

If you think sprouts taste bad, try watercress. However, the taste 'grows' on you, and it contains phenethyl isothiocyanate; this compound blocks CYP1A2 and 2E1, and inhibits the activation of a number of tobacco-related carcinogens, so again, eat it quickly and live longer. Glucobrassicin, found in sprouts, also inhibits these isoforms. Some studies have been carried out with raw garlic. It would be expected that consumption of sulphides related to garlic and onions would affect CYP2E1 or 1A2, however it had no visible effect, although N-acetyl transferase was stimulated. Consumption of vegetables leads to an alkaline, rather than acid, urine and this is beneficial in maintaining the stability of a number of Phase II metabolites of aromatic amines and preventing their degradation to the parent metabolite in the bladder, an organ not exactly renowned for its detoxification capability.

Diet – general effects

It is clear that diet can substantially modulate Phase I and II metabolism – the consumption of high levels of cooked meat induces CYPs 1A1/2, but prior established consumption of cruciferous vegetables and watercress, for example, can negate the carcinogenic effects of the cooked meats. This is why in the Mediterranean, the local diet is sufficiently rich in stimulators of Phase II detoxification and inhibitors of Phase I oxidation, that it is possible to eat what you like, drink everything in sight and smoke pounds of shockingly pungent tobacco and live to be 116 years old. As to the effects on prescription drugs, this is more difficult to measure reliably, although abrupt changes in a person's diet may significantly alter the clearance of drugs and lead to loss of efficacy or toxicity.

7.5 Gender effects

For many years, there was a very large scientific literature on the sex differences between rats and other animals in their clearance of drugs. In humans, this was less well investigated, however a number of differences have been found. In hindsight, it should be glaringly obvious that the highly sophisticated control system for menstrual steroid metabolism, one of the *raisons d'etre* of Phases I–III, should indicate that women are likely to clear drugs differently from men and that drugs which modulate Phases I–III are more likely to lead to adverse effects on female metabolism than male.

In general, experimental or 'probe' drugs such as antipyrine, which are used to study the activities of a number of CYPs, are metabolized more quickly by women than men. This is allowing for differences in weight, fat distribution (body mass index), volume of distribution, but not necessarily mood. This effect was most pronounced at the time of ovulation and the luteal phase of menstruation. So pre-menopausal women clear CYPs 1A2, 3A4 and 2C9/19 substrates (theophylline, prednisolone and anticonvulsants) more quickly than men. There are some contradictions, such as with CYP1A2, where women demethylate caffeine more slowly than men. Most 3A4 substrates such as erythromycin are cleared more rapidly in women than men.

It appears that CYP expression is controlled by growth hormone (GH) and about the same amount is secreted over 24 hours in both sexes. In animals the pattern of release of the hormone is crucial to the effects on the CYPs; in females, GH is secreted in small but more or less continuous pulses, while males secrete large pulses, then periods of no secretion. The system is thought to be the same in humans.

In female epileptics, phenytoin metabolism is significantly accelerated just before the beginning of their period. This can cause the drug levels to fall out of the therapeutic window. The effect can be so pronounced that carbamazepine must be used instead. Anticonvulsant metabolism can be accelerated in pregnancy also. This suggests that some CYPs (2C9/19) could be more sensitive to female sex-hormone cycles than others (3A4), although this could be a reflection of the much greater expression of 3A4 compared with other CYPs. Little is known of the effects of the menopause and hormone replacement, where steroid metabolism changes dramatically. It is highly likely that these events could have profound effects on female drug clearance.

It is also apparent that females in general are more susceptible to drug adverse reactions than males. This may be a reflection of their increased formation of reactive or toxic metabolites, although there are also pharmacodynamic differences in drug sensitivity. Women are much more likely to develop torsades des points, or dangerous lengthening of the QT interval (section 5.5). This is because endogenous oestrogens lengthen the interval anyway and it does not take a great deal of a QT-lengthening drug to cause a severe and rapid effect in women; indeed, many more females died from terfenadine-induced torsades des pointes than males, before the drug was withdrawn from OTC status.

7.6 Smoking

Smoking tobacco still has a very strong hold on humanity, although its use is declining in Western countries. Not surprisingly, the tobacco manufacturers have exploited the general aspirational tendencies of Third World economies to market smoking as highly attractive and this has resulted in expanding tobacco consumption worldwide. As far back as the 1860s, it has been known that cigarettes are toxic (there is a tirade against the dangers of cigarettes in Dostoevsky's *Crime and Punishment*), so it is frankly bizarre for anyone today to be unaware of tobacco's toxicity. Although incomprehensible to non-smokers, it has been said to be easier to give up heroin than cigarettes. Tobacco smoke contains around 4000 chemicals, of which around 45–50 are carcinogens. Practically the only compounds proven to be human bladder carcinogens, beta naphthylamine and 4-aminobiphenyl, are present in tobacco smoke. Most of the aromatic hydrocarbon carcinogens induce CYP1A1 and 1A2 as well as GSTs Mu and Alpha. CYP1A1 contributes little to the clearance of drugs as it is extrahepatic and is subject to polymorphisms, so it is not inducible in all Caucasians. CYP1A2 is inducible to a high extent in about 45 per cent of Caucasians and this metabolizes a considerable number of drugs that are cleared more quickly in smokers compared with non-smokers. Clearance of caffeine is about 1.6 times faster in the smokers. CYP2E1 is inducible by a number of small heterocyclic carcinogens found in tobacco smoke and is likely to be induced in smokers. However, since smokers who do not drink coffee are unusual, it is difficult to prove this beyond doubt in humans. Interestingly, nicotine is metabolized by CYP2A6, and in individuals with polymorphisms for this CYP (20 per cent of Asians), it is said that they can give up smoking easily and do not smoke so much, presumably because they cannot clear nicotine easily to cotinine and the nicotine effects are pronounced, although these studies are controversial. Apparently, using tranylcypromine or methoxsalen to block this CYP can facilitate giving up tobacco.

7.7 Effects of ethanol on drug metabolism

Around 10 per cent of men in the UK regularly exceed the healthy limits of alcohol intake and probably half of those are fully dependent on alcohol. Increasing proportions of women are also becoming dependent on high alcohol intake. More than half of all violent crime and a similar proportion of fatal road accidents are linked to alcohol. The vast majority of the population drinks regularly and the alcohol industry is exceedingly keen to bring to our attention more imaginative ways to consume it, although less effort has gone into an effective hangover cure. Since alcohol use is all-pervading in most societies, whether it is legal or not, it is important to consider its effects on real-world prescription drug usage.

The question to whether alcohol intake can affect the clearance and efficacy of prescribed drugs does rather depend on patient honesty – the difference between what a patient tells a doctor he drinks and what he actually consumes can be considerable. The range of alcohol consumption is correspondingly wide, from a couple of glasses of beer per week, to bottles of spirits per day. Since drinking habits are built up gradually, many patients are genuinely unaware that they are exceeding the limit for what is generally considered healthy, i.e. approximately two spirit measures worth per day. Around 10 spirit measures per day, or 5 pints of reasonable strength beer, is bordering on dependence.

Ethanol is an inducer of CYP2E1 and the degree of induction will be dependent on the patient's usual consumption. The main route of metabolism of alcohol is hepatic alcohol dehydrogenase (ADH), although the enzyme is found in the stomach and other organs. ADH oxidizes ethanol to acetaldehyde that is normally converted by aldehyde dehydrogenase (ALDH) to acetic acid and water. Acetaldehyde is extremely toxic and if ALDH is inactivated for any reason, acetaldehyde causes a severe flushing/vomiting/sweating and nausea effect. This is why patients are told not to drink when they take metronidazole, isoniazid, sulphonyl ureas and several antibiotics, as they inhibit ALDH and cause acetaldehyde toxicity. Antabuse, or disulfiram, is intended to block ALDH, so causing acetaldehyde toxicity to help alcoholics stop drinking (Chapter 5).

ADH has no bearing on drug clearances, although CYP2E1 is responsible for the clearance of a number of anaesthetics, paracetamol, isoniazid and chlorzoxazone. In non-drinkers, in the absence of alcohol, or in occasional drinkers, ADH metabolizes the vast majority of ethanol and only a small fraction is cleared by CYP2E1. Consequently, their clearance of 2E1 substrates is not likely to be affected by their alcohol intake. When alcohol is consumed in considerable quantities (a good night, but not a total 'skinful'), then CYP2E1 substrates will have to compete with the ethanol for the enzyme, their half-lives will be lengthened and their CNS effects pronounced. This effect will be seen through the standard intoxicating effects of ethanol. So a single moderate drinking session will change the pharmacokinetics of prescribed 2E1 substrates. Moderate drinking can also reduce the first pass of tricyclic antidepressants but even small doses of ethanol can affect warfarin metabolism, reducing first pass and leading to excessive bleeding. Warfarin patients should not drink alcohol at all.

Alcohol and antibiotics

Patients usually believe that they should not drink when given antibiotics. This is only true for drugs that block ALDH, such as metronidazole, cefoperazone, cefamandole, griseofulvin, chloramphenicol, nitrofurantoin and sulphamethoxazole. Tuberculosis patients should definitely not drink when on isoniazid, as CYP2E1 converts this drug to several reactive species. Isoniazid (INH) is not that well tolerated in otherwise healthy individuals and it does cause high liver enzymes in heavy drinkers and can lead to severe liver damage in those cases. If the patient can stop drinking, then their CYP2E1 induction will fall and their problem with INH may diminish. Of course, many who contract tuberculosis in Western countries are at the margins of society and are highly likely to be very serious drinkers indeed. So they are more likely to sustain liver damage due to the INH/alcohol problem, which means they stop the INH, and the disease reignites, this time resistant to the drug.

Heavy alcohol usage and drug clearance

For those chronically dependent on alcohol their CYP2E1 levels can be tenfold higher than non-drinkers and they would clear 2E1 substrates extremely quickly if they chose to be sober for a period of time. This may lead to the accumulation of metabolites of the substrates. It is apparent that alcoholics that are sober can suffer paracetamol-induced liver toxicity at overdoses of around half that of non-drinkers. This is due to the induction of CYP2E1. However, it is less than likely that the overdose would be washed down by anything other than a heroic amount of ethanol, so in reality, the situation is complicated by the state of induction of the CYP and the strong competitive effect of the alcohol preventing the CYP-mediated formation of the hepatotoxic metabolite. It may be that as long as the alcoholic keeps drinking, they may well escape fatal liver injury from paracetamol overdose.

When alcoholics are 'maintenance' drinking, that is, enough alcohol to be able to feel 'normal', but not intoxicated, reduced clearance of CYP2E1 substrates will be seen, although when alcoholics drink to become intoxicated, they consume staggering amounts. This means that ethanol will fully occupy 2E1, so any other substrates will barely be cleared at all. As a result, toxicity could occur, that is, if the alcoholic notices. Certainly, warfarin metabolism is accelerated in alcoholics and higher doses must be given for the drug to show efficacy.

Ethanol – general hepatic effects

Social drinking is of little direct effect on hepatic metabolism, but in chronic heavy drinking, long-term disruption of the liver results. As you probably know, the liver is the toughest organ in the body biochemically. It is by far the best-protected organ in terms of detoxification systems, and very high 6–10 mM levels of GSH are maintained intracellularly. Consequently, it takes enormous quantities of ethanol to damage the liver beyond repair. An estimate of how much alcohol is needed to kill the liver is interesting: assuming the average alcoholic drinks heavily for 20 years prior to liver failure and drinks about a bottle and a half of spirits per day, this amounts to about 2000 litres of pure ethanol ranged against a 1.5 kg liver.

In chronic drinkers, the high activity of ADH results in an excess of NADH formation, which deranges fat metabolism and leads to 'fatty liver'. Glucuronidation can be disrupted, as the sustained high NADH levels affect UDP-glucuronic acid formation. Hepatic GSH maintenance is put under stress by the high demand for thiols to detoxify reactive species formed by acetaldehyde and gradually GSH maintenance is compromised. In the early stages of alcoholism, liver enzymes, such as serum ALT and AST, climb from three to ten times the normal limits. Chronic acetaldehyde toxicity leads to hepatocyte death and the simultaneous stimulation of collagen formation that leads to a scarring effect in the liver. During the scarring process, there is progressive replacement of hepatocytes with fibrotic connective tissue. This is cirrhosis, where nodules and lumps of this fibrous tissue appear all over the liver and disrupt its blood circulation and the removal of bile. Cirrhotic liver damage is permanent, but if the drinker can stop, what liver function is left is usually retained, unless it has been left too late. Although there are other causes of cirrhosis (hepatitis, drug therapy, genetic conditions), over 90 per cent of cases are sustained by alcohol consumption. Biochemically, the liver fights a losing battle as production of essential proteins gradually falls as the drinking progresses the disease and cholesterol, sugar and triglyceride metabolism is compromised.

Elsewhere, the gut is damaged by ethanol intake to the point that it becomes excessively porous and even undigested food particles enter the blood, which are recognized by the immune system. This leads to virtually permanent gut inflammation and variable drug absorption.

Women are much more vulnerable to ethanol damage and on average die in half the time it generally takes for a male alcoholic to drink himself to death. Ethanol distributes in total body water only, so in women their greater fat content means that blood ethanol levels are higher than men of similar weight and age. In addition, their stomach ADH is less effective than men's, which also promotes the entry of more ethanol into the blood, although the role of stomach ADH in ethanol clearance is disputed.

As cirrhosis progresses, hepatic back pressure becomes so high that the blood from the portal vein has difficulty in entering the liver to the point that blood starts to leave the liver and run back down the portal vein. This causes swollen varices, or varicose veins in the oesophagus and stomach. Fluid is forced out into the tissues, causing abdominal ascites. By the time the alcoholic sustains this level of damage, there is no way back and death usually results. Alcoholics in end-stage liver failure have particularly poor outcomes in hospital intensive care units, especially in hepatorenal syndrome, where kidney failure occurs as a result of the liver disease. Approaching end-stage liver failure, serum ALT and ASP levels are in the thousands and bilirubin appears in the blood in quantity leading to severe jaundice. Once the liver packs up, the only therapy is a new liver, provided the alcoholic has been 'dry' for six months or more, or is exceedingly rich and famous.

Effects of cirrhosis on drug clearance

High extraction drugs

The main effects of cirrhosis on the liver include the reduction in blood flow (indeed, the total derangement of the portal system) and the loss of functional hepatocytes. So in high extraction drugs, where blood flow is the major determinant of clearance, clearance of these agents will be severely compromised. The clearance of beta-blockers (propranolol, metroprolol, labetalol), as well as pentazocine, lignocaine and opiates such as pethidine and morphine can fall by between 30 and 50 per cent. The key issue here is that this results in major increases in bioavailability after an oral dose, which in turn means plasma concentrations increase by two- to sevenfold, or in the case of chlormethiazole, 17-fold. So for alcoholics, it is recommended to reduce oral dosing by five- to tenfold and *IV* dosing by around twofold.

Low extraction drugs

Clearances fall by more than 50 per cent in drugs such as naproxen and cefoparazone, but may fall by 70–90 per cent in theophylline and sulindac, whilst paracetamol clearance falls by around 20 per cent. Again, plasma levels may double or quadruple. Protein binding is much less in cirrhotics due to the failure of the liver to make enough albumin and the various fluid accumulations affect drug distribution. The net effect is to increase levels of unbound drug, which also contributes to the general two- to fourfold increase in drug plasma levels.

Overall, the extent of cirrhosis can be judged from general indices of hepatic health and usually the more severe the disease, the greater impact on drug clearance will occur. Mild cirrhosis generally does not significantly impact drug clearances. Interestingly, cirrhosis has less effect on some drugs that are cleared by Phase II processes only, such as lorazepam.

MARS

This innovation was developed at the end of the 1990s and it stands for molecular adsorbent recirculating system. This is an extracorporeal liver support system that works on a similar principle to renal dialysis. MARS uses a combination of albumin and activated charcoal to bind and remove drugs, hepatotoxins and accumulating metabolic waste (bilirubin and ammonia). The system is still under intensive experimental and clinical evaluation and it seems strange that nobody thought of it sooner. In a study in pigs, it was shown that the MARS system could remove midazolam and fentanyl. In humans, the system was shown to be beneficial in renal problems caused by cirrhosis. This system will be useful in patients suffering from overdoses and is likely in the future to be valuable in modulating the concentrations of drugs such as anaesthetics, analgesics and antibiotics in patients awaiting liver transplants.

7.8 Effects of disease on drug metabolism

There are number of conditions and their treatments that influence CYP activities and expression. Interferon (IFN-2b) treatments for melanomas can selectively impair CYP metabolism, with CYP2E1 unaffected and 1A2 significantly inhibited. Some alcoholics have been shown to express auto-antibodies to CYP2E1 and to 3A4. Chronic hepatitis C and autoimmune hepatitis antibodies have been found against CYP2D6 and 2A6, as well as anti-UGT antibodies.

Over 2% of the US population have the antibodies to the Hepatitis C virus. This can result in chronic liver disease, such as cirrhosis or even liver cancer. It is usually, but not always, associated with a history of intravenous drug usage. Few studies have been carried out, but some evidence suggests that CYP expression (such as CYP3A4) declines as the disease progresses, although in liver cancer induced by hepatitis C, some CYP isoforms' expressions increase. This coupled with the previously described effects of cirrhosis indicate that hepatitis C patients may show reduced clearance of many of the major therapeutic drugs.

It has emerged that hepatitis B infection appears to suppress some hepatic detoxification processes, such as GSTs, and interfere with thiol metabolism. This appears to result in the increased susceptibility of hepatitis B sufferers to acute liver toxicity, as well as cancer. It is likely that in hepatitis B patients, the time 'window' where reactive species generated by Phase I metabolism of drugs and environmental toxins have the opportunity to bind irreversibly within cells before they can be detoxified may well be considerably longer in these patients, thus predisposing them to greater hepatotoxic risk compared with healthy patients.

7.9 Summary

Overall, there are a large number of factors that can influence drug metabolism, either by increasing clearance to cause drug failure, or by preventing clearance to lead to toxicity. In the real world, it is often impossible to delineate the different conflicting factors which result in net changes in drug

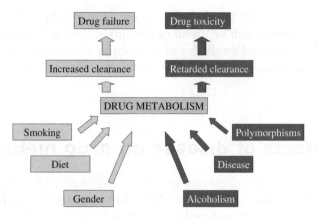

Figure 7.4 Generalized scheme of factors which influence drug metabolism, leading to changes in clearance, which are responsible for extremes of drug response

clearance which cause a drug to fall out of, or climb above, the therapeutic window. It may only be possible clinically in many cases to try to change what appears to be the major cause to bring about a resolution of the situation to restore curative and non-toxic drug levels. Figure 7.4 tries to form a summary picture of the major influences on drug clearance.

8 Role of Metabolism in Drug Toxicity

8.1 Adverse drug reactions: definitions

It is important to see the role of metabolism in drug toxicity as a component of the bigger picture of all adverse reactions suffered by patients during drug therapy. One view of this picture is on Figure 8.1. Different authors and textbooks classify these effects in various ways, but a convenient way to look things can be to resolve all drug adverse effects as either reversible (Type A) or irreversible (Type B). At this point, it is worthwhile being more precise over the terminology of drug adverse reactions. The term 'toxicity' is a loose one and it has been used flexibly in this book so far. However it is useful in looking at drug-metabolism-mediated effects to define toxicity more accurately for the cell in particular:

Irreversible change in structure leads to irreversible change in function.

The key here is 'irreversible'; it follows that a process that is not irreversible is not actually 'toxicity' in the strict sense of the word. There is not really a precise term for reversible systemic disruption to homeostasis, but perhaps the phase 'adverse effects' is useful for describing a Type A patient adverse reaction that is reversible, but not exactly toxicity. There are, of course exceptions: this strict definition of toxicity is fine for the cell, but is not so clear for the relationship between the patient, their organs, tissues and individual cells. Obviously, the effects of an anti-cancer alkylating agent are irreversible and toxic to a cell, but could ultimately save the life of the patient. Conversely, a heroin overdose reversibly inhibits central control of respiration, but this leads to death, which is about as irreversible as it gets. In general though, it is probably fair to say that cumulative irreversible damage at the cellular level usually leads to patient morbidity and mortality.

Human Drug Metabolism, Michael D. Coleman
© 2005 John Wiley & Sons, Ltd

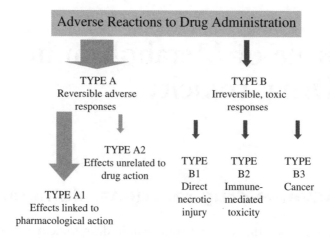

Figure 8.1   Summary of reversible (Type A) and irreversible (Type B) drug effects

8.2   Reversible drug adverse effects: Type A

Type A are the vast majority of adverse effects (Figure 8.1) and are experienced by patients in direct proportionality to the quantity of the drug and/or its metabolites in their tissues. These effects are sometimes described as 'toxic' but these are not usually irreversible effects. They can be resolved into two main causes, as follows.

Intensification of pharmacologic effect: Type A1

This is proportional to drug concentration and happens if drug levels climb above the therapeutic window. Anticonvulsants are membrane stabilizers, so at high concentrations they cause sedation and confusion. Similarly, high concentrations of anticoagulants cause excessively long clotting times. Some drugs may display a series of known pharmacodynamic effects at therapeutic window levels, but exert other unwelcome effects at high concentrations. Some beta-blockers at higher doses cause central effects such as nightmares. When drug levels fall, the excessive pharmacodynamic effects subside also. These adverse effects, also known generally as 'side effects', are mostly an intensification of the 'main effects', and are thought to be the cause of more than 80 per cent of patient problems with drug therapy. Many patients will experience an unpleasant concentration-dependent drug effect at some point in their lives. As we have seen in earlier chapters, drug metabolism-related changes in clearance caused by induction or inhibition of Phase I–III systems can have profound and occasionally lethal effects on the patient. Other reasons for the intensification of drug effects include renal problems, over-dosage, and problems with dosage calculations, or being too old, too young or too sick.

Reversible adverse effects – methaemoglobin formation – Type A2

During the metabolism of any given drug, it is possible that at least one or other of the metabolites may disrupt cellular function in a way that is un-related to the pharmacological effects of the drug, but the disruption is reversible and predictable. This situation is again dose related, in that the more drug is absorbed, the more is cleared though the pathway which forms a 'problem' metabolite. This type of adverse effect, though reversible, has the potential to make a drug almost intolerable to take from the patient's view-point and can even be lethal. A good example of a reversible adverse effect is methaemoglobin formation, where the appearance of the patient's blood becomes a passable impression of chocolate milk.

To see the link between a product of drug metabolism and an adverse drug effect, it is first necessary to understand the endogenous system involved. Haemoglobin is a molecule that becomes reversibly oxygenated, rather than irreversibly oxidized. Our continued existence depends on the difference between those two terms. Haemoglobin, as you know, is oxygenated to trans-port the gas from lung to tissues and release it where required. It is a tetramer, which means it has four protein subunits, each of which contains an iron molecule as Fe^{2+}. The iron molecules bind the four oxygen molecules. The oxygen binding is dependent, like many enzymes, on the ability of the metal to gain and lose electrons, rather like charging and recharging a battery as mention previously. It is clear that a molecule like haemoglobin is potentially reactive and is going to need protection from oxidation so it can continue to function, so the erythrocyte is designed to maintain haemoglobin so that it carries oxygen and is not damaged or changed in structure. It accomplishes this with the second highest level of GSH in the body after the liver and a series of protective enzymes, more of which later. Normally, the haemoglo-bin iron molecules (Fe^{2+}) bind the O_2 and form superoxoferrihaem complexes ($Fe^{3+} O_2^-$). These dissociate at the tissues and 99 times out of 100, the Fe^{2+} is restored and O_2 is delivered to the tissue. The one time out of 100, the oxygen retains the electron and becomes superoxide (O_2^-) and the Fe^{2+} becomes Fe^{3+}. This is very bad, as Fe^{3+} will bind anything but oxygen, such as anions. So the Fe^{3+} means that this haemoglobin monomer is now methaemoglobin and useless for oxygen carriage. Since this is a natural consequence of transport-ing a reactive gas with a reactive protein, the erythrocyte carries two systems for reducing the oxidized Fe^{3+} to Fe^{2+}, so restoring the function of haemo-globin. The systems are NADH diaphorase and NADPH diaphorase. The

NADH diaphorase operates for 95 per cent of the time, as the NADPH system is incomplete and requires an artificial electron acceptor for full operation. Why this is the case is unknown. If it were not for NADH diaphorase, methaemoglobin formation would be around 4–6 per cent per day, more if you smoke. If you measured your methaemoglobin levels now, they would be less than 1 per cent, so the system is adequate to maintain haemoglobin in normal circumstances.

It is possible for some xenobiotics to react with haemoglobin to form methaemoglobin. Nitrites are moderately efficient at this process, but the aromatic hydroxylamines are particularly effective in forming methaemoglobin. They oxidize haemoglobin to methaemoglobin in two stages. Initially, the hydroxylamine directly reacts with oxyhaemoglobin to form methaemoglobin. This is known as a co-oxidation, as the hydroxylamine will be oxidized to a nitrosoarene. This alone would not account for the speed at which methaemoglobin can form in patients with high levels of hydroxylamine metabolites in their blood (Figure 8.2). The nitrosoarene formed by the initial reaction is then 'helpfully' reduced to the hydroxylamine by GSH, so allowing the hydroxylamine to oxidize another oxyhaemoglobin molecule. The resultant nitrosoarene can then be re-reduced to the hydroxylamine and oxidize another oxyhaemoglobin and so on.

The initial oxidation is thus amplified by GSH and the presence of millimolar levels of GSH is like pouring fuel on a fire. Each hydroxylamine molecule can oxidize at least four oxyhaemoglobin molecules. The result is a very rapid process, where as soon as the metabolite is produced, methaemoglobin starts forming in significant quantity, in direct proportion to the level of the metabolite released by the liver, which is of course in proportion to the drug dose.

Clinical consequences of methaemoglobin

Methaemoglobin is measured as a percentage of haemoglobin. However, even modest levels exert a potent effect, due to the Darling–Roughton effect. You recall that haemoglobin is a tetramer and binds four oxygen molecules as oxyhaemoglobin. If an Fe^{2+} of one of the monomers is oxidized to an Fe^{3+}, then the remaining oxygen molecules are much more tightly bound and it is harder for them to escape and oxygenate tissues. If two monomers are oxidized then it is even harder for the oxygens to be released. This means that a small percentage of methaemoglobin, say 5–10 per cent, has a greater effect than just removing 5–10 per cent of haemoglobin. The effects on the patient of methaemoglobin formation are a reflection of increasing inability of their tissues to receive enough oxygen. So at low levels, 4–6 per cent, people of fair complexions may look slightly bluish and may have a mild headache. As levels increased to 10–15 per cent, this extends to headache, fatigue and

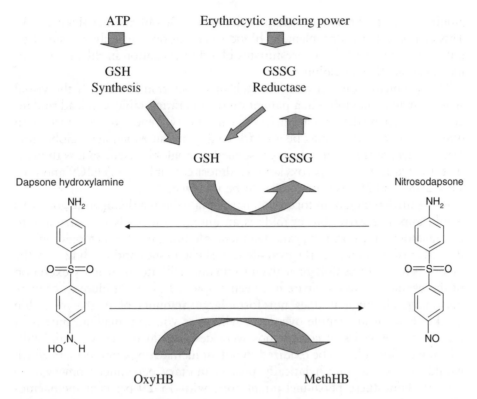

Figure 8.2 Basic process of methaemoglobin formation in the human erythrocyte. This is repeated many times per second in a futile cycle that is limited only by the levels of GSH in the erythrocyte

sometimes nausea. At levels of 20–30 per cent, hospitalization is usually required, with the intensification of the previous symptoms plus tachycardia and breathing problems. Higher levels (50 per cent plus) lead to stupor and loss of consciousness, with 70 per cent plus leading to death. Methaemoglobinaemia is a drug-dependent effect which may be either acute or chronic.

Acute methaemoglobinaemia

The most dangerous situation for methaemoglobin formation can be as a result of benzocaine usage in anaesthetized patients. The local anaesthetic is sprayed on the oropharynx prior to intubation, although not used much in the UK, it is still used in some countries. Many formulations of the drug are around 14–20 per cent and three 1-second bursts of the spray could deliver perhaps 600 mg of the drug. A number of reports have shown that methaemoglobin levels of 30 per cent or more can result in 30–40 minutes (Figure 8.3). This can be a serious problem, as blood oxygenation is usually measured by pulse oximeters and this overestimates blood oxygenation in the presence of increasing methaemoglobin.

This problem, coupled with the lack of recognition by staff of the visual signs of methaemoglobin in a patient on the operating table, can lead to dangerously high methaemoglobin levels without awareness of the staff. If in doubt, a CO oximeter must be used to reliably measure methaemoglobin formation. Benzocaine is unable to cause methaemoglobin itself, so it is thought that it is oxidized to a hydroxylamine, almost certainly by CYP2C9 and possibly 2C8. CYP2E1 is thought not to be involved.

Acute methaemoglobin formation has actually been a therapeutic goal: this would appear bizarre, but cyanide is an anion, so it binds very strongly to methaemoglobin, forming cyanomethaemoglobin. The methaemoglobin has the effect of 'vacuuming' the cyanide out of the tissues and holding it in the blood, before a thiosulphate is given to finally facilitate the urinary excretion of the cyanide. Sodium nitrite has been employed as an antidote to cyanide poisoning, although it does not form large amounts of methaemoglobin quickly enough in cyanide overdoses where, as you can imagine, time is of the essence. A series of compounds were designed in the 1950s and 1960s which were intended to be oxidized to potent methaemoglobin formers which would be used to prophylatically protect military personnel from cyanide toxicity. How these personnel might cope with 15–20 per cent methaemoglobinaemia and maintain their offensive capabilities seems difficult to imagine. However, cyanides remain in many countries' 'weapons of mass destruction' armouries. These compounds included phenones, such as 4-aminopropiophenone, which is also oxidized to a hydroxylamine and acts in a similar way to any aromatic hydroxylamine.

Chronic methaemoglobin formation

It is unlikely a new drug with an aromatic amine group would be approved for clinical usage today, on the grounds of toxicity. Sulphonamides retain their therapeutic place in HIV patient maintenance and their hydroxylamine metabolites are cytotoxic, and immunotoxic; fortunately, they form negligible levels of methaemoglobin. The sulphone, dapsone, is still the mainstay of the treatment of leprosy, dermatitis herpetiformis and conditions where neutrophil migration into tissues leads to inflammatory damage. Despite efforts to develop non-methaemoglobin forming analogues of these drugs, the market is just not large enough to sustain the development of replacements. So patients are essentially stuck with dapsone and its dose-dependent methaemoglobin formation. Dapsone is usually given at 100 mg/day for leprosy and anything from 25 mg/week to 400 plus mg/day for dermatitis

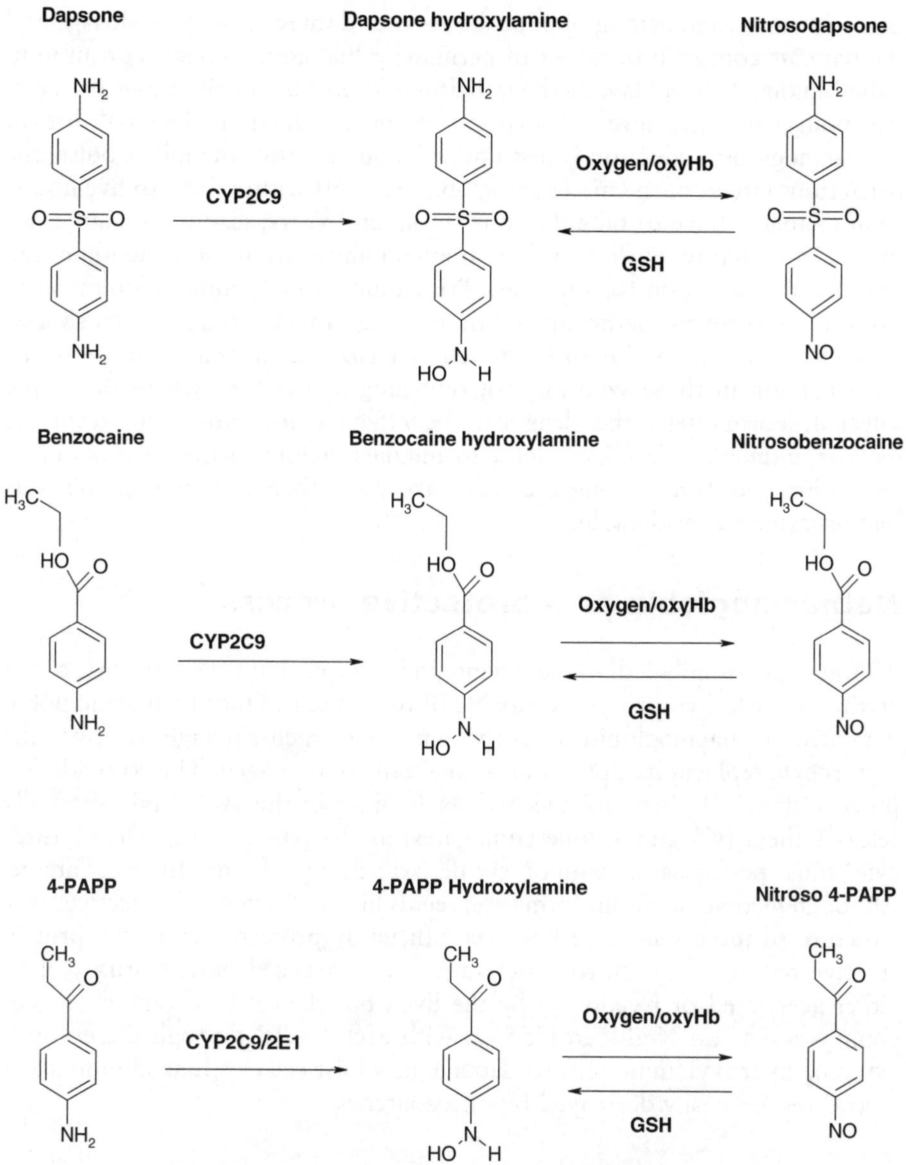

Figure 8.3 Production of various methaemoglobin-forming species from dapsone, benzocaine and 4-aminopropiophenone (4-PAPP). In each case, the hydroxylamine is formed from the parent compound by CYP-mediated oxidation and the presence of oxygen and/or oxyhaemoglobin (oxyHb) converts the agents to nitrosoarenes, whilst erythrocytic GSH re-reduces them to their hydroxylamines within the co-oxidation cycle

herpetiformis. Methaemoglobin peaks at around three hours post-dosage and the patients complain of a sort of permanent 'hangover' effect. For an individual taking 100 mg/day, methaemoglobin levels may peak at 5–8 per cent, depending on their level of hydroxylamine production. The half-life of methaemoglobin reduction is just under 1 hour, so after the initial pulse, the deleterious effects of the methaemoglobin wear off within three to five hours. Many patients have to take dapsone for several years, leading to significant impact on quality of life, although co-administration of cimetidine can improve this situation (section 5.6). Primaquine, the 8-aminoquinoline anti-malarial, also forms methaemoglobin, although this is used in much shorter courses for the elimination of *Plasmodium Vivax, Malariae* and *Ovale* (recurrent) malaria in those who are not returning to the area where they were infected. Fortunately, the drug can be effective in eliminating recurring malaria from a single 45 mg dose, so methaemoglobin formation is only a temporary problem. If longer courses are used, then methaemoglobin formation can be considerable.

Methaemoglobin as a protective process

Although potentially lethal, methaemoglobin formation is not toxicity, as the erythrocyte has two processes capable of reversing it. Once methaemoglobin is reduced to haemoglobin, it can resume its oxygen carriage function, the erythrocyte replaces its thiols and is physically undamaged. The co-oxidation process effectively 'ties up' the hydroxylamines in the cycle and eventually releases them (via glutathione conjugates) as the parent drug. The erythrocyte thus performs a temporary detoxification of the hydroxylamine. Although methaemoglobin formation seems like an 'own goal', effectively the structure of the erythrocyte has been efficiently protected from the protein reactive nature of the nitroso derivative. The released parent drug will be either acetylated or reoxidized by the liver, but then it has some chance of conjugation as an N-glucuronide, so with each 'cycle' through the erythrocyte, the hydroxylamine fails to damage it, whilst cells such as mononuclear leucocytes are easily destroyed by nitrosoarenes.

Glucose-phosphate dehydrogenase deficiency (G-6-PD)

In around 100 million people predominantly of Afro-Caribbean descent, the genetic polymorphism of G-6-PD is normally not an issue, except when the individuals are exposed to methaemoglobin forming drug metabolites. This enzyme supplies the majority of the reducing power of the erythrocyte and if it is poorly or non-functional, there is only sufficient reducing power available to supply GSH to protect erythrocytes from background levels of reactive species. As soon as the cells are exposed to high concentrations of hydroxylamines or primaquine metabolites, there is insufficient reducing power to tie up nitrosoarenes in the co-oxidation cycle and no detoxification occurs as little methaemoglobin formation happens. The nitrosoarene is then free to react with the structure of the erythrocyte. This causes the normal system of the erythrocytes' 'sell by date' to be prematurely activated (they usually last 120 days) and the spleen automatically removes them from the circulation. This can happen so quickly that anaemia can result in days, with associated hepatic problems with the processing of large amounts of now waste haemoglobin. G-6-PD patients that must take either dapsone or primaquine must only receive half or less than the recommended dosage of the drugs. G-6-PD effectively converts what would be a reversible drug effect into true toxicity.

8.3 Irreversible toxicity (Type B)

Although the vast majority of side effects that patients experience with drugs are related to (usually) reversible pharmacological effects, a much smaller proportion, perhaps less than 15 per cent of patient problems with drug therapy, are potentially much more dangerous, as they share several characteristics, as follows.

Type B1: necrotic reactions

- Fatal organ-directed toxicity can occur from a relatively modest overdose;

- Organ death can occur from the recommended dose;

- The organ/tissue affected is often not related to the pharmacological target of the drug;

- Onset may take days or weeks.

Type B2: immune reactions

- Reactions can be unexpected and unpredictable although they are most likely to occur within three months of initiating therapy;

- The organ/tissue affected is often not related to the pharmacological target of the drug;

- The effects can be severe, life-threatening and rapid in onset;

- The effects may lead to vulnerability to further injury on re-challenge.

Type B3: cancer

- Linked to antineoplastic drugs;

- Irreversible changes in tissues where cell growth is continuous;

- Future neoplasms may occur in tissues unrelated to the original tumour.

Type B1 irreversible reactions are related to either acute or chronic drug over-dose. This may be deliberate or reflect abnormal sensitivity to the tendency of the drug to cause irreversible tissue binding. Type B2 irreversible reactions are linked to the immune system and are often known as idiosyncratic or idiopathic problems.

Reactive species generated from xenobiotics which originate in diet, or tobacco or atmospheric pollution are strongly linked with damage to DNA which can lead to the development of Type B3 reactions, or neoplasms. In drug therapy, the only agents likely to lead to malignancies in patients are alkylating anti-cancer agents, which in some cases can lead to the development of lymphomas after therapy has apparently been successful.

However, these reactions all have one thing in common, in that the drug or toxin has caused irreversible changes in tissue structure and function. Figure 8.4 summarizes the consequences of irreversible damage due to reactive species formation. This can lead to necrosis, from which follows tissue damage and eventually organ failure. Reactive species are also the conduit by which drug-related material becomes bound to cells in such a way as to elicit an immune response. This could be either disseminated (widespread) or organ directed.

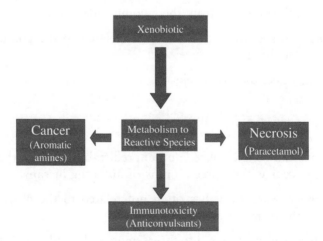

Figure 8.4 Main consequences of reactive species formation due to xenobiotic metabolism in different organs and tissues

How drugs can cause irreversible effects

It is important to understand the possible link between a drug and the potentially devastating effects in a patient of organ failure and toxic immune response. Normally, a drug functions by reversible interaction with a receptor system, which then modulates a specific function or group of functions. The key here is 'reversible'. If the drug is interacting reversibly, it cannot 'damage' a tissue, as it has not changed its structure, or its function irreversibly. Drugs usually exert their effects by reversible ionic interactions, the weakest of which are van der Waals' forces (could be likened to a child's toy magnet) or ionic bonds (like an electromagnet, strong but reversible).

For irreversible effects to ensue, the drug must somehow change cellular structure. The only way this can happen is if the drug reacts covalently with the cellular structures. A covalent bond could be likened to a piece of metal welded to another. For a covalent bond to form, the drug must have been made into a highly unstable and therefore chemically reactive species.

You might be aware that drug development costs hundreds of millions and takes around 8–10 years. This process ensures that there is no chance of a drug that is a highly unstable and reactive chemical getting through to the patient. Indeed, thousands of chemicals fail to reach the clinic, as they are too toxic or reactive.

So for drugs or toxins to cause irreversible effects, they must be chemically altered *in the patient* to form an unstable and reactive species. This reactive species then changes cell function irreversibly. Although cells in the activated immune system are capable of forming reactive species from some drugs through enzymes like myeloperoxidase, Phase I&II enzymes are more likely to form reactive species in sufficient quantity to damage tissues.

Role of biotransformation in causing drug reactivity

As you will have gathered, CYP enzymes can radically rearrange the structure of a molecule to make it more water-soluble and during this process molecular stability is usually reduced. Phase I metabolism can transform some molecules from innocuous agents to highly reactive species that are lethal to cells if formed in sufficient quantity. In general, the less stable a compound is, the more likely it is going to react with cellular structures.

The CYP enzymes function in a similar way that machine tools do, where, say, a robot welds a piece of bodywork onto a car. The metal is subject to an intense, concentrated assault in a specific area that is designed to form a product. You can imagine what would happen if a live grenade was subject to this treatment. That would be the end of the robot. Obviously the robot is pre-programmed to weld anything of the appropriate dimensions that it is presented with, even something that could destroy it. You might feel that this is an 'Achilles heel' in drug metabolism; however, 1 billion years of research and development has indicated that there is really no other way to metabolize otherwise stable chemicals and for the occasional reactive by-product, there are sufficient repair and protection systems (GSTs, GSH, etc.). The success of the Phase I–III system shows that the protective systems are effective in reducing the risk of organ damage to minimal levels.

On a molecular scale, some chemical structures that are subject to the rigours of CYP-mediated oxidation form reactive products because of unique inherent features of their structure. Examples include strained three-membered rings and epoxides. These structures are the chemical equivalent of the old explosive, nitroglycerine, which could be detonated by shock alone. Some reactive species, such as those mechanism-based inhibitors discussed in Chapter 5, can covalently bind to the active site and the enzyme is no longer functional. For biological function to continue, more enzyme must be synthesized. Drugs or chemicals that cause this effect are often termed suicide inhibitors and grapefruit juice and norfluoxetine cause this effect. The long period of inhibition of the CYPs that formed the metabolites reflects the time taken for more enzyme to be synthesized. These metabolites are so reactive that they are paradoxically no problem to the cell, as they just destroy the enzyme that formed them and cannot reach the rest of the cell. Indeed, after all the available CYP has been inactivated by these metabolites, no more metabolite will be formed until more CYP is synthesized (Chapter 5). The rest of the parent drug may well leave the cell by other pathways. At the other extreme are metabolites such as hydroxylamines, which are no immediate threat if they are stabilized by cellular thiols or antioxidants such as ascorbate. These metabolites are so stable they can travel through cells and leave the organ in which they were formed and enter the circulation. Erythrocytes can thus detoxify them as described previously. In certain conditions, they can spontaneously oxidize forming nitroso derivatives, which are tissue reactive and cytotoxic. Further metabolism is necessary before they can be detoxified. In between these extremes are metabolites that can react with any cell structures which are short of electrons and seek electron-rich structures. Potent electrophiles such as nitrenium ions (N^+) will react with nucleophiles, which are electron rich. If a CYP or any other enzyme forms a species that is missing electrons and seeks them, or is too electronegative, the net effect is a reactive species which has the potential to attack cellular proteins, DNA and membrane structures, forming covalent bonds, which can do sufficient damage to necessitate the resynthesis of that structure. It is important to consider also that reductive metabolism can form equally reactive species which are capable of causing similar cellular damage to oxidatively produced species. Whatever process forms reactive species, the likely result will be some form of irreversible binding to cellular macromolecules.

Cellular consequences of CYP-mediated covalent binding

The obvious question is how covalent binding is linked to cell damage and what are the processes that lead to cell damage. When a reactive species is formed in a cell, it can react with cellular organelles, enzymes, nuclear membranes, DNA, and the structure of the cell membrane. However, the hypothesis that a high rate of protein binding leads directly to cell death is an oversimplification. When animals have been treated with antioxidants prior to exposure to a reactive species, the animals survive, despite their levels of covalent protein binding, which are as high as untreated animals that have developed fatal organ toxicity. So the fate of the cell is subject to a competition between various factors:

- The rate, quantity and reactivity of the toxin formed;

- The extent of reactive 'secondary' toxins (superoxide, various free radicals) formed from the initial reactive species;

- The extent the cell can defend itself from the reactive toxin by rendering it harmless;

- The period of time which elapses before cellular defensive resources are overcome;

- Which specific molecules are damaged in the cell where irreversible damage occurs;

- Extent of possible repair and restoration;

- Whether the intra- and extracellular damage attracts the attention of the immune system.

These processes might lead to several cellular outcomes.

Sites of biotransformational-mediated injury

It is usually the case that although Phase I–III capability exists in all tissues to varying degrees, a specific xenobiotic will show biotransformationally mediated toxicity in a particular organ, tissue or group of tissues. These are often 'barrier tissues' that represent the front line against exposure to environmental toxins; these include the lung, the gut and the liver. These tissues are rich in Phase I–III enzyme systems and have at their disposal the full apparatus for the control and expression of these enzymes. Although these organs are well defended, reactive species generation can still cause irreversible damage, either locally or distant from the site of formation. This is partly due to the nature of our acute and chronic exposure to environmental and dietary xenobiotics that overtaxes the capability of our defences and partly due to our genetically differing capabilities to resist these toxins over our life-spans. The following sections give some examples of agents that can cause irreversible damage to a number of different cells, tissues and organs.

8.4 Type B1 necrotic reactions

General causes of necrosis

This process describes the effect where a cell sustains a great deal of damage to vital cell macromolecules in such a short time that it cannot either protect itself from the toxic species or repair its systems fast enough to keep pace with the damage. The fastest way for this to happen is if a toxin generates oxidant species such as superoxide, and all the species react with membrane lipids; this effect triggers a cascade effect where the lipids will generate their own radicals as they oxidize each other in a chain reaction. This process is like a 'forest-fire' effect on the membrane lipids and the structure of the membrane will eventually break down, causing cell contents to escape. This is like a 'blunt-force trauma' to the cell. Cell walls are thiol rich, but large quantities of a toxin will overwhelm the membrane's defences.

Alternatively, if mitochondria are gradually rendered non-functional, cell respiration ceases and there is insufficient ATP to support cell function and death results. Ultimately, the impact of a high concentration of toxin without protection and repair seems to be the equivalent of cutting as many cables as you can see in a running car engine. Eventually something vital is hit and the engine stops. Necrosis is typically a result of a high rate of toxic species formation, a particularly reactive species and damaged repair or defence mechanisms. After only a couple of hours or less in contact with the toxin the cell disintegrates. This releases toxic endogenous species, such as proteolytic enzymes into the interstitial fluid, which can damage other cells. If enough cells necrose, the organ or tissue becomes non-viable and failure results. Organ failure can mean the death of the organism. A good example of drug that has this effect in overdose, but not when taken at correct dosage, is paracetamol. The important feature of necrosis is that the cell is overtaken by events and cannot affect or change its fate.

Paracetamol

Although a number of compounds can cause liver necrosis and death in overdose, none of them are extremely cheap and available in virtually every retail outlet in the country. Every year in the UK, we get through around 1700 tonnes of paracetamol (acetaminophen in the US) in various formulations and approximately 70 000 people overdose on this drug. The drug still leads to around 300–500 deaths per year from liver failure in the UK. Paracetamol is the first choice for those who wish to use an overdose to end their lives, although paradoxically, as you can see from the figures above, they are highly unlikely to die from the experience. Less than 0.1 per cent of paracetamol overdoses result in death. It seems that intentional overdoses are less lethal than unintentional ones and children are less susceptible to fatal overdose than adults. The public are obviously aware that paracetamol can kill, hence the numbers taking it in overdose; however, despite more than 30 years of publicity, few are aware of the drawn-out and painful process that can lead to death with this drug. It is still used in suicide attempts because it works (if the patient does not find medical help) and it is freely available. It is possible that those who take overdoses feel that paracetamol is an ideal 'cry for help' drug, where there is time to reconsider. Indeed, paracetamol is, strangely enough, the 'safest' way to attempt suicide. The rescue therapy usually works, but if it fails there is always the fallback position of a new liver. However, it is worth considering that fewer than one-third of patients with hepatic failure fulfil the clinical criteria for a transplant. Even in the light of restricted paracetamol pack sizes, which have arguably made some impact in death rates, it remains incomprehensible to many health professionals that paracetamol is still available at all. Suicide is usually a result of the 'balance of the mind being disturbed', so it does not make sense to provide a readily usable method that can be obtained by the simple expedient to a trip to three or four convenience stores. It is interesting that a number of much more therapeutically valuable drugs have been withdrawn from the market after accounting for a fraction of the deaths attributable to paracetamol.

Mechanism of toxicity

In the kidney, paracetamol is metabolized (possibly by CYP2E1) in small amounts to 4-aminophenol, which is a nephrotoxin. In overdose, nephrotoxicity is much less pressing a problem than the effects in the liver. Around 95 per cent of paracetamol is cleared hepatically to an O-glucuronide and sulphate conjugates and about 2 per cent escapes unchanged (Figure 8.5). A small fraction, maybe between 1–3 per cent, is oxidized mainly by CYP2E1 (with a fraction cleared by 1A2 and 3A4) to the exhaustively investigated reactive species N-acetyl-*para*-benzoquinoneimine (NAPQI). Recent evidence suggests that CYP2D6 is also involved, which raises the question of the link between severity of liver toxicity and the polymorphic expression of this CYP

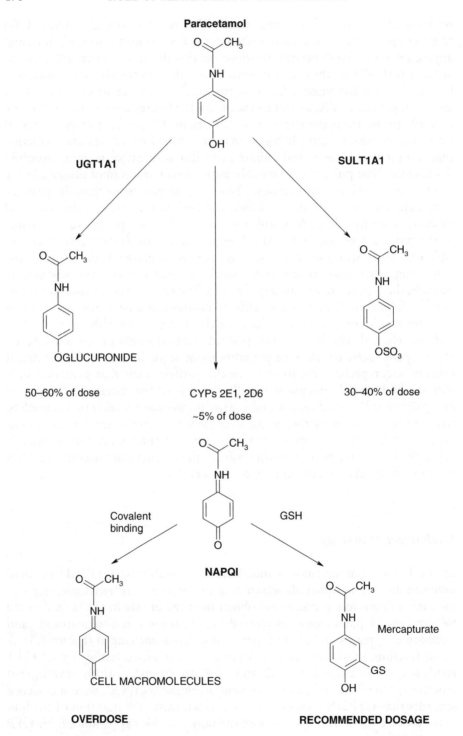

Figure 8.5 Main features of paracetamol metabolism. Aside from the toxic NAPQI (N-acetyl *p*-benzoquinoneimine), a 3-hydroxy derivative is cleared harmlessly by GSH to a catechol derivative. It is possible other reactive species are formed as well as NAPQI

(see Chapter 7). There are a number of other putative reactive species, such as dibenzoquinoneimines, but it is thought that NAPQI is the toxicologically important species. This compound is known to covalently bind to hepatocytes in various cellular areas, such as the cell wall. Normally, however, there is negligible binding as the NAPQI is efficiently conjugated to GSH. It was believed that GST Pi was responsible for catalysing this reaction, although it may be a combination of direct reaction with GSH and catalysis through other antioxidant enzymes. The net result is the excretion of NAPQI mercapturate in urine in small amounts. In its therapeutic dosage range, it must be stressed that paracetamol is harmless. The most a 70 kg adult can take a day without problem is about 4 g. For children, this is adjusted to 90–100 mg/kg in children, depending on which authority is cited. Most agree that no child should receive more than 4 g/day in total.

Overdose of paracetamol is considered to be around 7–8 g (100–115 mg/kg) in an adult and more than 150 mg/kg in children. In overdose, the same profile of paracetamol metabolism is maintained. The proportion of the dose cleared to NAPQI in overdose does not change much either, however the key here is that around 8–10 times as much NAPQI will be formed during overdose compared with a recommended dose. Obviously, the demand for GSH will be high to detoxify the reactive species, and you might recall from an earlier chapter that GSH is effectively 'thermostatically' controlled, in that if more is used, more will automatically be made to maintain organ concentrations at their normal preset level. Accelerated GSH consumption leads to an increase in the recycling of GSSG to GSH and the synthesis of more GSH from cysteine, glycine and glutamate. Up until 10–16 hours after the overdose, the GSH system responds to the increased load and GSH levels are maintained through recycling and resynthesis. The one component of GSH manufacture that is in limited supply in a hepatocyte is unfortunately the key one, the thiol-containing cysteine. More can be transported in and other sulphur-containing amino acids, such as methionine, converted to cysteine to meet the demand. Between 8 and 16 hours or so, GSH consumption by NAPQI gradually exceeds demand and cellular supplies of cysteine are exhausted. Since GSH is the cellular 'fire-extinguisher', this is the cellular equivalent of running out of foam in the face of a steadily encroaching fire. After 24 hours or so, there is nothing to prevent the NAPQI from binding to the hepatocytes and gradually killing them through necrosis. The key to the toxicity of NAPQI is which cellular macromolecules it binds. It is still not really clear (after 30 years of research) as to precisely which structures must be heavily bound before the cell necroses. Eventually, such numbers of hepatocytes are killed that the central area of the liver starts to die also. It is termed 'Acute centrilobular hepatic necrosis'. This translates clinically to a series of symptoms shown in Table 8.1.

Each of the three phases of paracetamol hepatotoxicity is reckoned to last around 24 hours. The first phase, up to 24 hours after the overdose, involves

Table 8.1 Time frame and clinical markers of paracetamol toxicity

Post-overdose Time (h)	Hepatic GSH (%)	Transaminases (units/litre)	Symptoms
6	100	Normal range	None
16–24	40–70	300–500	Anorexia, nausea/vomiting
24–48	10% or less	>1000–1500	Right upper quadrant pain, tenderness
48–72	Zero	>3000	Jaundice, bleeding, organ failure/death

nausea and vomiting and general reluctance to eat. Interestingly, some individuals do not show any symptoms at all during this time. Many do complain of a general 'sick' feeling and start to look very pale and 'washed out'. At this stage, the individual might be lulled into a false sense of security and might not think that he or she is in any real danger. In addition, many overdoses are accompanied by copious quantities of ethanol in various forms and the devastating hangover that ensues can effectively mask the hepatic paracetamol-induced symptoms. The second phase, 24–48 hours, involves the appearance of some physical pain in the area of the liver. Heart rate can rise significantly and blood pressure fall. At this point, the liver is sustaining serious cellular damage and liver enzymes such as ALT (alanine aminotransferase) and AST (aspartate aminotransferase) can be 30–50 times normal and this is an obvious sign of many disintegrating hepatocytes. In the third phase, the liver damage starts to become acute, although in less than 1 in 20 patients will this lead to organ failure. Symptoms of severe liver damage include jaundice, gut bleeding, general anticoagulation due to failure in clotting factor production and even encephalopathy. If organ failure does occur, then death follows within hours from cerebral oedema, renal failure and even blood poisoning.

Rescue therapy

Clearly the chances of survival depend on whether the patient undergoes treatment before too much liver damage occurs. If the individual does not seek medical help, then it is a matter of how much of the drug they consumed and their own liver's resistance to damage, as well as luck, as to whether they will survive. If the patient presents for treatment in less than an hour or so after the overdose, then it is likely to be worthwhile flushing out the stomach, as the entire drug dose will not be fully absorbed. If the patient appears within 3–4 hours of the overdose, then activated charcoal is sometimes given, which is controversial as to how effective it is and its effects on any subsequent anti-

dotes. Upon admission to hospital, a blood sample will be taken and paracetamol levels measured. Using a 'Rumack–Matthew nomogram', the amount
of hepatotoxicity that might occur is read off from the drug level. Hepatotoxicity is usually seen when paracetamol levels reach and exceed 2 mM. The
R–M nomogram is a product of data derived from hundreds of previous
patients, so it is fairly accurate in its prediction of liver damage, but not necessarily of liver failure. If the levels are above the upper line, then there is a
greater than 60 per cent chance of liver damage being sustained. Successive
blood samples track the elimination of the drug and as treatment progresses,
should show the patient gradually moving out of the hepatotoxicity 'danger
zone'. The nomogram tracking starts 4 hours after the overdose and ends
around 24 hours.

In any case, a confirmed overdose will be treated with N-acetyl cysteine,
which acts to supply cysteine to GSH synthesis, so that hepatic GSH levels
are maintained until all the paracetamol has been eliminated. This is not as
straightforward as it sounds, as orally, NAC tastes truly disgusting and the
smell can make patients vomit, so it can only be given as a 5 per cent solu-
tion in a fruit juice. The effects of NAC and the aftermath of a serious hangover from alcohol used to wash down the overdose must be exceedingly
miserable to the patient. If the patient vomits within one hour of NAC administration, then that one 'doesn't count' and must be repeated. The standard
treatment involves oral NAC every 4 hours for three days after the overdose.
As ever, it is imperative that the whole course is followed, even if paracetamol levels fall below toxic levels. Even though the stuff tastes so bad that
antiemetics are sometimes given for people to keep it down, it is preferable
to the intravenous route. Orally, the side effects include headache, diarrhoea,
skin flushing and can lower blood pressure in a small proportion of patients.
This is typical of the administration of any thiol and happens with radio-
protectant drugs also. Intravenously, in less than 10 per cent of cases, anaphylactic shock can occur, with severe hypotension and bronchospasm, so do
not try this at home. There is some confusion around the point that NAC is
effective and when it is less effective, but current studies have drawn some
main conclusions:

- If an individual presents for treatment at 8 hours or less after the overdose, then no matter how much paracetamol he or she has taken, no
  hepatotoxicity will be sustained.

- It is of particular importance to initiate the NAC therapy in pregnant
  women, as the NAPQI is very toxic to the foetus.

- If the NAC is started at 0–4 hours, there is no difference to the outcome;
  so early NAC treatment offers no advantage over later treatment up to
  the 8 hours 'cut off'.

- NAC is still effective up to 24 hours post-overdose, even though some hepatoxicity will have been sustained and can even be effective after this time, if paracetamol is still in the plasma and even if the liver is already damaged.

Methods for prevention of overdose

You might think that incorporation of a thiol with the paracetamol would solve the overdose problem instantly. It was first thought of in the early 1970s, soon after the mechanism of the drug's toxicity was discovered in the US. Unfortunately, nobody has ever determined the correct proportion of the thiol required to prevent liver damage in humans, nor are they likely to for ethical reasons. So to err on the side of caution, the only available product in the UK (paradote) contains methionine in a 1:5 ratio with paracetamol. It also means that everyone who takes this preparation would be ingesting methionine and there are some long-term concerns about its possible toxicity, as well as some mild side effects, such as drowsiness, flatulence and headache. Unless every paracetamol preparation (and there are hundreds of them) contains methionine, then the idea is unlikely to prevent lethal overdoses, due to the vast number of preparations that contain paracetamol without an antidote. The antidote/drug preparations are obviously much more expensive than plain paracetamol, which also means that they are unlikely to be commercially viable in the long run in the face of hundreds of cheap competitors.

Paracetamol use in children

Opinion is divided as to the value of paracetamol for children in treating fevers and mild discomfort. Certainly in children under three years old, there can be considerable reliance by parents on expensive liquid paediatric paracetamol preparations to counteract the often painful effects of various inoculations in babies and toddlers. In hospitals, paracetamol is often used for what is termed minor discomfort in mild infections and for post-operative pain, so reducing the opiate consumption. It is not always easy to demonstrate its effectiveness and children can easily be given repeated doses that exceed the 4 g/day limit. Although in general children are more resistant than adults to paracetamol toxicity, inadvertent overdosage in febrile children can lead to elevated transaminase enzyme levels and liver toxicity. This can occur where the doses of paracetamol have not been properly recorded, leading to hepatotoxicity from apparently low doses of the drug. Chronic paracetamol toxicity in febrile children is more likely to happen if they are less than three years old and are not eating or drinking enough fluid. Paracetamol is useful in cases of febrile children in heart and respiratory failure, but has little value in those who do not have heart or lung problems, as the fever can be beneficial. This is because viruses and bacteria have specific temperatures where they multiply most efficiently and the febrile response ensures that the body temperature is higher than the infectious agents' optimum temperature. This is borne out by observations that children do less well in cases of mild and severe infection when dosed with paracetamol. If it is used, then it is strongly recommended by a number of sources that paracetamol dosage should not exceed 90–100 mg/day in children with the risk factors described above.

Paracetamol: conclusions

This drug will always be a best seller, despite its toxicity in overdose. This is partly due to the toxicity of alternative drugs, such as non-steroidal anti-inflammatories, which cause severe gastric bleeding in overdose. There is no safe, mass marketed mild analgesic to replace paracetamol or aspirin, so it is important to be aware of the dangers of this drug and how it can lead to the destruction of the most resilient and best protected organ in the human body. Paracetamol's mode of toxicity is so obvious that if it had been submitted for testing in drug development systems over the last 30–40 years it would have been shown up as hepatotoxic and quietly dumped, alongside thousands of other failed agents. Interestingly, co-proxamol (325 mg paracetamol, 32.5 mg dextropropoxyphene) was withdrawn in the UK in early 2005. Many would say categorically that it would be almost impossible for a new drug to reach the mass market and cause necrotic hepatic damage, either from normal dosage of overdose.

Tacrine

Unfortunately, the above statement is proved completely wrong by the anti-cholinesterase and anti-Alzheimer's disease drug tacrine (1,2,3,4-tetrahydro-9-aminoacridine; THA). This drug underwent the normal battery of animal test systems (rodents and dogs) in its development and was not found to be toxic. In clinical trials it was found to be a potent dose-dependent hepato-toxin in humans and has since been found to be mutagenic in the Ames test (see Appendix A). However, development went ahead and the drug is currently part of the treatment of Alzheimer's disease and it is still not clear how it causes hepatotoxicity. The reason this drug was not abandoned is similar to the experience with other toxic drugs, such as the early anti-HIV agents. These drugs at the time filled a niche that was not being occupied by any other effective drug and there was a pressing therapeutic need to have something to treat patients, until a really effective agent appeared. Indeed, in the developed world, there may be as many as 12–14 million Alzheimer's sufferers. So in the face of such a huge and increasing therapeutic problem, the considerable expense of monitoring the drug's hepatotoxicity must be borne. The anti-Parkinsonian drug tolcapone was treated similarly. When liver enzymes exceed a value of about twice the normal range, the patient must cease therapy until the levels subside. Although tacrine was designed only to treat the symptoms of a reduction in CNS cholinergic transmission (by prolonging acetylcholine action) it has since emerged that it does have a number of other beneficial effects in Alzheimer's disease.

Tacrine toxicity

Initially it was discovered that between 30 and 50 per cent of patients suffered from elevated ALT and AST levels after 6–8 weeks on tacrine, which was reversible. If the drug is continued, it is capable of inducing fatal midzonal and pericentral hepatic necrosis. *In vitro* studies have shown that tacrine depletes GSH and it was logical to suggest that a reactive CYP-mediated species may have been responsible. In man, tacrine is cleared to a number of CYP1A2-mediated hydroxylated metabolites (1–4 hydroxy derivatives) that then undergo glucuronidation, although its metabolic fate has not been completely identified. The parent drug or its metabolites are capable of inhibiting the clearance of CYP1A2-cleared drugs such as theophylline. From a toxicological standpoint, the process of tacrine oxidative metabolism appears to be a 'red herring', as it was quickly established that liver injury is not related to metabolite levels of the drug, rather to blood parent drug levels. It seems that tacrine is toxic through several pathways, none of which are directly related to either Phase I or Phase II metabolism. Several studies in animals have tried to determine the route of tacrine-mediated necrosis, although this is somewhat ironic when you consider that studies in animals failed to predict the toxicity in the first place. However, work has also proceeded using human hepatic cell lines (Hep G2s, etc.) as well as animal models, so some of the hypotheses on tacrine toxicity may well be as close to the human situation as we are likely to get for some time. It is apparent that there are several potential routes to hepatotoxicity.

Tacrine causes an increase in reactive oxygen species formation, which can be ameliorated by the use of antioxidants such as vitamin E. Tacrine also causes hypoxia: the autonomic sympathetic nervous system controls liver microcirculation, so an increased in sympathetic output should shut down liver blood flow and cause hypoxia leading to necrosis. If you remember your basic autonomic pharmacology (adopt blank, slightly shocked expression at this point) then you will know that the sympathetic nerves all output noradrenaline, but they are different from the somatic (voluntary) nerves that are all one unit. Autonomic nerves have junctions (ganglia) that are cholinergic. Tacrine promotes cholinergic effects by preventing the destruction of acetylcholine, thus stimulating the cholinergic ganglia that in turn increase nora-drenaline release from the sympathetic nerves, so shutting off liver circulation. This also causes hypoxic reperfusion injury when circulation is resumed, as neutrophils and other immune systems are activated and cause tissue destruction, as seen in coronary thromboses. The tissue destruction is through reactive species release by the activated neutrophils, which will deplete GSH, as described above. In effect, this starts as a reversible adverse effect, which gradually turns into toxicity and is caused by the intended pharmacological mechanism of the drug.

Tacrine also increases hepatic membrane fluidity and damages various membrane-bound proteins and transport systems, leading to hepatic disruption. The drug can derange mitochondrial function as well as mitochondrial DNA replication. This is thought to be due to its ability to damage topoisomerase enzymes and disrupt DNA synthesis. This in turn triggers apoptosis in hepatocytes.

All these mechanisms are plausible, if not fully explained, and it is likely that future research may be more illuminating. Certainly the liver's unique susceptibility to tacrine toxicity is currently not clearly understood. Overall, this drug demonstrates:

- The vulnerability of the drug development system to 'stealth hepato-toxins', which do not affect animals in the standard context of a toxicity test;

- The likelihood that a deleterious pharmacological effect of a drug may be organ-specific only in humans;

- That even a manifestly toxic drug can be therapeutically valuable if sufficient investment in clinical monitoring is made to prevent the transition from reversible to irreversible toxicity.

Troglitazone

This drug was the first of three new thiozolidinedione insulin sensitizers that were originally developed by a Japanese drug company, for the treatment of the massive problem of Type 2 diabetes, a condition which is linked strongly to obesity. The drug was interesting because it had new mechanisms of action, one of which was the stimulation of glucose uptake by skeletal muscle. Soon after it was introduced, reports were received of several fatal incidents involving hepatotoxicity in Japan and the USA. There were 35 deaths after approximately 800 000 patients received the drug in late 1997. The FDA recommended that the drug should be monitored for hepatoxicity, but further clinical studies showed that the drug was causing threefold higher AST and

ALT levels than normal in nearly 2 per cent of those taking it, suggesting that there was a danger of significant hepatoxicity with the drug. Toxicity could occur within a couple of weeks of starting therapy, although liver failure could take as long as 6–9 months of therapy. In 2000, the drug was withdrawn worldwide. Unlike tacrine, the drug did not 'survive' its toxicity despite its usefulness. This was partly due to the availability of other effective anti-Type 2 diabetic agents, but it was also linked to the arrival of two sister compounds, rosiglitazone and pioglitazone, which were initially believed not to be subject to hepatotoxicity risks, due to structural differences. It is important to note that the tolerance of regulatory authorities to drug toxicity is strongly influenced by the intended disease target and the alternatives available. Hence the hideous toxicity profiles of anti-cancer agents can be accepted, whilst much less damaging and rarer effects in other drugs for non-life-threatening conditions where there are also many alternatives are withdrawn.

Troglitazone's toxicity is again subject to intense investigation in the very models that did not alert the drug company to its problems, that is, animal systems. However, studies with human hepatocytes, cell lines and clinical data have indicated that the drug is almost entirely cleared to a 6-O-sulphate. The sister compound rosiglitazone forms an N-desmethyl-*para*-O-sulfate as well as a *para*-O-sulfate. Over 70 per cent of troglitazone is sulphated by SULT1A3 (a phenol sulphotransferase) and to a lesser extent, SULT1E4, an oestrogen sulphation isoform. Around 10 per cent is cleared to a quinone and the rest is glucuronidated with only a few per cent excreted in urine unchanged. The main route 'out' for the sulphate is in faeces, which suggests that the bile is the major excretion route of troglitazone. Interestingly, rosiglitazone is cleared almost entirely in urine. In animal studies, those species that do not have the same high sulphation capacity as humans tend to eliminate the drug as glucuronides. This provides some clues as to why it is toxic in humans and not animals, although the mechanism behind its toxicity is not clear. The next section describes what is currently known from a variety of models, human and animal.

Troglitazone mechanisms of toxicity

It is apparent that the main metabolites, that is the sulphate, quinone or the glucuronide, are not directly toxic to human cells. This is perhaps surprising, as quinone metabolites are often protein reactive and some authors maintain that the quinone is the toxic metabolite, but this is believed unlikely. A study *in vitro* using expressed human CYP3A4 has shown that troglitazone can be oxidized to a reactive o-quinone methide. In addition, it is also possible for the thiazolidinedione ring to be cleaved, forming reactive alpha-ketoisocyanate or sulfenic acid derivatives. It is not known whether these GSH-reactive species would be formed *in vitro*, but the drug is a known inducer of CYP3A4, so it is certainly possible. Other cellular and animal studies show that toxicity seems to correlate strongly with parent drug concentrations and troglitazone itself appears to be able to curtail not only liver protein synthesis, but also its own sulphation in human hepatocytes. Perhaps most significantly, cholestasis has been reported in patients and this has been followed up with rat studies. These showed that troglitazone can cause a potent reduction in bile salt transport by inhibiting the various transporter efflux pumps. It is possible that there are a number of routes for troglitazone toxicity, but the cholestasis effect perhaps appears most persuasive at the moment. Interestingly, the sister compounds rosiglitazone and pioglitazone are metabolized in a similar fashion to troglitazone and it appears that both drugs are the subject of increasing reports of similar hepatoxicity to troglitazone. In one case, rosiglitazone caused severe liver injury in only two weeks of therapy. Future research will determine the exact mode of toxicity of these agents.

8.5 Type B2 reactions: immunotoxicity

Basic immune function

Most people are aware of the basic functions of the immune system in the detection and destruction of bacteria, viruses, infected cells and even malignant cells within the organism. The system in humans has evolved to protect us from relatively minor incursions of infectious agents as well as rapid and potentially overwhelming invasions. The immune system appears to operate on the 'better massively destructive than sorry' principle. Its responses are designed to eliminate all trace of the infectious agent, no matter how much 'collateral damage' may occur. This is on the basis that infections can and do kill in hours rather than days, so it is essential to control them now and thus be around to repair the damage at a later date. This is similar to the expectation that cancer patients will withstand severe toxicity during therapy, on the basis that survival should be attained at any cost. With the immune system, this means in practice that it is capable of destroying cells, tissues and whole organs, which can inadvertently lead to death of the organism. The immune system can be awesomely destructive and it must be reined in by a strict gradation of response to avoid huge overreaction to minor amounts of infectious agent. If you look at just one component of the immune system, a single activated neutrophil can generate enough oxidizing agents to kill 160 bacteria in one second. Lesions seen in diet-induced autoimmune diseases like dermatitis herpetiformis show what several thousand activated neutrophils can do to non-infected tissue. However, drug therapy is capable of triggering far more graphic and lethal examples of immune-mediated tissue destruction. Stevens–Johnson syndrome can lead to toxic epidermal necrolysis; this condition can destroy a patient's entire skin. Anticonvulsant hypersensitivity syndrome can cause severe, widespread tissue and organ damage. Other reactions, such as agranulocytosis, are more specific and lead to the complete shutdown of neutrophil production and death from sepsis. These reactions occur in a very small minority of patients, but they are exceptionally severe and have a high fatality rate. Doctors treating patients suffering from these reactions are often faced with extremely limited treatment options and a rapidly deteriorating patient. In addition, withdrawal of the causative drug does not always lead to amelioration of disease progression. Obviously the immune system should not respond in this way, but predicting whether a new drug might cause a catastrophic immune reaction in a small number of patients is still a long way off. This is because these reactions might affect maybe $1:5000$, or even $1:10000$ patients. It is not realistic to organize clinical trials with numbers high enough to hope that these reactions can be detected. Great progress has been made in the understanding of the immune system's normal operations, but we are still learning how drugs become immunogenic. There are conflicting theories and views as to how some immune reactions occur and it is possible to challenge many of these ideas, as they are still under development. This is mainly due to a lack of useful animal and *in vitro* models and difficulties in studying the reactions in patients, due to their understandable reluctance to be rechallenged by the drug that might have recently nearly killed them.

Mechanisms of immune-mediated drug toxicity

The immune system's activities could be resolved into three functions:

- Detection of non-self, or foreign material at a specific site, or sites;
- Initiation of an appropriate response which will lead to the destruction of that material;
- Retention of the 'memory' of that material.

Most immune problems start with the faulty recognition of 'self' as 'non-self'. There are millions of small molecules in living systems at any one time and they should logically be controlled by enzymatic systems such as CYPs, rather than the immune system, so small molecules of molecular weight of less than 1000–2000 daltons should not concern the immune system. Generally, bacterial and viral proteins or fragments are much larger, perhaps from 20000 daltons upward. However, as far back as the 1930s, with the studies of Landsteiner, it was established that the immune system would recognize small molecules if they were to become covalently attached to much larger ones (40000–50000 plus). These molecules were termed 'haptens' and their binding to cell macromolecules 'haptenation'. Injection of the hapten itself does not result in any reaction: the essential feature is that the hapten is bound to protein. There are many examples of chemicals and metabolites that spontaneously react with proteins, and the degree of binding depends on the balance of 'activation' and antioxidant status. The immune system then senses the hapten as non-self and initiates some form of attack. Why the immune system should respond to haptens at all is not clear, although it may be another case of 'better massively destructive than sorry', in that chemicals of bacterial or fungal origin could conceivably become bound to protein and could be indicative of a more widespread infectious presence, therefore it would be logical to attack to be on the safe side. Certainly, successful infectious agents use some unbelievably clever strategies all the time: for example, schistosomes blatantly sit unmolested in the portal circulation causing havoc for 30 years or more. These nematodal worms can be an *inch* long. At the other end of the scale, intracellular pathogens are extremely adept at escaping the immune system, and some of the most successful human pathogens of all such as viruses, malaria and even tuberculosis evade the immune system and often thrive in its presence. So perhaps we should forgive the human immune system some measure of paranoia, as everything 'out there' really is out to get us.

Antigen processing and presentation

Given that some form of a drug, either degradation product or metabolite, has reacted with cell structure, the obvious question is how does the immune system become aware of the existence of the haptenated protein and why does it then decide it is antigenic and form antibodies against it. Infectious agents can be found within cells as well as 'outside' in the interstitial fluid. B and T lymphocytes cannot mount a response to an antigen if they are not aware of its existence. However, there must be a system which contains and focuses the destructive power of these cells. So the antigen must be *processed* into a form where it can be *presented* to the B and T cells in such a way that they will recognize it as foreign and not self. The process is designed to prevent excessive recognition of self and can be resolved into intracellular and extracellular antigen detection and presentation.

Intracellular antigen detection and presentation

Normally within any given cell, there is a continuous process where various proteins are removed, shredded and then loaded onto a molecule known as MHC I, or major histocompatibility complex I (Figure 8.6). A protein called TAP handles this loading process and it happens in the rough endoplasmic reticulum of the cell. MHC I is related to immunoglobulins and can bind

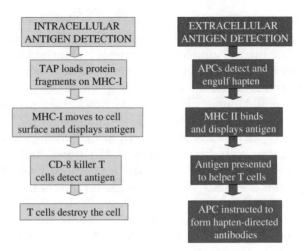

Figure 8.6 Basic events of intra- and extracellular antigen processing

practically any peptide, so it can carry any given piece of protein to the cell wall, where it expresses the protein on the surface. This is a form of constant quality control, a monitoring or sampling of the presence of self inside the cell followed by a clear presentation of 'self' at the exterior of the cell. The MHC molecular system is a vital link in the process that alerts the immune system to possible internal foreign antigens. In the case of a viral infiltration, the viral proteins are picked up and shredded, loaded onto the MHC I which then exhibits them. Cytotoxic T cells (CD8+) recognize the MHC I as self (self MHC restriction), which means they will then automatically accept the foreign material bound to the MHC I as non-self and then destroy the cell. This recognition by the T cell of the self of the MHC I before antigen recognition prevents the T cell from indiscriminately attacking anything in sight and channels their cytotoxicity to where it is needed. The weakness of this system is that it is a sequential multi-stage process like a production line; jam one stage and it all goes 'out of synch'. A number of infectious agents exploit this to evade detection. Whether haptens bound to internal proteins trigger this system based on MHC I is controversial, although there is no real reason why they should not, particularly if a very high density of haptens occurred to sufficiently alter internal cellular protein structure.

Extracellular antigen presentation and detection

Most bacteria and toxins are extracellular and viruses must be extracellular until they find a victim cell, so a series of antigen presenting cells (APCs) cruise the interstitial fluid around cells hunting for antigens. These include B lymphocytes, macrophages and dendritic cells. These cells carry Immunoglobulin (Ig) molecules on their surfaces and they detect smaller entities than whole proteins, such as nucleic acid fragments, lipopolysaccharides, lipids and the haptens. A surface IgG will recognize the hapten, but not the protein of the hapten carrier complex. At this point the APC cells engulf the whole hapten protein complex, dismantle it and tie up the protein of the complex to MHC II, which is only found APCs. This migrates to the APC surface as with the previous MHC I system, only this time the APC cell will present its processed MHC II protein fragments to helper T cells (CD4+), rather than the cytotoxic (CD8+) ones. The helper T cell activates and instructs the APC to make antibodies to the hapten, exactly the same as the initial IgG that first detected it. It also instructs B cell proliferation (memory cells), ensuring that the next time the hapten–protein complex appears there will be a much more rapid and intense response. Essentially, the APC reacts to the hapten, while the T cell reacts to the protein it has been bound to. This B cell amplification system is designed to 'buy time'. The immune system can respond to virtually any pathogen, provided it has the time to make enough cells and antibodies. This time period must not be slower than the proliferation rate of the infection, or death results by weight of numbers and secreted toxins. The memory pool of cells provides the ability for rapid response to the pathogen when it is next encountered.

Hence, the immune system can recognize small molecules and after an initial sensitization, mount a rapid immune response to the molecules and the macromolecules to which they were attached. The APC cells, such as the B lymphocytes, might detect haptenic antigens as a result of cell necrosis or perhaps binding of the hapten to the surface of other cells and structures. The key here is the immune system mostly does not react to haptens and only in certain individuals does the full force of immunocytotoxicity become unleashed. The most difficult problem in immunotoxicity is why certain individuals are susceptible and how to predict this situation in particular patients.

Nature of drug-mediated immune responses

As to what actually happens to patients during hypersensitivity reactions, these can be resolved by time of onset, severity of symptoms and lethality and particularly the site of the reaction. The first two types of reaction, anaphylaxis and anticonvulsant syndrome, lead to widespread reactions throughout the body. The second probably involves a more localized cause, such as a systemic loss of neutrophils (agranulocytosis). Other reactions are confined to particular organs or sites in organs, leading to hepatotoxicity and skin toxicity.

Anaphylaxis

This can happen in response to a variety of foodstuffs (particularly nuts), food colourings, handling latex, contact with animals, insect bites and stings as well as drugs such as penicillins, NSAIDS and some intravenous preparations. The symptoms include: fainting, swelling of the throat (laryngeal oedema), asthmatic symptoms as well as difficulty in breathing, rashes, swelling, vomiting and diarrhoea.

If anaphylaxis progresses to anaphylactic shock, blood pressure plummets, tachycardia and arrhythmia occur alongside a racing pulse, coupled with extreme bronchospasm. Anaphylactic shock can be lethal in minutes.

This condition is caused by some exposure to an antigen that provokes the formation (by B lymphocytes) of a unique Immunoglobulin E (IgE) for that antigen. The IgE sits on the surface of mast cells and basophils, rather like a primed grenade. Another exposure to the antigen, or something *similar in structure*, and the IgE causes the cells to release massive amounts of vasoactive substances such as histamine. This process is known as degranulation. Since mast cells are found in all the tissues, particularly the vasculature and bronchi, blood vessels are relaxed causing the fall in blood pressure and the spaces between cells widen, leading to swelling in the tissues. The constricting effect on the bronchi is basically dependent on the amount of these agents released. Subsequent exposure to the antigen raises many more antibodies that cause more and more violent and widespread reactions through the body. This is the worst form of immunological 'own goal' as it is grotesquely out of proportion to the threat involved and can lead to death of the patient. The treatment is immediate injection of 300 micrograms (150 for a child) of adrenaline, which should control the metabolic mayhem, although recovery times can be considerable.

Since haptenation is thought to be a possible route to the immune system recognition of self as non-self, it would appear to be a bad idea to market drugs that were directly protein reactive, but penicillins spontaneously degrade into a number of reactive derivatives in all patients that take them. The result of these species binding covalently to proteins leads to the formation of various haptens such as the penicilloyl derivatives. The B lymphocytes form IgEs in response to these groups and the next administration of the drug to the patient could be their last. This is essentially a disseminated reaction, i.e. a reaction that occurs in many areas of the body, including crucial ones such as the blood vessels and the lungs. As many as 10 per cent of the population could be at risk from this type of reaction from penicillin or related antibiotics. Around 75 per cent of fatal anaphylactic shock cases are linked to penicillin and its related drugs. Concurrent usage of beta-blockers makes anaphylaxis much worse as they prevent the beneficial effects of catecholamines released in response to the condition as well as those administered to treat it. Animal studies suggest that only a minuscule fraction of the dose needs to bind to provoke a reaction, so the degree of covalent binding itself is not the issue, rather it is the shape of what is bound and where it is bound. Penicillin originated from a eukaryotic organism (mould) and many fungus-type organisms are pathogenic to humans. Therefore it is not really surprising that the structure of the penicillin-related material is so intensely antigenic. What is also interesting is that penicillin is protein reactive in everyone without exception, but only a minority of patients develop anaphylaxis.

Anticonvulsant hypersensitivity syndrome

This multi-organ syndrome is similar to that seen with allopurinol and sulphonamides. It affects a small proportion of epileptics taking the older anticonvulsants, such as phenytoin, phenobarbitone and carbamazepine and even affects those using lamotrigine, a relatively new drug. It is not as rapid in onset as anaphylaxis, but can begin within 2–12 weeks of starting therapy. Virtually all patients present with fever, which often persists for weeks after the drug has been withdrawn. A rash affects the trunk and limbs; the face and lips may swell and blister appreciably. Around half the cases also have hepatitis; this is the most dangerous area of the reaction and up to a third of patients die from liver failure. High white cell counts are also recorded, with general haematological disruption. A serious clinical problem arises when the patient recovers, as the reaction may occur again with another anticonvulsant. The reaction will be much worse the second time, so patch testing is recommended before another anticonvulsant is started.

All the drugs responsible for this syndrome are extensively cleared by CYPs, often to reactive arene intermediates that are cytotoxic and tissue reactive *in vitro*. It is believed that a cytotoxic T cell response is behind the reaction and this is likely to be linked with MHC I intracellular antigen presentation.

Blood dyscrasias

These conditions usually are characterized by the loss of a group of cells within the blood system, such as erythrocytes, platelets or discrete white cell populations. However, some of the conditions seem to follow the classic hapten route, whilst others appear to have more than one cause. The loss of cells can be either due to damage or destruction of the organ that manufactures them, cell destruction in the vasculature alone, or both together.

Haemolytic anaemia

The premature intravascular destruction of erythrocytes can be caused by many circumstances, from physical damage to the cells (passage through surgical life-support systems) through to immune-mediated causes related to drug therapy. A number of drugs are associated with immune-mediated erythrocytic loss, such as methyldopa, penicillin, cephalosporins, quinidine and some NSAIDS. In the 1960s it was shown that haptenation of the cells' membranes by penicillin-related material led to recognition by B cell-mediated immunoglobulins, which led to complement activation. It is likely that the other drugs are also activated to reactive species which haptenate the cells. As mentioned previously, red cells already have a 'sell-by date' system, where normal wear and tear (red cells can be reversibly deformed to an amazing degree) induces the appearance of various wear indicator molecules on their surface. The spleen 'reads' the number of these molecules and when the number corresponding to the 120-day lifespan appears, the spleen removes and destroys the cell. Clearly haptenation of these molecules could accelerate the spleen's removal of the cells, as well as alerting other cytotoxic immune cells. Clinical presentation involves jaundice and dark urine, due to the liver struggling with the disposal of so much haem in such a short time. Symptoms appear that are related to tissue hypoxia, such as fatigue, shortness of breath and tachycardia. Usually once the drug is stopped, the liver will recover and transfusions can tide the patient over until normal red cell production eventually replaces the lost erythrocytes.

Aplastic anaemia

This condition is due to destruction of the bone marrow, which can be caused by radiation, infections or by an immune-mediated process. This results in the gradual reduction of vascular levels of all blood cells, including white cell populations, erythrocytes and platelets. The symptoms include those for haemolysis, alongside those of immune deficiency, such as oral thrush. Several drugs have been shown to cause aplastic anaemia, which include anticonvulsants, anti-cancer agents, chloramphenicol and phenothiazines. Interestingly, the chronic use of illegal drugs, such as opiates and cocaine, increases the risk of aplastic anaemia. Aromatic organic solvents such as benzene and toluene are also linked with this condition as well as a number of insecticides. The prognosis is poor, as even after a bone marrow transplant, survival over five years can be less than 60 per cent. Again, it is thought that haptenation of the bone marrow cells is responsible for the damage and failure of the stem cells to differentiate into new blood cells.

Agranulocytosis

There are many causes of neutropenia, where neutrophil levels fall to low levels in cycles, but agranulocytosis is characterized by the 'one-off' decline to the point of almost disappearance of neutrophils in the circulation. The condition is stealthy, in that it is symptomless until cell levels fall below

0.5×10^9 per litre. Agranulocytosis underlines the importance of neutrophils, as in spite of the existence of so many other immune cell types, life is only possible for a few days without neutrophils. The first symptoms are of a serious infection, with fever, malaise and chills, leading to acute sepsis. The type of bacteria that infect the patients in this context includes *Staph. Aureus* and various pseudomonads.

A considerable number of drugs cause this condition, such as clozapine, sulphonamides, dapsone, antithyroids and phenothiazines. It is an uncommon reaction and the overall rate for most drugs is very small. Clozapine is about the most dangerous drug in this respect, with a frequency of more than 1 per cent.

The condition usually appears from 8 to 14 weeks after initiation of drug therapy. Agranulocytosis is unusual, as it is the loss of a separate population of cells. Once the causative agent has been withdrawn, neutrophil production resumes as if nothing had happened. A combination of intravenous antibiotics and stimulation of bone marrow with filgrastim should attenuate the infections. Normal neutrophil blood levels should be attained in less than 14 days. Examination of bone marrow shows no actual damage, although myeloid precursor cells may be absent. That cell production resumes so quickly after the withdrawal of the drug reinforces the idea that agranulocytosis in some cases is not really toxicity, more a reversible interruption in the cell assembly line. The first drug to show this effect was in the 1930s, but was atypical. Aminopyrine therapy caused antibodies to be formed to neutrophils and they were destroyed in the circulation, but not in the bone marrow. The condition occurred within a week and would occur even earlier on rechallenge. Drugs such as dapsone and clozapine, which cause agranulocytosis, show the 8–14 week latency, which in the case of clozapine does not change on rechallenge. If the immune system were involved, the pool of memory cells would cause an effect in less than half that time. This suggests that the effect is probably not connected to the immune system. It may be that agranulocytosis is less to do with reactive species and more to do with some form of a direct switching effect on neutrophil maturation. Since so many small molecules are so crucial in the modulation of cellular responses, it would not be surprising that a drug could act on certain individuals' receptors that were atypical in some way due to genetic variation.

Site-directed drug-mediated immune responses

Most other drug-mediated immune reactions are either targeted at an organ, such as the skin or the liver, or at a cell population such as those in the blood. These reactions in general appear to be related to some form of covalent binding which has attracted the attention of APC cells, usually in the form of deposition of various immunoglobulins (IgA, IgG and IgM). For a covalent bond to occur in the first place, some form of reactive species must have been formed. It is likely that the species will have been too reactive to travel very far, so it is reasonable to suggest that the species was made close to where the binding occurred, which is where the immune reaction takes place also.

Hepatic immunotoxic reactions

For the immune system to be linked with hepatotoxicity, it is generally accepted that some symptoms of hepatitis should be present, which involves organ-wide inflammation, presence of inflammatory cells in the sinusoids as well as disruption of normal hepatic processes which lead to jaundice and high liver enzyme levels. Viral hepatitises generally show these symptoms, but it can be difficult to distinguish an infected liver from a drug-hypersensitivity affected liver. A case of hepatitis without indication of viral or bacterial causes could well be due to drug hypersensitivity. Although the liver can form many different types of reactive metabolites, it also possesses the most comprehensive and effective protective systems against reactive species-mediated damage in the entire body. These systems should minimize hepatic covalent binding. In addition, the paracetamol story, with its high degree of reactive species generation and covalent binding, is not normally associated with hepatitis. So clearly, highly specific covalent binding must be taking place for the immune system to detect antigen and then attack the whole organ. There are number of agents which have been associated with drug-induced hepatitis, particularly the anaesthetic halothane, isoniazid, statins and several anticonvulsants, such as phenytoin. Other hepatitis-like effects are more likely to be the result of interruptions in bile flow, rather than of immunological origin (steroid and chlorpromazine hepatitis). All of the drugs described above undergo metabolism to reactive species; indeed, isoniazid hepatitis is much more likely in CYP2E1-induced heavy alcohol users.

If a reactive species is formed that has such a short half-life it destroys the CYP enzyme that formed it, then it is possible for covalent binding to occur which evades the normal protective mechanisms of the liver. It is then possible that the normal cellular MHC I quality control might pick up the degraded CYP and process and present it as an antigen. Another way this could happen is if the drug causes a focus of severe liver cell necrosis, leading to the release of a number of haptenic proteins which are then detected by the APC system. Either way, it is conceivable that the immune system in some individuals becomes sensitized to drug-related antigens which are only likely to be formed in the liver, and nowhere else, on the basis of the site of enough of the appropriate CYP enzyme which activates the drug to the binding species.

Skin-directed immunotoxicity – sulphonamides

As previously mentioned, these drugs can cause a range of mostly skin hypersensitivity reactions which make patients, particularly those with a high risk of reaction and little clinical alternative, intolerant of the drugs. Sulphonamides are aromatic amines, so they undergo the classic CYP (usually 2C9) oxidation to hydroxylamines that then spontaneously oxidize to nitrosoarenes which are very short-lived and reactive. Sulphonamide hydroxylamines are poor methaemoglobin formers, and they are not concentrated by erythrocytes like some other aromatic amine hydroxyl derivatives. So they can be formed in the liver and apparently circulate in blood, so they could theoretically reach any organ. Sulphonamide-related material has been found bound to proteins in a number of areas, and binding occurs in human keratinocytes in cell culture. Sulphonamides and other related amines, like the now obsolete procainamide, can be oxidized through extrahepatic metabolism. Neutrophils use the iron-based enzyme myeloperoxidase to generate hydrogen peroxide, as well as hypochlorous acid to attack bacteria. It is established that these oxidants can form reactive species of sulphonamides and other drugs, which can covalently bind to tissues as well as form other reactive oxygen species. It is necessary for a neutrophil to be activated before it will form high levels of oxidant species, so it might be reasonable to suppose that APC cells had already found some form of the sulphonamide-related material antigenic and formed antibodies against it. This in turn attracts the neutrophils. It is very difficult to show this happening *in vivo*.

However the reactive species are formed, sulphonamide-related material is certainly strongly immunogenic in up to 5 per cent of patients. There is a wide range of reaction, ranging from rashes caused by similar pathways to penicillin (IgE-mediated mast cell disruption) to the triggering of cytotoxic T cell destruction. This is usually associated with the MHC I intracellular system for antigen detection and is likely to be what happens in the most severe hypersensitivity reactions, such as Stevens–Johnson syndrome. Again, the obvious question is if everyone metabolizes sulphonamides into reactive species, why do most of us escape any immunological consequences of this?

Summary of mechanisms of drug-mediated immunotoxicity

It is generally accepted that covalent binding of drug-related material must occur, prior to the immune reaction, which is related to antioxidant status and activation of the drug by an oxidative (or possibly reductive) system. It has been suggested that some drugs can directly bind to MHC molecules without prior activation and elicit an immune response.

The sensitivity of any given individual's immune system must be a combination of many genetic factors, as well as diet and general health. In the case of dapsone-mediated agranulocytosis, the condition is very rare in immunosuppressed leprosy patients, around 1:8000 in 'normal' individuals when used as an antimalarial and 1:250 in patients with dermatitis herpetiformis.

Agranulocytosis might not be a good example of a classic hapten-related response, but the role of immune sensitivity in these reactions should probably be the focus of future research into immune-mediated drug reactions.

8.6 Type B3 reactions: role of metabolism in cancer

Sources of risks of malignancy

It has become clear that oxidative and reductive metabolizing enzymes are responsible for the generation of some reactive species that interact differently with cellular structures than immunogenic or necrotic agents. Carcinogenic reactive species have exquisitely precise structural characteristics that are necessary to react with individual nucleotides of DNA. This can lead to cross-linking the DNA, preventing transcription, or causing transcriptional errors.

One of the chief defences against the propagation of damaged DNA is apoptosis. Whether specific or non-specific binding is responsible for initiating the process, controlled and ordered cell death results, where reactive endogenous systems are shut down or made safe and DNA is destroyed and the cell dismantles itself. Apoptosis is a very complex process, but in terms of a response to reactive species, it is an attempt by the organism to contain damage and limit its consequences for other cells and most importantly, the organism itself. The destruction of the stricken cell's DNA prevents faulty DNA from being propagated in cell division. The survival of the cell in this context could mean eventual death of the entire organism from a future neoplasm. If apoptosis is not triggered, the organism will rely on gene repair to prevent possible future malignancies. Gene repair in dividing cells is an endless process, like roadworks on motorways. The balance between enzymatic reactive species generation, degree of detoxification of the species, DNA damage, as well as the efficiency of DNA repair ultimately dictates an individual's risk of malignancy.

Risks of malignancy and drug development

Regarding drug development, there is a theoretical risk that a drug designed to treat a condition for perhaps many years could be metabolized to reactive species that might trigger a neoplasm. The drug industry is required to examine this possibility with carcinogenicity tests with new drugs. After *in vitro* studies, such as the Ames test (Appendix A), have shown a drug not to be mutagenic *in vitro*, the animals are exposed to the drug in carcinogenicity studies for their whole lifetimes with doses that greatly exceed the likely therapeutic level. These studies are often still going on while the drug is in Phase I and II (human volunteers and patient) trials.

The common ground in carcinogenicity between animals and humans is usually the local formation of a reactive species, either in the liver, lung or perhaps the kidney. The particular reactive species may interact with human and animal DNA in a similar fashion. However, animal models may diverge from the human situation strongly as to which CYP enzymes actually form the reactive species. In the case of aromatic amines like sulphonamides, dapsone, aniline, β-naphthylamine and 4-aminobiphenyl, different enzymes between the species form the same hydroxylamines. The recent examples of troglitazone and tacrine underline the problem that humans are more susceptible to certain toxic events than animals. So the drug industry is aware that there is the danger that a drug might be metabolized to a reactive and carcinogenic species in humans which does not happen in an animal model. This can be addressed by the use of human liver CYP enzymes to activate the compounds prior to inclusion in the Ames test, followed by the animal lifetime carcinogenicity studies. These studies can be backed up by the many DNA damage/repair assays (sister chromatid exchange, Comet etc; Appendix A) that can detect genotoxicity in human primary and cultured cell systems. Overall, it is likely that the chances of a new drug causing cancers in humans are virtually non-existent. The main causes of human cancers where drug-metabolizing enzymes are involved in the formation of DNA-reactive species include smoking, diet, occupation and atmospheric pollution.

Environmental carcinogenicity risks

Although there is a vast literature on carcinogens in animal species, there are surprisingly few proven carcinogens in man. It is perceived that our greatest risks of exposure to carcinogens lie in what we eat, what we breathe (or inhale, if it is tobacco) and where we work. The earliest hard information about human carcinogenic risk came from occupational sources. The first documented example (eighteenth century) was the detection of scrotal cancers in young chimney sweeps, followed by polycyclic aromatic-mediated disease in the early twentieth century. Aromatic amine-mediated bladder cancer risks in the dye and rubber industries were established well before the 1950s. This real-life 'experimental' system is from the human standpoint tragic and costly and from the scientific standpoint, relatively uncontrolled and incomplete. Exposure to carcinogens is varied and confounded by factors such as genetic predisposition, age, smoking habits, changes in recommended exposure levels and working environments. Individuals are often exposed to carcinogens for up to 40 years and in some cases, their exposure is relatively brief and the latency period before the cancer appears can be several decades. It is also increasingly clear that protective mechanisms that maintain DNA are also extremely sophisticated and vary in their effectiveness between individuals. So what is perhaps remarkable, is that so many thousands of individuals smoked heavily, worked in the rubber or dye industries and died of old age.

Occupational carcinogens

Aromatic amines: introduction

To understand why aromatic amines are so toxic and carcinogenic, it is first useful to look at some basic amine chemistry. It is easiest to see these compounds in terms of existing mostly in the environment as two main forms, both of which are essentially non-toxic, that is, they are stable and non-tissue reactive. The first form is the amine itself and the second is the nitroderivative (Figure 8.7). From Figure 8.7 you can see that the amine can be oxidized at stage 1 to the N-hydroxy, or hydroxylamine. This usually requires some

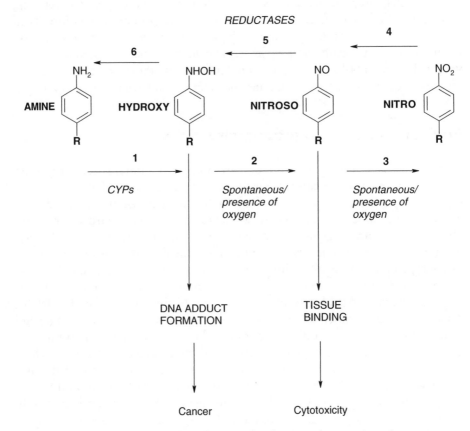

Figure 8.7   Stages of oxidation and reduction of aromatic amines

serious oxidative energy, which is supplied by CYP isoforms. The product hydroxylamine varies in stability according to the rest of the structure of the molecule. Stage 1 (Figure 8.7) essentially converts a stable entity into a relatively unstable one, in true CYP tradition. Two electrons are lost in the process. The hydroxylamine can now be conjugated, but this can lead to the formation of even more unstable products, which split, leaving a reactive nitrenium group (more later) which attacks DNA. The other alternative is the spontaneous oxidation (stage 2) and loss of two more electrons to form a nitrosoarene, which can often be highly tissue reactive and rapidly cytotoxic, although some are much more stable. Nitrosoarene stability again depends on the structure of rest of the molecule. The further spontaneous oxidation and loss of two more electrons (stage 3) forms a stable nitro derivative, which is usually not a problem unless it meets a reductase enzyme, of which there are a large number, in the liver (NADPH reductases), erythrocytes (NADH reductases) and the cytosol of most cells. These return the electrons and form the (stage 4) nitroso and (stage 5) hydroxylamine and then the (stage 6) amine in turn. At each point, the same dangerous intermediates, the nitroso and the nitrenium ions, can be formed. So aromatic amines are a problem because they are so easy to oxidize or reduce, but essentially the same toxic intermediates are formed. So many different enzyme systems can activate them anywhere in the body, not just the liver. This explains their ability to cause toxicity and cancer in widely differing types of tissues.

As mentioned above the pattern of toxicity caused by aromatic amines depends very much on the stability of their hydroxylamines (Table 8.2). This is a generalization, but usually the more stable the hydroxylamine, it is less immunogenic, a poorer methaemoglobin former and the more carcinogenic it becomes.

Hopefully you can see how aromatic amines can be so toxic, so the following examples should be easier to understand. It is highly unlikely that a new drug would appear on the market which contained an easily oxidized aromatic

Table 8.2 The relationship between the stability of aromatic hydroxylamines and their mode of toxicity

Parent drug	Hydroxylamine half-life (pH 7)	Methaemoglobin formation	Immunogenicity	Carcinogenicity
S'onamides	<10 min	+	++++	No
Chlor'col	<20	++	+	No
Dapsone	<60 min	++++	++	No
4-ABP	>3 h	++++	No	++++
BNA	>10 h	No	No	++++

S'onamides (sulphonamides); BNA (β-Naphthylamine); 4-ABP (4-aminobiphenyl); Chlor'col (chloramphenicol).

amine, or a free nitroaromatic group, as it would be toxic like chloramphenicol, where its nitro group is reduced to a hydroxylamine which caused methaemoglobin in babies in the 1950s (grey baby syndrome). This drug only survives today as a topical preparation for minor eye infections, so its systemic absorption is virtually zero. Interestingly, a number of other drugs in the last 20 years have failed in clinical trials because they were metabolized to amines that were then toxic. There are many aromatic amines consumed as foodstuffs (overcooked burgers), environmental pollutants and occupational agents. I have cited some examples below, but there are many more in the scientific literature. As mentioned previously, there are two main ways aromatic amines can be metabolized to carcinogens: through oxidative or reductive means.

Aromatic amine carcinogens – oxidative metabolism

β-Naphthylamine (BNA) was used in the rubber industry for many decades as an antioxidant to maintain pliability in rubber products, such as tyres. It could be found in levels that exceeded 1 per cent. It was employed as an anti-rust additive in various oils used to coat metals between manufacturing stages. BNA was also used in the dye industry and it has been established as one of the few compounds that are accepted to be a human carcinogen even in a court of law, provided exposure can be documented. Benzidine, aniline and o-toluidine were all aromatic amines used along with BNA in the manufacture of various colourfast dyes. The pattern of aromatic amine carcinogenesis is interesting: it appears that in any given population of workers that were exposed to this agent, up to 10 per cent may develop bladder cancers. This may be from a relatively short exposure of as little as 1–6 years. Up to 30 years after exposure ends, the bladder tumours appear and often the first realization that something is wrong for the patient is blood in the urine (haematuria), although many tumours are symptomless until quite late stages.

The following factors influence whether a worker might develop aromatic amine-related bladder cancer. If they:

- Are slow acetylators;
- Are heavy smokers;
- Have a diet low in vegetables and high in meat;
- Work in a hot environment with poor fluid intake.

Mechanism

It seems that aromatic amine carcinogens all share a similar metabolic profile and it is possible to trace the metabolites formed and determine which are carcinogenic and which are not. It is also possible to explain each of the risk factors above. What is not easy to explain and is beyond the scope of this book, is why it takes 20–40 years before irreversible changes in the bladder lead to the appearance of a tumour.

From Figure 8.8, it is possible to see that there are several metabolic products of aromatic amine clearance. Usually low levels of parent amine are found in urine, but the main fate of these compounds is Phase I and II metabolism. The hydroxylamine derivative is usually too unstable to be able to proceed through the bloodstream to be filtered by the kidneys to reach the bladder. It is much more likely to form an O- or an N-hydroxy glucuronide. The parent drug can also form an N-glucuronide. Free parent amine in the bladder is probably not a problem, as the bladder is unlikely to be able to activate it to its hydroxylamine in quantity. The acetylated derivative is not a problem, provided it is not deacetylated to the parent drug that can then be oxidized to the hydroxylamine. The fact that slow acetylators are more likely to develop bladder cancers suggests that the acetylation process does 'hold up' the amine and protects it from oxidative clearance. Some aromatic amines are excreted in urine as acetylated derivatives, but these may also be glucuronidated and oxidized to form the N-hydroxyacetylated derivative, although this usually a relatively minor pathway.

The majority of the dose of aromatic amines undergoes oxidative metabolism and the various glucuronides are stable in blood, but not in acid urine. Most people in the developed world eat too much meat and not enough vegetables. This leads to acid urine, which accelerates the decay of these metabolites to only a few minutes in some cases. In addition, men working in hot environments often do not drink enough fluid. They might have a flask of tea or coffee, but the caffeine in these drinks causes a net dehydration throughout the day. This coupled with possible restricted access to water due to the work environment means that often men's urine is very concentrated throughout the working day, so leading to high levels of the various aromatic amine metabolites in the bladder. The decomposition of the glucuronides leads to the formation of parent amine, hydroxylamine and possibly nitrenium ions through a number of different pathways (Figure 8.9).

Nitrenium ions (sometimes called aminylium ions) can be formed when a nitrogen/oxygen bond is broken, which leads to the formation of a positively charged nitrogen with two unshared electrons. This makes for a very reactive species that seeks to find its missing electrons from a rich source of them, perhaps DNA or other cellular macromolecules. The first pathway where these ions could be formed is by the decomposition of the aryl-hydroxy-O-glucuronide. There are other ways where nitrenium ions could also be formed (Figure 8.9), involving decomposition of the aryl-hydroxy N-glucuronide to yield the hydroxylamine. Nitrosoarenes would form in the presence of oxygen from the hydroxylamine and be protein reactive, although it is not clear whether they would be carcinogenic. It is suspected that nitrenium ions can be formed from reactions involving the hydroxylamine, but it is also

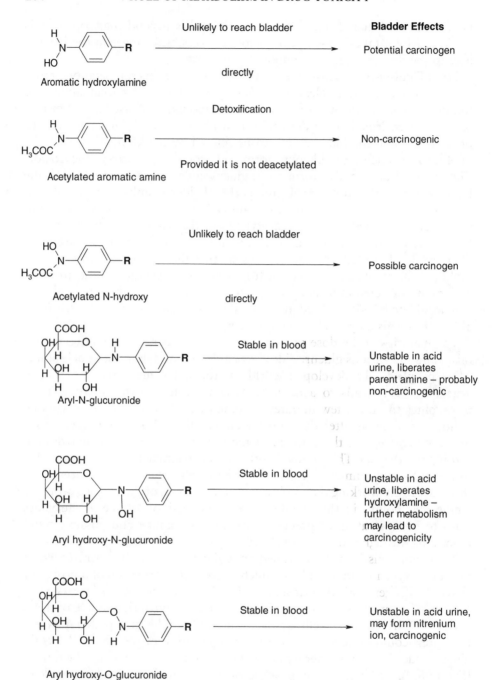

Figure 8.8   Some major metabolites of aromatic amines and their possible role in bladder carcinogenesis

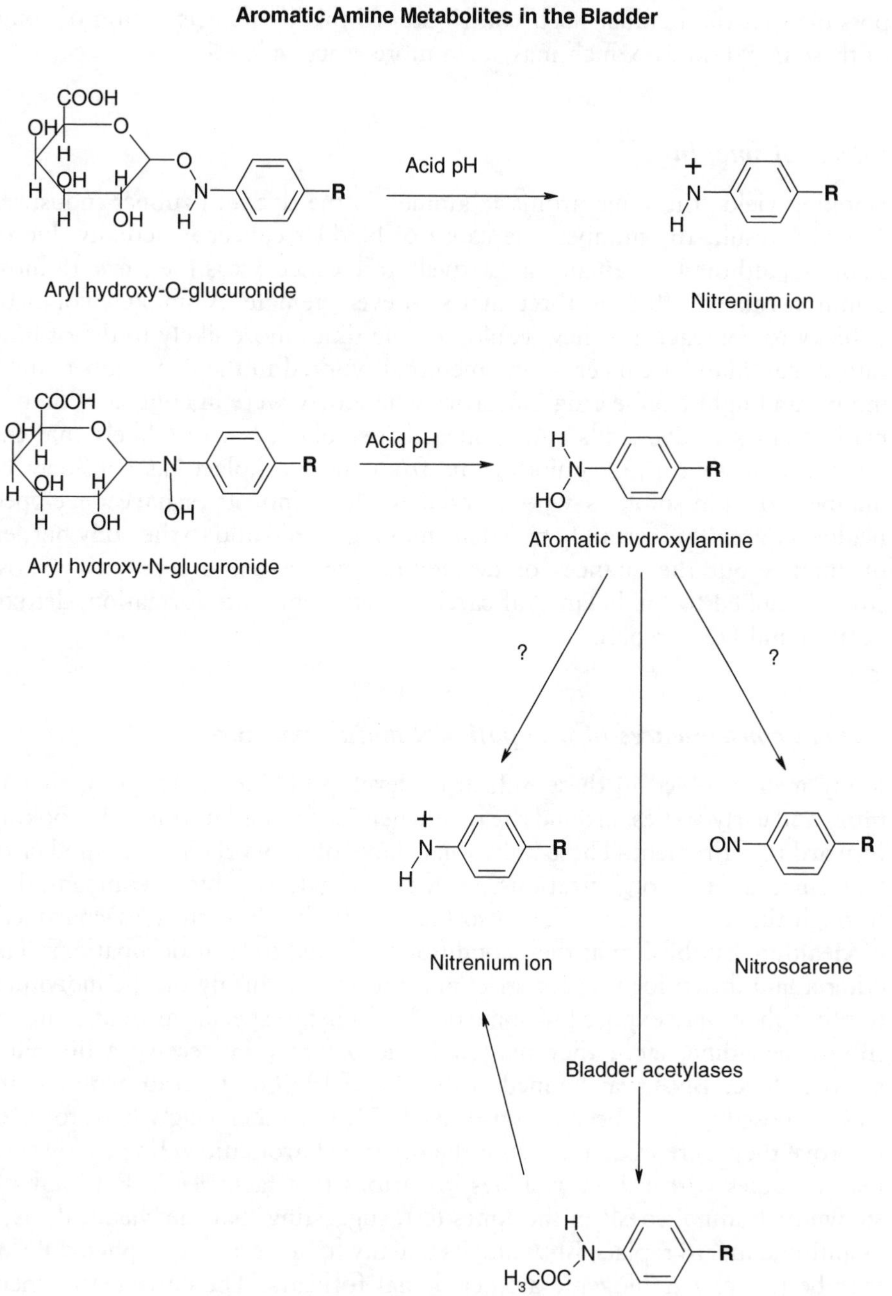

Aromatic Amine Metabolites in the Bladder

Figure 8.9 Final formation of aromatic amine-derived carcinogenic metabolites in the human bladder

possible that the bladder itself contributes to this by its acetylation of some of these metabolites, which may form more reactive species.

Effects of smoking

Smoking yields the same aromatic amines as the dye and rubber industries and as a result, the number one cause of bladder cancer is actually due to smoking, although it remains a relatively rare cancer; it is the eleventh most common cancer, affecting three males to every female. A smoker would be unlucky to contract it – they would be nine times more likely to die of lung rather than bladder cancer. Many men that worked in the dye, rubber, automotive and light engineering industries where they were in contact with aromatic amines in dyes, oils and rubber also smoked, but it is likely that the greatest contribution of amines came from the workplace, as considerable numbers of non-smokers who worked in these industries have developed bladder cancer. It is certainly true that smoking would add to the body burden of amines, but the chances of developing the disease are probably most strongly linked to the balance of carcinogenic metabolite formation, detoxification and DNA repair.

Human consequences of occupational amine exposure

Many men involved in these industries develop bladder cancer in their late fifties and early sixties, around the time when they would normally be looking forward to retirement. These individuals have often worked for a number of long-since defunct organizations, so they struggle to obtain compensation through the legal system. They also face a long battle with the Department of Health to establish that their condition is related to their occupations. The criteria laid down for this are strict and the onus is firmly on the individual to prove they were exposed to some or all of a list of specific aromatic amines (BNA, benzidine, etc.); they may well die before they receive a disability pension. Since BNA was banned in the UK in 1949 and world manufacture was supposed to have been curtailed by 1971, it is increasingly hard for men to prove they were in contact with the described aromatic amines. However, recent studies with rubber residues in various tyre factories in Europe have shown high mutagenesis in the Ames test, suggesting that the chemicals used as antioxidants to replace BNA and its equally toxic derivatives (phenyl BNA) may be just as carcinogenic as their lethal forbears. The current treatment for bladder cancer is removal of the bladder; five-year survival for bladder cancer is between 35 and 40 per cent and it is improving with earlier diagnosis and awareness. However, the pain and discomfort that these patients can suffer make their quality of remaining life relatively poor.

Aromatic amine carcinogens: reductive metabolism

Nitroaromatics

As you know, most of atmospheric pollution is the result of burning fossil fuels. In general, the lighter the fraction of crude oil that is burned, the lower the polycyclic aromatic emissions become. Among the fractions used in transport, diesel is seen as a 'greener' fuel than petrol, in that it contains more hydrocarbons so you can travel further on a given volume of fuel, with lower carbon dioxide emissions. Early diesel engines put out seriously loathsome fumes, which contained large amounts of carcinogenic polycyclic aromatics alongside the particulates, and many studies over the last 25 years or so have shown the very high mutagenicity of diesel emissions. Although cleaner than they were, it seems that no matter which future emission standards they are said to be compliant with, diesels still smoke and stink. They remain one of the main sources of mutagenic polycyclic aromatics in the atmosphere – indeed, the most mutagenic substances yet measured have been found in diesel emissions. Although there are many mutagens in diesel, the nitroaromatics are the most potent and are discussed below.

Nitropolycyclic aromatics

These compounds are formed during the combustion of many fuels, but they appear to be produced in the greatest amounts in diesel exhausts, particularly when the engine is under high load and hard acceleration, such as in fully, or overloaded trucks. The previous record holder for the most mutagenic compound ever, 1,8 dinitropyrene, was supplanted in 1997 by 3-nitrobenzanthrone (3-NBA; Figure 8.10), which supplied 6 million mutations in the Ames test (Appendix A) per nanomole, compared with the 4.8 million caused by 1,8 dinitropyrene. The metabolic fate of nitroaromatics is a useful example of the conflicting roles that different enzymatic systems have in detoxifying, activating and excreting these toxins. They also illustrate the effects of reduction, rather than oxidation, which is a minor route in drug metabolism, but an important route in carcinogenesis.

Reductase enzymes are found all over cells in the cytosol and you might (or not) recall that they are the 'fuel pumps' for CYP isoforms, as they supply electrons that 'power' the enzymes. They are found in tissues that are most likely to meet significant levels of 3-NBA and other nitropolycyclics, such as the lungs and the gut. Since these compounds are thought to be lung carcinogens, it is likely that the reductases form the hydroxylamine which either hits DNA itself through oxidation to a nitrosoarene, or more likely, undergoes Phase II sulphation and GST conjugation reactions which lead to the formation of esters and sulphates which decompose, leading to the forma-

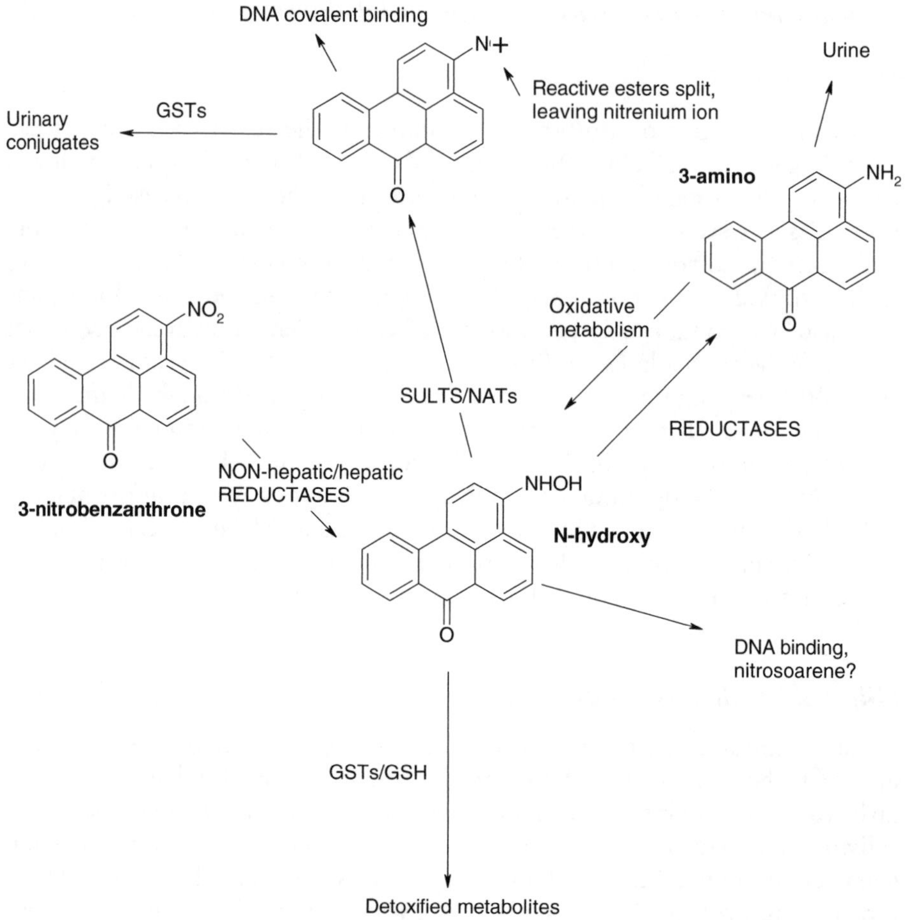

Figure 8.10 Processes of possible activation of 3-nitrobenzanthrone by reductive metabolism

tion of DNA reactive nitrenium ions (Figure 8.10). Whatever reactive species is formed, it certainly binds DNA but does not seem to be formed by CYP enzymes, so it appears that most of the activation is through reduction, followed by conjugation. All the enzymes necessary to activate these compounds (reductases, SULTs and GSTs) are found in the lung and the gut. Human reductases are particularly adept at this nitroreduction and many have suggested that nitropolycyclics are responsible for many cases of lung cancer in those exposed to diesel fumes, which, unfortunately, is most of us. The interesting feature of 3-NBA activation is that essentially the penultimate stage in carcinogenesis is the same as that for all aromatic amines, the formation of the hydroxylamine, which can then lead to nitrenium ion formation, via an unstable conjugated product. It is important to see the process in terms of varying stages of oxidation and reduction from aromatic amine to nitro derivative and back again.

Other occupational carcinogens: 1,3 butadiene

This chemical is among the top 50 chemicals manufactured in quantity in the developed world. It is derived from the petrochemical industry and it is used in the manufacture of styrene-butadiene synthetic rubber in the automotive industry, as well as for making belts, hoses, seals and gaskets, among many products. It has dozens of other uses in the electrical and plastics industries. As this agent is used in such quantity, it is manufactured in many facilities and significant numbers of individuals are exposed to 1,3 butadiene. It is now considered a human carcinogen, responsible for cancers of the lymphatic system, such as lymphosarcoma and reticulosarcoma. The compound has also been less strongly linked to stomach cancers. 1,3 Butadiene itself is capable of causing intoxication, as many organic solvents such as toluene and benzene can, but its carcinogenicity is rooted in its oxidative metabolism.

1,3 Butadiene is oxidized by CYPs 2E1 and 2A6 in human liver predominantly to a butanediol, which is not thought to be DNA reactive and is more polar than the parent and is conjugated by GSTs with GSH to form highly polar mercapturate-like derivatives, which are Phase III cleared from the hepatocyte. However, there are several minor pathways that involve attempts by CYPs and systems such as epoxide hydrolase to clear the compound to polar derivatives. What is interesting about 1,3 butadiene is the considerable number of highly DNA reactive products that are formed during its metabolism. These include epoxybutene, diepoxybutene, butenediol and epoxybutenediol (Figure 8.11). There is also evidence that crotonaldehyde is also formed, which is also DNA-reactive. All of these potential carcinogens can be dealt with by GSTs to reduce the possibility of their reaction with tissue macromolecules and it is probably significant that liver cancer is not associated with this compound, despite the number of potentially reactive species it forms. The liver is known for its highly efficient protective systems, and it is possible that 1,3 butadiene is carcinogenic to the lymphatic system and the stomach because various extra-hepatic cell systems can oxidize drugs (either by CYPs or activated neutrophils) to toxic metabolites, but the local protective cellular systems are insufficient to detoxify these species, leading ultimately to neoplasms. The liver also maintains high thiol levels (see paracetamol) and it usually takes very high GSH consumption before critical components of the thiol (cysteine/methionine) are exhausted. Extra-hepatic tissues, with the exceptions of the lung, gut and kidney, are likely to exhaust their thiol supplies much earlier than the liver, making them more vulnerable to DNA damage from reactive species such as those generated from 1,3 butadiene.

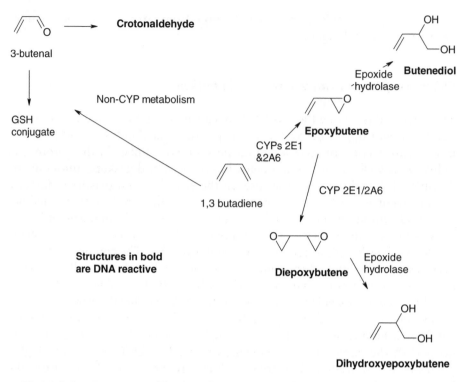

Figure 8.11 Formation of 1,3 butadiene into potential DNA-reactive carcinogens

Dietary carcinogens

Many carcinogens are thought to be present in foods, although they should be less likely to affect the developed world, due to the degree of processing which occurs in the food industry. Banned carcinogens such as the colouring Sudan I occasionally still appear in foods in the developed world due to oversights, stupidity and greed. Polycyclic aromatic amines are known to be a high risk in the cooking of meat products, however there are several classes of carcinogens that are found in foodstuffs that have been contaminated by moulds and fungi. The most potent are included in the general class of mycotoxins and these are known as aflatoxins.

Aflatoxins: introduction

This class of difuranocoumarins was unknown until 1960, when a bizarre disease wiped out over 100 000 turkeys in the UK. Eventually the disease was found to be caused by contamination of the birds' feed by *Aspergillus* fungus. These fungi grow on peanuts, corn, wheat, maize and many other oilseed crops. It is now believed that some form of mycotoxin contaminates perhaps a quarter of world grain production. *Aspergillus* grows best where conditions of storage are excessively damp and there is a lack of ventilation. The fungus forms dozens of different aflatoxins, which range from merely extremely, to ferociously toxic. They are unusual in that they are mutagenic, immunogenic and carcinogenic to anything living, from birds, animals and fish to humans. Their effects can be resolved into acute and chronic toxicity.

Aflatoxins: acute toxicity

Since the 1960s threat to the UK's Christmas lunch, there have been much more serious outbreaks of human acute aflatoxin effects, which are termed aflatoxicosis, particularly in India. This has been due to poverty, where rural people had to eat mouldy cereals or nothing at all. The effects of aflatoxicosis include rapid and massive liver damage, shown by severe jaundice, portal hypertension, abdominal ascites and a condition similar to the effects of cirrhosis, which is quickly fatal in 60–80 per cent of cases. Only a few milligrams per day of the aflatoxins is necessary for these toxins to induce liver failure in days or weeks. In some of the areas in India affected, all the domestic dogs died of the disease just before the humans developed it. These toxins can also cause a disease similar to Reye's syndrome, which is rooted in damage to mitochondria. This complaint is usually fatal and has been described widely. This is rare in the developed world, but the risk of eating food contaminated with aflatoxins and other mycotoxins imported from the Third World is a recognized one for developed countries and monitoring of samples of potentially affected imported foodstuffs is carried out for mycotoxin contamination.

Chronic toxicity

Aflatoxins are potent inducers of hepatocellular cancers and this has been shown in a variety of environments, such as in workers in peanut processing plants in the developed world, as well as in diets in Third World areas. High liver cancer rates have been correlated with the presence of aflatoxin metabolites in urine of affected individuals. These compounds are found in human and cows' milk, as well as in various dairy products, so there can be considerable exposure to these agents in human diets in many countries. Liver cancer rates in the developing world are far higher than developed areas and it is thought aflatoxins play a considerable role in these statistics. Aflatoxins are reasonably chemically stable, but roasting peanuts apparently decomposes them, so now you know. Aflatoxins affect growth in children and make them more susceptible to bacterial and other infections through immunosuppression.

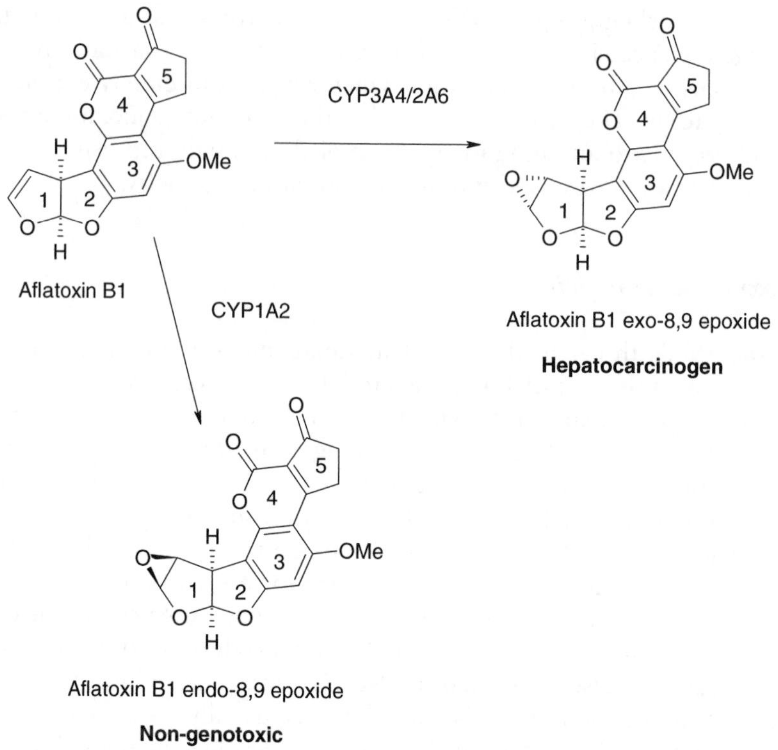

Figure 8.12 Structure of aflatoxin B1 and its carcinogenic and non-genotoxic metabolites

Aflatoxins: activation

The most toxic all these molecules is aflatoxin B1 (AFB1), followed by G1, B2 and G2 in terms of acute toxicity. The reason AFB1 is so dangerous is the presence of a double bond at the 8,9 position in ring 1 (dihydrofuran; Figure 8.12) as well as other substituents of the coumarin (rings 4 and 5). These compounds are thought to rely on CYP activation for their toxicity and the major isoform involved appears to be 3A4, but 1A2 and 3A5 may also be involved. Many metabolites are formed, but the key carcinogenic and general macromolecule-reactive agent is the 8,9 exo-epoxide, formed only by 3A4. If you look at Figure 8.12, the best way to visualize the shape of the molecule is to imagine that rings 2–5 are basically planar (flat) while ring 1 sticks up at an approximately 45° angle to the horizontal. The term 'exo' for the epoxide means that the oxygen dips away from you as you look at the molecule on the page. There is an 'endo' epoxide, where the oxygen would be oriented towards you as you looked at the molecule.

The reason the 8,9 exo-epoxide is so dangerous is the precision where it interacts with DNA. It binds at the N7 position of guanine residues. This is obviously a direct consequence of the three-dimensional shape of the molecule, as the 8,9 'endo' epoxide and other aflatoxin metabolites do not intercalate with DNA in this position and are not as genotoxic. This intercalating effect of the epoxide causes a transversion of guanine and thymidine at codon 249 of the p53 gene of the liver. This may be linked with the route of induction of hepatocarcinoma.

Detoxification of aflatoxins

It would be expected that processes would detoxify the 8,9 exo epoxide and the most obvious candidates would be epoxide hydrolase, GSH and GST enzymes. The detoxification of this metabolite is not completely understood; although its half-life is so short (around 10 seconds), epoxide hydrolase may well not have a significant role in the formation of the diol, which apparently has an even shorter half-life. GSH does not react directly with the epoxide at pH 7, so an important route of clearance from the cell is likely to be via GST catalysed thiol conjugation. GST Alpha, Mu and Theta are thought to be involved with aflatoxin 8,9 epoxide clearance. The fate of the genotoxic metabolites of aflatoxins is the subject of much current research.

Prevention of aflatoxin damage

Since these toxins make a massive impact in developing world health, the major concern is to educate ordinary food producers about the dangers of poor feed storage. In addition, the alleviation of poverty, although highly unlikely, would be invaluable in preventing the situation where there is no choice but to eat contaminated food. On a more realistic preventative level, it is known that it is possible to decontaminate feedstuffs with ammonia treatment, which has been shown to reduce the capability of aflatoxins to cause tumours in animals, most likely by chemical decomposition of the toxins by the ammonia under reduced pressure. For the food consumers themselves, inhibitors of CYP3A4 should be protective, although it is difficult to see how this would practically be applied to prevent aflatoxin carcinogenicity in everyday diets. A more promising idea has been tried with the chemopreventative agent oltipraz. This dithiolthione was originally designed to kill schistosomes (you remember, the vile human parasitic trematodes), but it is a potent chemopreventative and inhibits carcinogenesis in aromatic amine-mediated bladder cancers and other neoplasms. It operates by increasing GSH synthesis and inducing GST enzymative performance. Detoxification of reactive species is thus stimulated by this drug. A large-scale Phase II clinical trial in China has shown some encouraging results, where 500 mg of

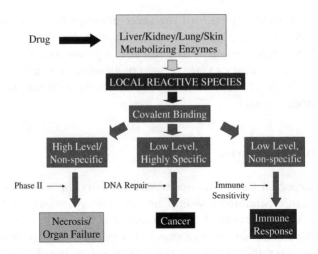

Figure 8.13   The links between drug metabolism, formation of active species, covalent binding and irreversible damage to the organism. Phase II defences are crucial to prevent organ failure from high levels of covalent binding, whilst Phase II defence mechanisms as well as DNA repair are crucial to avoid carcinogenicity as a result of specific DNA binding of reactive species. For an immune response, the sensitivity of the individuals' immune system may be the major determinate of whether a response occurs

oltipraz weekly for two months showed a reduction in aflatoxin adducts in urine. Knowledge of the process of aflatoxin carcinogenicity, as well as the use of various regimes for diminishing the formation and effect of the toxic species plus useful urinary biomarkers for monitoring of beneficial effect, should reduce the death toll from these 'natural' toxins.

8.7   Summary of biotransformational toxicity

Although irreversible toxicity is seen in several guises, such as necrosis, immunological damage and malignancy, the common thread is the formation of unstable and damaging species from a xenobiotic compound (Figure 8.13). Ultimately, virtually all of us form these species, but the combination of our net exposure to these toxins and our individual detoxification and repair mechanisms decide whether we will suffer Type B toxicity or tolerate and clear the agent without ill effects.

Appendix A
Methods in Drug Metabolism

A.1 Introduction

When a new chemical entity has shown potency in a biological test system and the decision is made to develop it as a drug, the next stage must be the determination of its metabolic fate. Drugs are designed and selected for their pharmacodynamic performance and what happens to them metabolically is in effect 'pot luck'. Clearly, a drug is only effective if it is in contact with its target tissue and can be maintained within the therapeutic window, so several metabolic factors will contribute to its success as a therapeutic entity:

- *Rate of its metabolism*: drugs which are very rapidly, or very slowly, cleared can present problems in accurate control of plasma levels, and with very long half-life agents, the risk of toxicity can be considerable.

- *Multiple CYP metabolism*: this is a very positive attribute, as if many CYPs can clear the drug and one or two are inhibited by co-administered drugs, there will usually be a route of metabolism to prevent serious accumulation.

- *Likelihood of 'DDI's*: if a drug is likely to inhibit a major CYP isoform, or its metabolism is blocked by a known series of inhibitors, then the likelihood of DDIs or drug–drug interactions will be high.

- *Single CYP clearance*: this can be seen as vulnerability, as inhibition of the CYP will easily lead to accumulation and potential toxicity. Conversely, induction of this CYP will lead to treatment failure.

- *Polymorphisms*: if the metabolism of the drug is dependent on a CYP isoform that is polymorphic, this erodes the mass-marketability and safety of the drug. Clinically, a drug that was subject to a single poly-

Human Drug Metabolism, Michael D. Coleman
© 2005 John Wiley & Sons, Ltd

morphic CYP clearance may well be restricted in its usage or would require close medical supervision, as the risks of toxicity and drug failure would be considerable.

- *Linearity of metabolism*: most drugs are cleared at a rate proportional to their intake (linear metabolism). Some (ethanol, phenytoin) are cleared at a constant rate, irrespective of intake (non-linear metabolism). If the metabolism of the drug is non-linear, then it will be difficult to predict plasma levels with ascending dose, which will also make the drug difficult to use and subject to toxicity and potential failure.

- *Metabolism to toxins*: drug metabolism may lead to the formation of toxic products in some or the entire target patient group.

Although any one of the above factors can cause a drug to be abandoned as a therapeutic option, there are several drugs available clinically where all the factors above apply. The reason these agents have entered clinical practice and other less problematic drugs were abandoned is strongly dependent on the condition targeted and if there are any alternative agents currently available. Clearly, a new beta-blocker which has some mild toxicity will have little chance of success; however, a toxic but effective Alzheimer's disease or anti-cancer agent will pass the 'risk versus benefit' evaluation made by regulatory agencies, as there is little else available.

In most countries it remains a legal requirement for basic toxicological whole animal studies to be carried out with a new drug, and the hepatic metabolism of the drug will be determined *in vitro* using the same animal model. Although these initial 'pre-clinical' studies evaluate the potential toxicity of the drug in terms of target organs and tissues, it is essential that some estimate of the metabolic fate of a drug must be made in man. This is because both the distant and recent history of drug development is littered with examples of potent and safe drugs in animals that became toxic in humans – and in the case of drugs such as tamoxifen, the other way around. Although drug studies in human volunteers cannot take place before pre-clinical (animal studies) work has been carried out, there are various systems which can be used to determine at least the structure and possible therapeutic and toxic effects of drug metabolites using human tissues.

A.2   Human liver microsomes

The most basic tool for the determination of the metabolic fate of a candidate drug is the fractionation of human liver through differential centrifugation. The liver is homogenized on ice and centrifuged at around $10\,000\,g$ to remove cellular and nuclear membranes, as well as larger cellular organelles. The supernatant is then centrifuged at $100\,000\,g$ to provide a pellet that contains the smooth endplasmic reticulum (Chapter 3) where the CYP isoforms and UGTs reside. This is termed a 'microsomal' pellet and it is then stored at least $-70°C$ until the content of the total CYP content is measured using a standard method that exploits the ability of carbon monoxide to bind the CYPs. Every human liver also has a unique profile of individual CYP isoforms and the livers are usually characterized in terms of their ability to metabolize certain substrates that are known to be cleared by particular CYP isoforms. As there is so much variability in human liver microsomal systems, in trying to determine the metabolic profile of a candidate drug, it will be studied using many human livers to build up a picture as to which isoforms predominantly oxidize the drug. The products of the oxidation are usually extracted and purified, then analysed by a variety of techniques such as nuclear magnetic resonance (NMR) where a chemical structure can be assigned to particular metabolites. This assumes that the metabolites are stable enough to survive the analysis, which is not always the case. It is possible to confirm which CYP isoforms are oxidizing the drug by the use of specific CYP inhibitors as well as antibodies which have been raised to CYP isoforms, which also block their activity. It is also possible by using specific substrates of various isoforms to determine if the new agent has any inhibitory effects on the main CYP isoforms.

Once the CYP or CYPs have been identified which confirms the oxidation of the drug, other microsomal studies can be carried out using human lung, kidney and gut to determine what contribution these organs will make to the overall oxidative metabolism of the drug. The addition of UDGPA as a cofactor will activate the UGTs in the liver to provide a preliminary evaluation as to the degree of glucuronidation that may occur. Human liver cytosolic fractions (S9 fractions) can also be used to determine levels of sulphation and GSTs. In addition, cytosolic and microsomal epoxide hydrolase activity can also be measured.

Supplies of human liver have dwindled somewhat, happily because liver transplants are now more common and more successful than in previous years. The disadvantages of human liver homogenate preparations include the wide variation and the detailed observation of only some parts of a complex system of metabolism. If a very reactive oxidative metabolite is detected which is cytotoxic, this suggests that the drug could be a hepatotoxin or may be reactive elsewhere. However, what cannot be determined with human microsomes is that detoxification and transport systems might just as well avidly clear the toxic metabolite and no systemic or organ-directed toxicity occurs. Essentially, liver microsomal and cytosolic fractions are not a complete system and may not always bear much resemblance to the drug's clearance *in vivo*.

A.3 Human hepatocytes

For obvious reasons it is very difficult to obtain human liver suitable for the preparation of hepatocytes; however, hepatocyte preparations are still the

'Holy Grail' of human drug metabolism. They provide an opportunity to study the completed metabolic 'treatment' the new drug is likely to undergo in the patient. The cells can be separated from the liver tissue matrix by treatment with collagenases in calcium-free media. Depending on the amount of tissue obtained, several million cells can be isolated. Although the same interindividual variation problems occur as in microsomal human liver systems. Problems where CYP expression would tail off within a few hours of isolation have been alleviated by the use of various additives such as drugs and co-cultured cells, which maintain stability in hepatocyte CYP isoform expression. In addition, the cells can be cultured between two gel layers (sandwich cultures), which sometimes maintains CYP expression. Hepatocyte cell lines have been immortalized and will express a variety of CYPs and other metabolizing systems. Hepatocytes provide the closest representation as to which metabolites are likely to be formed *in vivo* and they are also the first indicator of whether a drug is likely to act as an inducer of hepatic metabolism. There is now a strong literature on the relationship between CYP induction in hepatocytes and how this corresponds to *in vivo* induction in humans. Other disadvantages of hepatocytes include the aforementioned difficulties in obtaining human cells, the labour-intensive nature of the preparation, the variable results that occur on cryopreservation, as well as loss of the hepatic cellular matrix. This latter point can be addressed by using hepatocyte couplets, which are cells in collagen matrixes. This facilitates the study of hepatic drug and nutrient transport. Hepatocytes are at least as predictive of future drug clearance as liver slice systems, which require much more complex equipment to operate. Overall, hepatocytes retain a vital role in drug metabolism screening and culture systems will continue to be developed.

A.4   Heterologous systems

In the late 1980s and early 1990s, the technology for the excision of complete human CYP genes as well as their reductases and their insertion into bacterial, eukaryotic or viral vectors was perfected. This allowed the almost unlimited expression of specific human CYP isoforms, as well as many UGTs, SULTs and GSTs. This facilitates the detailed study of how a particular isoform metabolizes a candidate drug, along with inhibition studies and detailed kinetic measurements, such as K_i's and the rate of formation of the metabolite. Often a new drug will be cleared to some extent by the major CYPs, such as 1A2, 2C8/9/19, 2B series and 3A4/5. Occasionally, a drug will be cleared by only one CYP preferentially and metabolism by other isoforms may be slow or non-existent. At this stage, there will be concern if the drug is cleared by CYP2D6, which automatically ensures that a considerable group of patients will have impaired drug clearance and this might lead to toxicity. If no other CYPs or Phase II systems can clear the 2D6 substrate, then it would be less likely to proceed further towards the clinic, due to the problems the route of clearance would cause. Similarly, if the drug were to be a potent inhibitor of the major CYPs, there would be problems co-administering it with other agents. In addition, inhibition of the endogenous steroid-metabolizing CYPs in drugs that are to be used chronically would lead to unacceptable disruption of steroid metabolism. The protease inhibitor anti-HIV drugs are mostly potent inhibitors of CYP3A4 and are difficult to co-administer with other drug regimens, which can be complex in HIV patients. It is probably unlikely that these drugs would have been adopted had they not been the only real alternative for the therapy of a lethal disease.

Studies with specific oxidative and conjugative enzyme isoforms do provide the possibility of estimating how much of a drug might be cleared in humans, although allometric (related) studies in animals are also employed for such estimates. There are limitations to the use of single expressed CYPs for the study of the metabolism of a candidate drug. There is an assumption that the gene cloned and expressed is identical to the CYPs in all patients, which may not necessarily be true. Although a drug may be avidly cleared by a particular CYP *in vitro*, there is no guarantee that this will occur *in vivo*, due to a host of different factors, such as degree of absorption, gut first pass and Phase III egress by P-glycoprotein and similar transporters. In addition, the basic heterologous systems have no mechanisms for the estimation of the potential of a drug to cause enzyme induction.

Induction can be studied through the expression of the control systems for human CYPs, which include the complete xenobiotic response elements (XREs) and PXR/RXR systems. Binding of candidate drugs to human PXR as well as CAR systems can provide a strong indication of which mechanism is operating in the induction process that would have been first discovered from human hepatocyte work. Studies with 'knockout' transgenic mice which have had human CYP control systems inserted into their genes can also illustrate the potential operation of the compound in an *in vivo* setting with the human genes operating.

A.5 Toxicological metabolism-based assays

For an experimental drug, much work will obviously focus on the particular metabolizing system that might form reactive metabolites. However, it is also important to visualize what these species will actually do to a cell. So, in the last 30 years, considerable efforts have been made to determine what effect toxic metabolites might have on human cells or tissues. This requires the design of in vitro systems that can model the balance between the formation of toxic species and their effects on a human target cell. The simplest test of all is probably trypan blue exclusion, where recently dead cells cannot exclude the dye and swell as well as looking bloated and grotesque.

To study the effects of a reactive species, there are a number of assays that can showcase damage to DNA, cellular respiration, or other functional aspects of a target cell.

Ames Test

Although originally developed in the 1970's to determine if a chemical was mutagenic, it was quickly realized that the effects of reactive species could easily be incorporated into the test to make it relevant to drug development. Briefly, the test uses *Salmonella typhimurium* bacteria, which have been altered to make them dependent on supplied histidine in their media. If they are plated out onto media without histidine they will not grow. If a mutagenic agent is added, it causes reverse mutations and the bacteria grow on the deficient media as they can now make their own histidine. The more colonies that appear, the more mutagenic the chemical. The addition of human microsomes and S9 fractions made the test useful for new drugs. Indeed, all the major human CYPs can currently be expressed in separate strains of Salmonella to determine if the test agent has the potential to form a mutagen. It is important to carry out this test before a large investment is made in a compound, as if it fails, then it's 'dead'. Interestingly, several older drugs do fail it, such as isoniazid. Aflatoxins obviously fail, as do diesel emissions.

Comet Assay

Detects DNA damage in cells by subjecting the DNA to an electric current in a gel (electrophoresis) in solutions of different pH. The DNA moves through the gell forming a characteristic 'comet' like shape and DNA strand breaks are visualized using fluorescent dyes.

Micronucleus Test

This test can be carried out *in vivo* or *in vitro* and this detects micronuclei, which are formed during mitosis when a chromosome is lagging behind and may be lost (aneugenic event) or when a chromosome is broken (clastogenic event). These faults prevent the chromosomes integrating into the daughter nuclei and can be counted. The more of these events, the more toxic the agent.

DNA Microarray

These assays depend on amplifying the mRNA from cells or tissues exposed to toxic agents and comparing it with control mRNA expression. This can create enormous amounts of data that has required the rapid evolution of software systems to process it all. The data can be difficult to interpret out of context and most may not have immediate meaning. Some recent studies with liver tissue microarrays after treatment with NSAIDS in mice have shown cellular responses that usually occur after exposure to bacterial lipopolysaccharides. This was eventually reconciled with the clinical effects of these drugs in gut wall perforation and the microarray was found to be picking up the liver's reaction to the presence of gut bacteria.

Other Cell Assays

Flow cytometry can be used to study the effects of a toxin on the cell cycle, both from the apoptotic and necrotic viewpoints. Various dyes are used, which either bind DNA or become activated within metabolically active cell areas, such as mitochondria. The MTT test indicates whether a cell is broadly capable of oxidizing a dye to a blue product which is easily measured by a plate reader.

Combination Models

Once the assays have been selected to study a particular aspect of drug toxicity, the next stage is what method to use to bring the source of the reactive species close enough to the target cell to cause cell damage. Current recombinant technology allows two major options to study this relationship between toxin former and 'victim'.

'One Compartment' Models

The simplest system here is the mixture in one sample tube, of victim cells such as human mononuclear leucocytes, or adherent cell lines grown on a matrix with human liver microsomes, hepatocytes or even expressed human CYPs. After a period of time, the human cells would be separated from the mix and assayed for toxicity as detailed above. A more sophisticated version of this method is also used where human CYP systems are inserted heterologously into human cell lines, such as HepG2 cells. A reactive species could be made by the particular CYP and the degree of toxicity measured. These systems are very efficient at modelling short-lived species that cannot escape a cell, or tissue before reacting with a macromolecule.

'Two Compartment Models'

Toxins which are relatively stable like hydroxylamines, are better modelled in multi-compartment systems which separate the source of the reactive species from the victim cells by a porous barrier, which keeps cellular material apart, but allows small molecules to pass through. Dialysis systems comprising Teflon disks are useful for adapting to this purpose. The victim cells can be aseptically assayed and the ability of a toxin to travel some distance and still inflict toxicity can be evaluated. Modular systems like those described above can be used with virtually any cell type and many different sources of reactive species.

Summary

Although all in vitro systems have their limitations, they are growing in sophistication and can yield important insights into the metabolism and toxicity of current and future therapeutic drugs. It is highly controversial whether they will eventually replace animal models in drug metabolism. The main reason why humans suffer drug toxicity from agents tested in animals is related to the lack of variation of animal models, which are too reproducible (for regulatory purposes) and do not reflect the enormous heterogeneity of the human race. Some animal models are undergoing development using recombinant technologies that will effectively 're-create' diversity so as to more closely model the human system. Both animal and human in vitro systems will continue to be developed to find the most reliable systems for predicting human drug toxicity. Data from these systems has been the mainstay of the development of *in silico* predictive systems that are currently under development.

A.6 *In silico* studies

In the past five years, rapid advances in the availability of specific software packages designed to design new drugs combined with easy access to extremely cheap and fast PCs have widened access to some serious 'laboursaving' in drug discovery. The older laborious methods of synthesizing thousands of probably useless drugs have been supplanted by software packages that can exploit huge databases accrued by either commercial or academic institutions to search for pharmacophores, i.e. specific areas of molecules which have high pharmacodynamic activity, and toxophores, i.e. areas which are likely to lead to either direct toxicity or the propensity to be metabolized to something unpleasant. This software design process is evolving extremely quickly and has been combined with a process known as combinatorial synthesis. This involves using a form of chemical 'mass production' to exploit many basic chemical structures, like modular platforms seen in the car industry. This means that hundreds of analogues can be designed and then synthesized in days using robots that make small quantities of not very pure compound. These can be rapidly screened and if there is a 'hit', i.e. pharma-codynamic activity, the effect can be fine-tuned in days rather than years. Software-directed combinatorial synthesis did at first create 'bottlenecks' where thousands of potential drugs were designed and made in days, which would then take months to test. Much investment has accelerated pharma-codynamic test systems to 'catch up' with the potential flow of useful compounds. *In silico* drug metabolism software has matched this targeted drug design by incorporating large databases on human CYP metabolism of hundreds of thousands of structures and systems such as the simCYP (University of Sheffield). This system contains vast amounts of data on human genetic, physiological and metabolic systems, which is combined with the *in vitro* clearance data. This provides a platform where the likelihood of a new entity to cause problems in the clinic can be modelled with a greater degree of certainty than has been the case to the present. Due to the volume of data available on the liver, hepatotoxicity has been most successfully predicted using these systems. Drug development is a famously expensive and risky process, and the drug industry is investing strongly in *in silico* systems to minimize costs and accelerate the time frame for candidate agents to reach the clinic. One problem that cannot be changed is the enormous 'leap of faith' which is made when a drug which has been tested on perhaps 10 000 individuals in 4–5 years, but then enters the marketplace and within 6 months is in use in half a million patients. Considerable expectation is being placed in the predictive powers of *in silico* systems to reduce the potential for drugs to be withdrawn due to unforeseen toxicity and treatment failure due to metabolic processes.

Appendix B
Metabolism of Major
Illicit Drugs

B.1 Introduction

It is certain that the use of various plant and animal sourced chemicals by humans for their pleasurable effects predates recorded time. These agents have been and continue to be directly ingested, smoked, extracted, inhaled and manufactured using a variety of processes. Often it is the case that drugs that are abused have vital clinical roles, such as the opiates; however, others, such as cocaine, amphetamines and PCP, are of little or no current clinical use. In general, those seeking some form of chemical stimulation will pay any price and often go to any length to obtain it. Virtually every culture in history has used a particular favoured drug or group of drugs, based on availability and tradition. It is only relatively recently that the use of chemicals for pleasure has been subject to legal restraint, to the end that nicotine and alcohol are the only freely available drugs to the public in most Western countries. Most other 'hard' drugs are illegal and although judicial tolerance to milder agents such as cannabis is gradually building, developed world societies expend vast resources to stem their own unquenchable thirst for mind-altering substances.

The ethical and moral implications of illegal drug usage are clearly outside the scope of this book; however, scientifically, it is informative to discuss the metabolic fate of some of the more commonly used and interesting abused drugs and how this might impinge on their pharmacological effects and those of prescription drugs.

B.2 Opiates

These agents include opium, morphine, diacetyl morphine (heroin), methadone, codeine and dihydrocodeine. Several other prescription drugs have

Human Drug Metabolism, Michael D. Coleman
© 2005 John Wiley & Sons, Ltd

opiate-like effects, which include fentanyl, meperidine, pethidine, buprenor-phine and oxycodone. With the morphine derivatives, essentially they are all converted to morphine and its metabolites once they are absorbed.

Morphine

Morphine and its relatives act on mu-opioid receptors and are the most effec-tive agents of relief available for most types of pain, although interestingly, around a third of patients receiving these drugs do not receive adequate anal-gesia. It remains controversial whether this is due to inadequate dosage and all pain should respond eventually, or whether some types of pain (e.g. neu-ropathic pain) are insensitive. The euphoric aspects of morphine and its deriv-atives effects have been the basis for their abuse and they induce tolerance and dependence. Addiction to morphine-like compounds is a worldwide problem, which is as acute in the countries that grow opium poppies as it is in the developed world. During opiate addiction, aside from dangers associ-ated with the lifestyle and the particular attendant dangers of the intravenous route of administration, fatal respiratory depression is a consequence of overdose.

The pharmacological potency of morphine resides in several aspects of its structure (Figure B.1). The tertiary nitrogen and its methyl group are required for analgesic activity and changes to either moiety will reduce activity – indeed substitution of the methyl group with larger groups yields antagonists. Sub-stitutions to the 3-hydroxyl group on the phenolic group usually result in loss of activity, whilst changes to the 6-hydroxy group can increase activity.

Morphine metabolism

Morphine is cleared mostly by conjugation to 3- and 6-glucuronides and these are the major plasma and urinary metabolites, with less than 5 per cent of a 3-sulphate and around 10 per cent of the dose appearing in urine unchanged. A diglucuronide and a 3,6-glucuronide is also formed in small quantities. Less than 1 per cent of morphine is methylated to codeine (3-methoxymorphine) and there is some N-dealkylation at the tertiary nitro-gen, forming an N-oxide as well as the formation of normorphine. It appears that virtually no gut wall metabolism occurs in man, although the main metabolites are formed in a number of other organs as well as the kidney and liver. The liver is probably the major site of morphine metabolism, as cirrhotic patients show a substantially increased half-life of the parent drug. Renal failure also increases morphine half-life in man and when renal func-tion declines, the drug and its 6-glucuronide accumulate unless the dose is reduced. Although the 3-glucuronide has no analgesic activity (but some

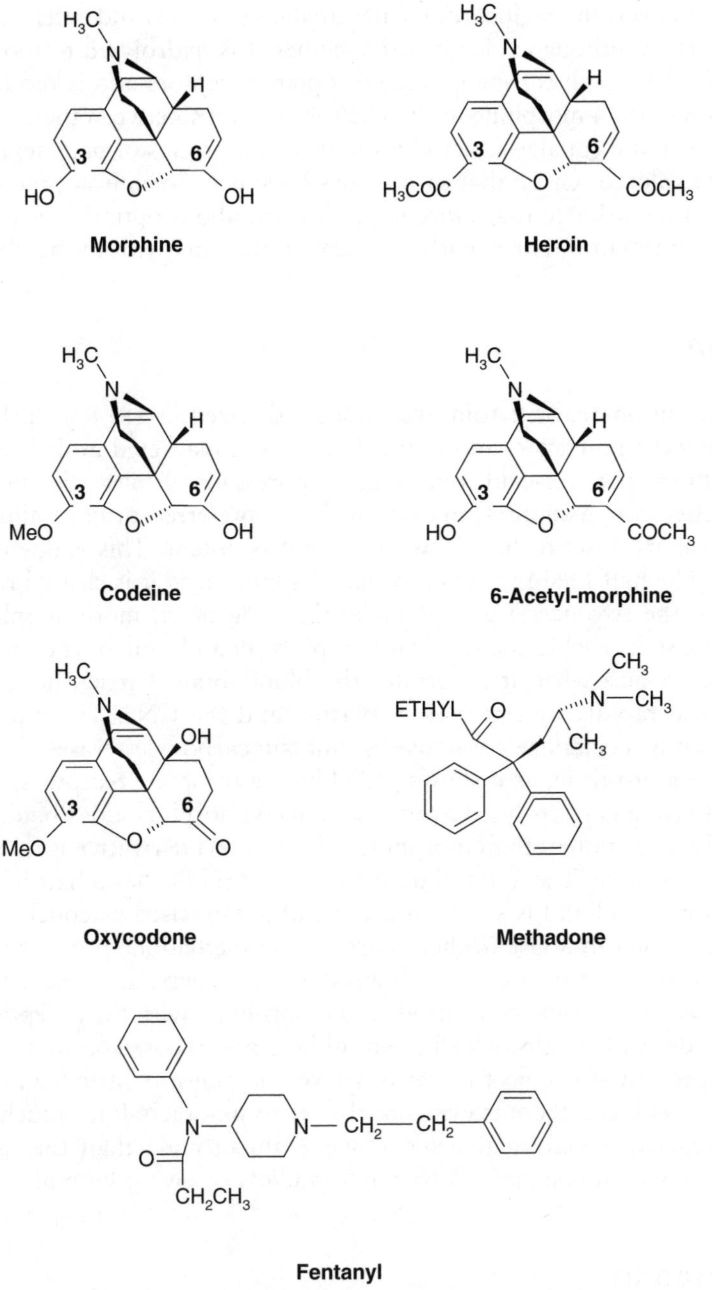

Figure B.1 Structures of morphine-based opiates and the synthetic opiates, methadone, oxycodone and fentanyl

stimulant effect) the 6-glucuronide has analgesic actions and enters the blood-brain barrier, although it is unclear whether it is hydrolysed to morphine in the brain. The 6-glucuronide binds to opiate receptors and is thought to be more potent than morphine itself. The relationships between the clearance of morphine and its analgesic activities in different groups of patients remain to be fully explored. Given that these drugs have been in clinical practice for so long, it is remarkable that more is not known about optimizing their therapeutic performance, particularly in terminal patients with intractable pain.

Heroin

Diacetyl morphine, or heroin, was first synthesized in 1874 with the aim of increasing the potency of morphine; it was even marketed in the early twentieth century as a non-addictive cough suppressant. Whilst it is undoubtedly an effective cough suppressant, heroin is the preferred drug of abuse of the opiates, as its onset or 'hit' is as rapid as it is potent. This is due to several factors. The half-life in man is less than 5 minutes, so it is cleared rapidly. In addition, the two acetyl groups make the drug much more lipophilic than morphine so it reaches the CNS more rapidly. In addition, during its progress to the CNS and when it penetrates the blood–brain barrier, heroin can be hydrolysed rapidly by esterases in plasma and the CNS. The most studied and recently crystallized esterase is human carboxylesterase-1, or hCE1. Heroin is a pro-drug, as it shows little binding to opiate receptors, but if the 3-acetyl group is hydrolysed away, the 6-acetylmorphine does bind, and it is probably more potent than morphine. The 6-acetyl derivative is then hydrolysed to morphine. The 6-acetyl derivative of morphine has a half-life of 6–25 minutes in blood and is stable in urine and is thus used as conclusive proof of relapsed heroin abuse in those enrolled on methadone programmes. This is because no other opiate is metabolized to the 6-acetyl derivative. The metabolic profile of heroin use is the same as morphine, with the exception of the 6-acetyl derivative. Although heroin addicts are exposed to many different substances and are subject to various systemic abnormalities (e.g. effects on glucose tolerance), there is evidence that heroin addicts form much more of the pharmacologically active morphine 6-glucuronide than the non-active 3-glucuronide, in comparison with non-addicts receiving heroin.

Methadone

This synthetic opiate was first synthesized in Germany during the Second World War in response to opiate shortages. Although it does not resemble other opiates chemically, it does act on opiate receptors and is cleared relatively slowly. Its best-known use clinically is as a substitute for heroin, so

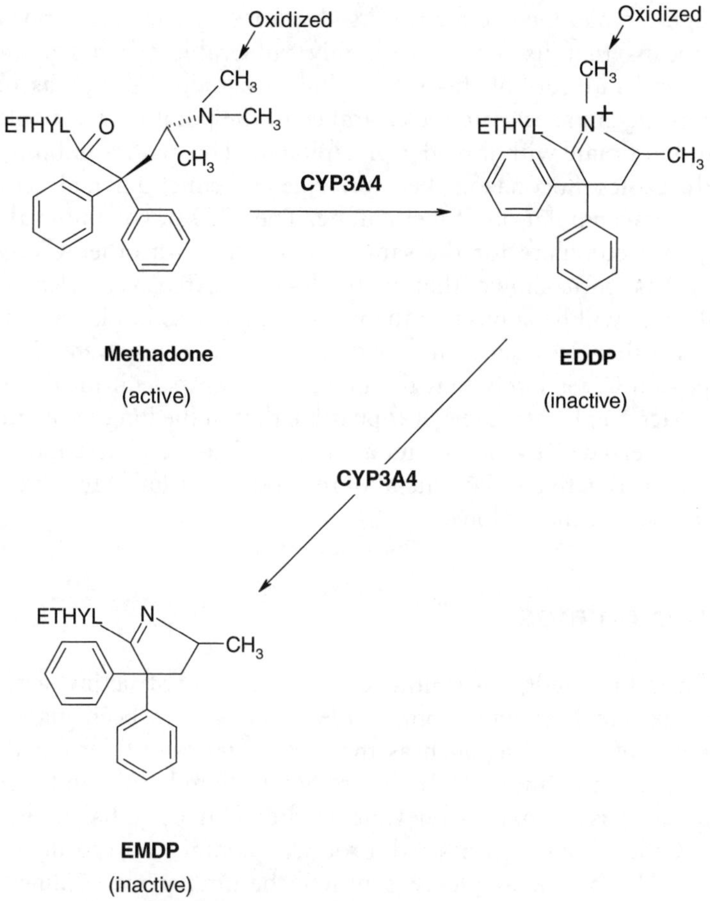

Figure B.2 Dual, sequential N-demethylation of methadone to inactive products by CYP3A4 in the gut and liver

aiding gradual withdrawal from addiction. It can fulfil this role, as its half-life is much longer than other opiates, at around 24 hours in man. The drug is very effective orally and is very cheap, so it is finding increasing use in pain control in cancer. The process of methadone clearance is a very good example of how CYP isoforms can carry out a simple operation on a compound that causes a marked change in structure and subsequent loss of function. Methadone undergoes two sequential CYP3A4-mediated N-demethylations (Figure B.2); the first methyl group is removed from the tertiary nitrogen and the molecule essentially reacts with itself and immediately cyclizes forming EDDP (2-ethylidene-1,5-dimethyl-3,3-diphenylpyrrolidine) which is then demethylated again to form EMDP (2-ethyl-5-methyl-3,3-diphenylpyraline). Both metabolites are inactive.

Although methadone is effective, its clearance by such an important CYP as 3A4 means that its levels are highly vulnerable to change caused by inhibitors and inducers of this CYP. Clinically, inducers such as phenytoin and rifampicin can accelerate the clearance to the point that not only is analgesia lost, but opiate withdrawal is precipitated. The major inhibitors of 3A4, such as the azoles (fluconazole, ketoconazole and cimetidine), all retard clearance causing accumulation of methadone. The SSRI fluvoxamine also causes the drug to accumulate for the same reason. As with other CYP3A4 substrates, it has been shown that methadone is extensively cleared by gut CYP3A4, so it will be subject to the marked increases in plasma levels associated with other 3A4 substrates that undergo high pre-systemic clearance like terfenadine. It is likely that the presence of grapefruit juice may have a potent impact on plasma levels. It is possible that in the long term, methadone might be superseded by one of its analogues, l-α-acetylmethadol, which is demethylated to active opiate metabolites and has a half-life which is more than twice that of methadone.

Designer opiates

With a basic knowledge of synthetic chemistry and structure–activity relationships, extremely potent 'home-made' opiates have been made over the last 30 years or so. Some, such as the methylated and fluorinated fentanyl derivatives, are thousands of times more potent than heroin and their metabolism/clearance is virtually irrelevant as they can be lethal in less than 5 minutes. Other home-synthesized products contain extraordinarily toxic impurities. The best example is 'synthetic heroin', a meperidine analogue known as MPPP (1-methyl-4-phenyl-4-propionpiperidine). When the synthesis is poorly managed, MPTP (1-methyl-4-phenyl-1,2,5,6-tetrahydropyridine) appears, which causes a permanent Parkinsonian condition, as it is metabolized by MAO-B to MPP+, a potent and selective neurotoxin.

B.3 Cocaine

Cocaine originated in South America and 70–90 per cent of the world's supply still comes from Colombia alone. The drug is a potent inhibitor of presynaptic dopamine and noradrenaline reuptake by transporter systems and the pharmacological effect is through the persistence of the neurotransmitters. Judging from its popularity and the cravings that it causes in addiction, to classify the drug merely as a stimulant is a spectacularly inadequate description. The drug also acts to block sodium channels and inhibit action potentials in peripheral nerves. During its use for its local anaesthetic effects, its vasoconstrictive actions are useful to restrict bleeding. However, many other

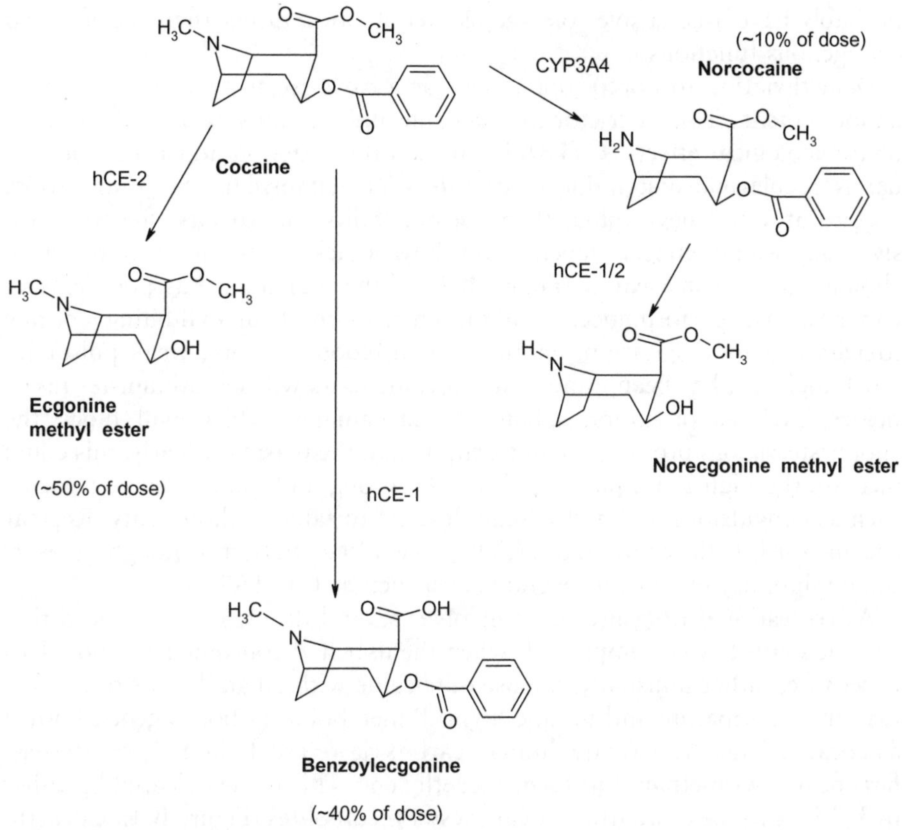

Figure B.3 Cocaine metabolism, showing the role of CYP3A4 in demethylation (toxic pathway) and human carboxylesterases (hCE-1 and 2) known as butyryl or pseudocholinesterases

safer analogues can be used which do not have the attendant cardiotoxic effects. Although its stimulant effects when smoked as the base (crack) or when injected intravenously occur within 10–15 seconds and are intense, this does not last more than 5–10 minutes. This is due to the extremely rapid clearance of the drug.

As with heroin, human cholinesterase/carboxylesterases (mainly hCE-1 and hCE-2) metabolize most of the drug (Figure B.3) as they are found in quantity in the plasma as well as most other organs, particularly the liver. The hCE enzymes are high capacity, low affinity and are found in the endoplasmic reticulum in the liver. Drugs like cocaine are subject to widespread and rapid attack by these enzymes, hence its short half-life. About half the dose is de-esterified to ecgonine methyl ester, which is low in toxicity, as it has little vasoconstrictor effects or cardiotoxicity. The hCE group of enzymes are thought to be capable of metabolizing a very wide variety of substrates and probably have a defensive role against xenobiotics, rather than specific vital endogenous functions.

Demethylation to norcocaine is seen as a toxic pathway, as norcocaine is a more potent vasoconstrictor than cocaine and it retains the rest of cocaine's pharmacological effects. CYP3A4 catalyses this reaction and if the individual is regularly using inducers of this CYP (rifamycins, St John's wort, barbiturates and nevirapine) then the possibility for toxicity due to excessive norcocaine effects depends on how quickly the hCEs and serum cholinesterases can clear it (Figure B.3). If the individual has poor plasma cholinesterase performance, then the chances of them exhibiting cocaine toxicity (tremors, agitation, paranoia, high blood pressure, weak pulse) are much higher. It has been known that cocaine users will self-administer insecticides, such as organophosphates or carbamates, which will block the cholinesterases to prolong cocaine's survival in the plasma. Clearly, this could increase the high but equally go horribly wrong and induce severe toxicity, such as convulsions and arrhythmia, leading to fatal cardiotoxicity. Regular cocaine use is believed to induce CYP2B1, whilst acutely, it is thought to exert some inhibitory effects on several CYPs, such as CYP1A2.

As recreational drug use often involves several drugs, it was noticed that cocaine's effects were 'improved' when the user had consumed ethanol. This is because, rather unusually, the use of cocaine with ethanol leads to the formation of a separate and unique 'hybrid' metabolite of both agents, known as cocaethylene. Apparently, human carboxylesterase 1 (hCE-1) transesterifies cocaine with ethanol to form cocaethylene. This is then cleared by either hCE-1 or 2 to the more usual cocaine ester metabolites (Figure B.4). Cocaethylene is thought to induce a more potent state of euphoria than cocaine and the dysphoria (down) is much less unpleasant. Cocaethylene seems to be able to retard the clearance of cocaine and prolong its effects. The downside is that it is more cardiotoxic and can induce convulsions at lower concentrations. Although any drug of addiction can be destructive, cocaine in all its forms is particularly efficient at destroying its victims remorselessly, both physically and mentally.

B.4   Hallucinogens

LSD

Lysergic acid diethylamide (D isomer) was first synthesized by Albert Hofman in 1938, who then consumed it and attempted to ride home on his bicycle with predictably hilarious results. The US military flirted briefly with the drug as a non-lethal weapon and entertainment figures such as Cary Grant used it under supervision as part of various experimental psychiatric treatments in the 1950s and 1960s. Increasing abuse led to its proscription in the late

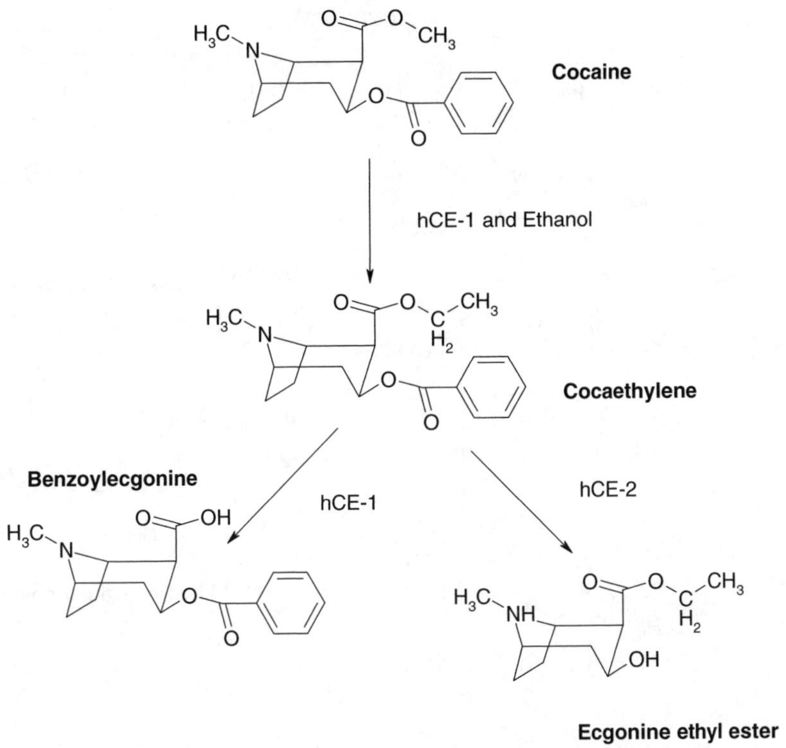

Figure B.4 Formation of cocaethylene by esterification with ethanol and the metabolism of the product to other cocaine esters and metabolites by esterases (hCE-1/2)

1960s. It is more than 100 times more potent than psilocybin and 5000 times stronger than mescaline. The D-disomer is active and the rest of the usually racemic mixture that is synthesized illicitly (iso-LSD) is inactive. The drug is usually taken in very low doses (50–100 micrograms) and is extensively metabolized, so is difficult to detect and is not usually included on standard laboratory drug screening systems. Excessive use quickly leads tolerance within only a few doses, although the chief danger from the drug is not really from direct toxicity, but from accidents during intoxication. The effects of LSD begin within 1 or 2 hours and may last for up to 12 hours. It has been likened to a 'mental rollercoaster' that you cannot get off. Despite its long period of effect, it is rapidly metabolized, primarily by dealkylation, or de-ethylation, to be precise (Figure B.5). The main metabolite in the urine of individuals who have used the drug is 2-oxo-3-hydroxy LSD, which is not found in the plasma, presumably as it is rapidly filtered by the kidneys. This metabolite is found in much greater quantity than the parent drug in urine. Aside from the de-ethylated derivative (lysergic acid ethylamide) a demethy-lated metabolite (nor-LSD), the side chain and the top phenyl ring (13/14

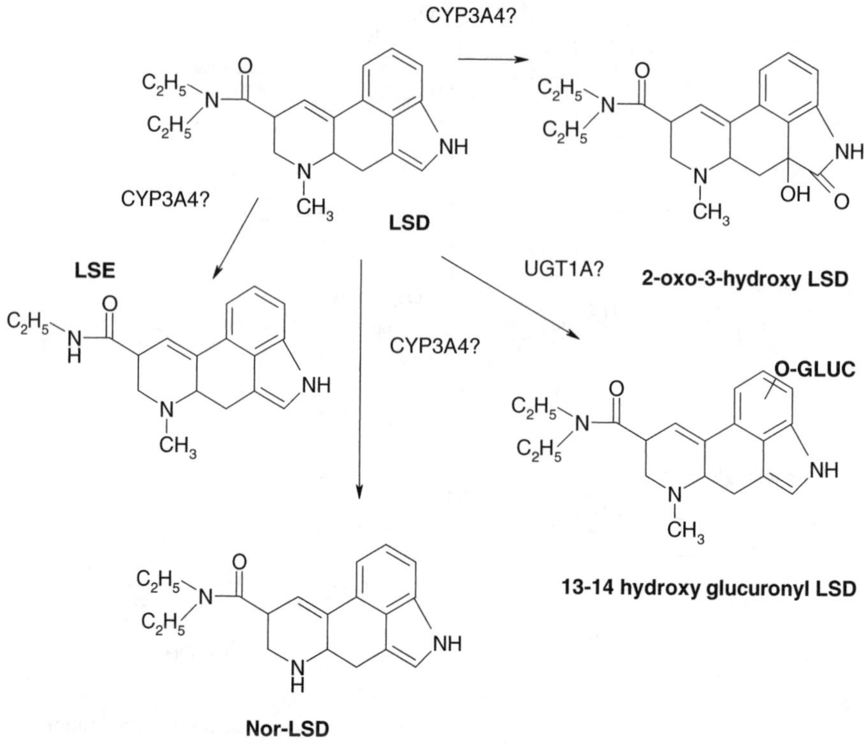

Figure B.5 Metabolism of LSD: formation of lysergic acid ethylamide (LSE), nor (N-demethylated) LSD and its hydroxylated derivatives

position on the molecule) can be hydroxylated and at least one glucuronide is formed from the 13/14 hydroxylated derivative. Presently, no CYP has been assigned to these products, although the molecule is quite lipophilic (log P of 1.3) and vaguely resembles a steroid shape, so it would not be unreasonable to suggest that CYP3A4 and possibly 2C9 and 2D6 might be involved in the hydroxylation and dealkylation of LSD.

Serotonin-based hallucinogens

The Sonoran desert toad, or Colorado river toad (*Bufo alvarius*) found in Arizona, as well as many other species such as the Australian cane toad, are much sought after in some circles for the hallucinogenic properties of their skin secretions. These secretions are exuded when frightened or alarmed to deter predators. It is not generally realized that toad venoms contain many other exceedingly toxic agents, such as bufagins (bufendienolides) that have cardiac glycoside-like effects and catecholamines. The net result is heart

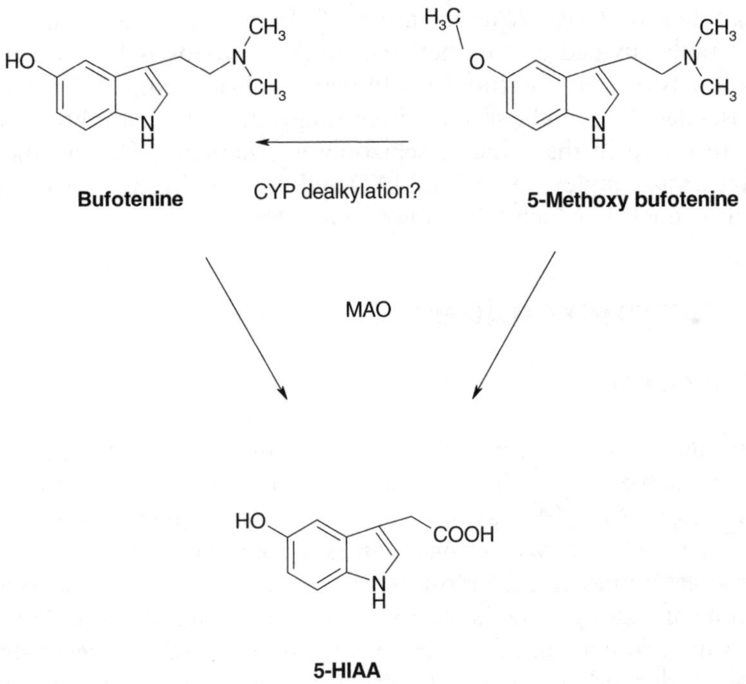

Figure B.6 Some routes of dimethyltryptamine derivative clearance leading to 5-hydroxyindole acetic acid (5-HIAA)

failure, seizures and vasoconstriction leading to death in animals and at least some recorded cases of seizures in children. The collective effect from an entire toad skin can be lethal to the average weight adult. The hallucinogenic fraction of the venom contains a series of serotonin-like compounds, the indolealkylamines, which are commonly named bufotenines. Bufotenine itself (5-hydroxy-N,N-dimethyltryptamine) is a weak hallucinogen, which has potent cardiodepressive effects, sufficiently severe to induce circulatory crises. 5-Methoxy-N'N' dimethyltryptamine (known also as 5-MeO-DMT, O-methylbufotenine and 5-methoxy bufotenine; Figure B.6) is a very potent hallucinogen. Orally, they have no effects, as MAO clears dimethyltryptamines to 5-OH indole acetic acid in the gut, although the 4-hydroxy substitution of the close structural analogue psilocybin (O-phosphoryl-4-hydroxydimethyltryptamine) makes it orally active. 5-Methoxybufotenine was first identified in the 1930s but it was not until the late 1960s that it was found in the toad exudates. 5-Methoxybufotenine is highly active when inhaled as an aerosol through smoking the dried toad exudate as well as intravenously. Due to the variability of the active 5-methoxybufotenine content of the venom exudates, the effects have been described as 'from bliss to horror'. Chemically synthesized bufotenines are now available illicitly, although they are Class 'A' drugs in the UK. In the US and Australia, opinion is predictably divided as to whether licking the toads is harmful to them, although it is certainly harmful for humans to lick them, as the toxicity as previously detailed, can be severe. Interestingly, the dimethyltryptamine derivatives are found in the urine of schizophrenic patients. The metabolism of these agents is complex, involving MAO and methylation as well as demethylation. It is unclear which CYPs may be involved.

B.5   Amphetamines

Introduction

Amphetamines have been popular drugs of abuse for more than forty years. They retain some slender clinical uses, such as in narcolepsy and some weight control effects. MDMA may well be their most popular manifestation in current usage (see below). Amphetamines are known by the usual litany of tedious street-names and the most popular variant of the more serious forms at the time of writing is methamphetamine, known mainly as 'ice' or 'crystal meth'. Amphetamines and their derivatives can be dosed intravenously, orally or smoked, depending on the physical form of the drug and the speed of effects onset desired. They act to cause CNS and peripheral biogenic amine effects to be strongly potentiated by preventing their re-uptake and destruction. These sustained elevated amine levels, (particularly dopamine) lead to the characteristic stimulatory effects, which include feelings of well-being, euphoria, and boundless energy; they may also cause hallucinations. The effects are similar to that of cocaine, but with an important difference. Cocaine is a very transient 'high', perhaps only a few minutes, whilst amphetamines can maintain their potent effects over more than half a day. The dysphoric effects of the drugs once they have been cleared are notoriously bad, due to severe synaptic biogenic amine depletion. Of course, the tight neuronal regulation of biogenic amine adapts rapidly through mechanisms such as receptor down-regulation. These erode the pharmacological effects over time, leading to tolerance and dependence with repeated usage. Addicts escalate their doses and try to beat the tolerance and the dysphoria by taking the drug for days alongside depressants such as ethanol or heroin. 'Tweaking', as it is known, leads to continuously wakeful states that may exceed two weeks and can make these individuals exceedingly dangerous to themselves and others. Amphetamines can cause a long list of toxic effects, from hypertensive crises to strokes and seizures. They can even induce paranoid schizophrenia in some individuals. The effects on the physical appearance of serious addicts over time are genuinely shocking.

The variety in amphetamine clearance routes reflects their closeness in structure to endogenous biogenic amines. Their main route of metabolism seems to be ring – hydroxylation by CYPs 3A4, 2D6 and 2B6. Potent inhibitors of 3A4 such as some of the HIV protease inhibitors are thought to be capable of causing fatal amphetamine accumulation from normally safe dosages as a consequence of inhibition. Amphetamines can also be N-oxidised by flavin monooxygenases (FMO-3) and deaminated (chapter 3) by various enzyme systems such as the MAOs. A good example of how the metabolic fate of an amphetamine has been gradually unravelled and how this might relate to the long-term consequences of its usage is with MDMA.

Ecstasy (MDMA) mode of action and acute toxicity

This drug has undergone a dramatic increase in popularity in the youth of the developed world over the last 5–10 years, with estimates of weekly usage in the UK as high as 300 000 individuals. MDMA (Figure B.7) is the best-known representative of a group of N-substituted methylenedioxyamphetamine derivatives, which also include the N-ethyl derivative ('Eve') and MDA, the primary unsubstituted amine derivative. These agents are stimulants, although they are also reputed to induce feelings of empathy and warmth towards oneself and others; the word that has been coined to describe them is 'entactogen'. MDMA analogue toxicity can be resolved into acute and chronic toxicity – acute toxicity is well understood and described. Overdose of these agents can lead to hyperthermia, high blood pressure, rhabdo-

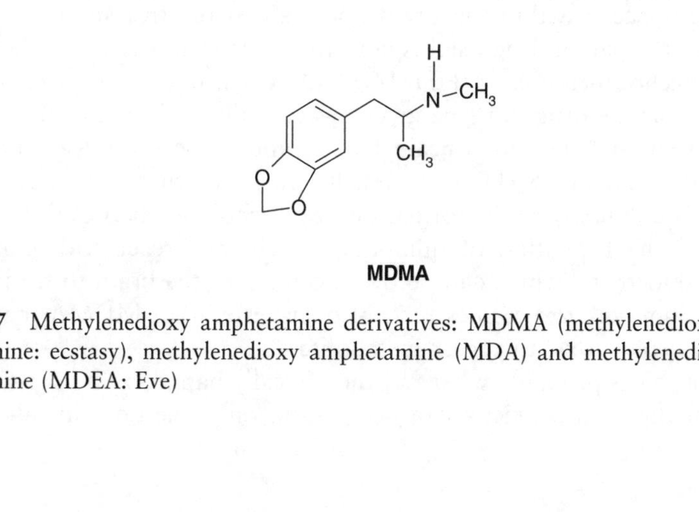

Figure B.7 Methylenedioxy amphetamine derivatives: MDMA (methylenedioxymethyl amphetamine: ecstasy), methylenedioxy amphetamine (MDA) and methylenedioxyethyl amphetamine (MDEA: Eve)

myolysis and kidney failure. Deaths attributed to these drugs are sometimes exacerbated by repetitive violent physical activity (some call it dancing) and its attendant dehydration. Overall, deaths due to MDMA are rare, although the chronic toxicity is still far from completely understood.

Unfortunately, there is a strong perception among users that MDMA derivatives are generally much safer than other drugs. However, these MDMA users blithely trust someone they met in a Club to sell them unadulterated and high quality MDMA which is free from unpleasant impurities. A number of sources have also reported the sale of 4-methylthioamphetamine as 'ecstasy' and this agent is much more toxic than MDMA and has been fatal in a number of cases. In response to these problems of purity and adulteration, in some European countries MDMA testing facilities are available where the drug is sold to guarantee a reasonable standard of purity.

Chronic toxicity and metabolism

There is some evidence that moderate or sparing use of MDMA may not lead to permanent neural impairment, although some studies have also highlighted a much more serious effect at lower doses in younger users below the age of 18. However, it is difficult to evaluate the true risk of neurotoxicity caused by these drugs due to problems estimating accurately how much is taken and how often. It is generally agreed that around 10 per cent of MDMA users could experience serious long-term neurotoxicity as a result of their high regular intake of the drug.

The metabolism of MDMA has been hotly pursued (Figure B.8) as it was discovered in the mid 1990s that these agents were specifically demethylenated by CYP2D6, forming a catechol product. The ethyl side-chain in 'Eve' and the methyl group in MDMA can also be dealkylated by CYP2B6, although this route is a minor one in humans, as MDA levels are around only 5 per cent of parent drug in plasma. In man, the major route is 2D6-mediated demethylenation, and initially it was thought that catechol formation might occur within the brain and lead to reactive species formation. However, the parent drug itself is not directly neurotoxic and neither are any of its catechol metabolites (HHMA/HHA) when injected into rat brains. It appears that the drug must be given systemically and the metabolites make their way across the blood-brain barrier and cause the release of reactive species that damage 5-HT neurones. It is believed that in rats the route of toxicity is due firstly to the formation of catechol metabolites (HHMA), followed by the formation of quinones, which then react with glutathione-derived thioethers, which can be transported into the brain to form reactive species. Some *in vitro* studies have also suggested that MDMA may be oxidized to nephrotoxic thioether metabolites.

Whilst this is probably what *can* theoretically happen in humans, it is also apparent that neurotoxicity can occur from only one dose in rats and this

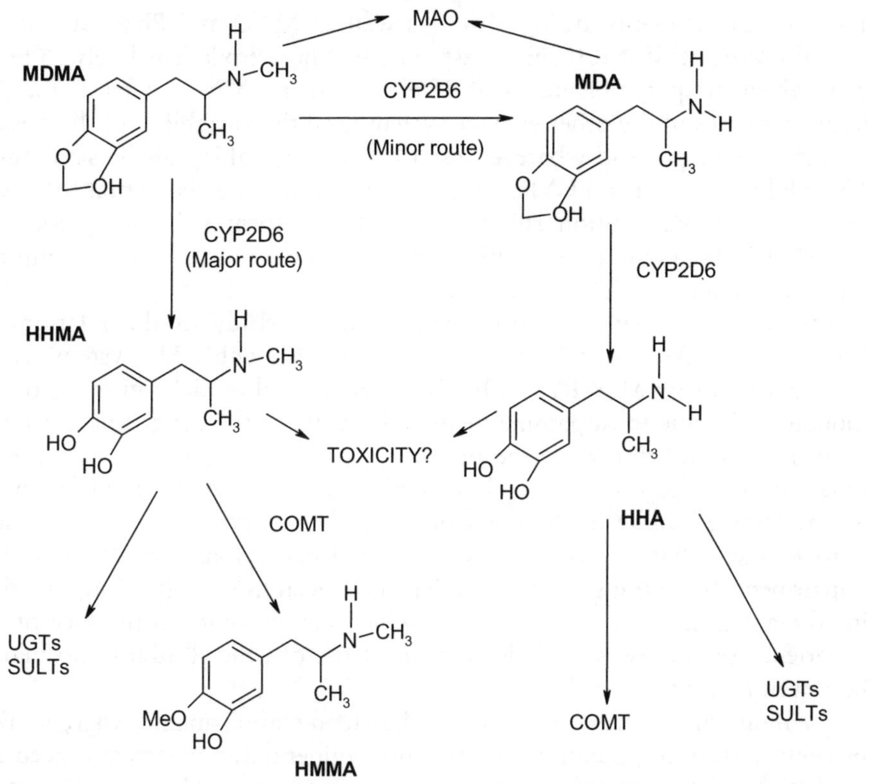

Figure B.8 Metabolism of MDMA: the main route of clearance is initially via CYP2D6 to HHMA (3,4,dihydroxymethamphetamine), which is cleared either to Phase II conjugates or may be methylated by catechol-O-methyl transferase (COMT) to HMMA (4-hydroxy-3-methoxymethyl amphetamine). The demethylated MDA may then be demethylenated to HHA (3,4 dihydroxyamphetamine) which can also be methylated and undergo Phase II clearance. MAO may also oxidize MDA, or MDMA

does not seem to occur in man. The role of 2D6 in the human clearance and toxicity of these amphetamines quickly led to the prediction that the polymorphism in the expression of this CYP might lead to dramatic effects on the plasma concentrations and the level of toxic catechol precursors, as well as the clinical effects of these drugs. However, it was then discovered in 1999 that MDMA causes a mechanism-based irreversible inhibition of CYP2D6, which occurs after one or two consecutive doses. The effect could be to partially block 2D6 capability and make all chronic users poor metabolizers for the isoform. This suggests that if demethylenation was the main route of toxicity through catechol formation, then bizarrely, repeated dosage of the drug might reduce the potential neurotoxicity. In practice, the 2D6 blockade does cause the drug to show non-linear kinetics, i.e. it accumulates on repeated dosage. It also takes about 10 days for the inhibition of 2D6 to disappear. However, there are several other CYPs such as 2B6, 3A4 and even

1A2 that can demethylate the drug, as well as MAO and Phase II systems that also clear it. It is difficult to estimate just how toxic it is likely to be in man, given the polymorphisms of 2D6 and other CYPs, as well as the differing activities of the other enzyme systems and the variability of the dosage in each ecstasy pill and whatever else the users are taking at the same time. The inhibitory effects on CYP2D6 are so potent that it is likely that the clearances of any prescription substrates of this isoform will be significantly extended: this might occur with antipsychotics (chlorpromazine), antidepressants (SSRIs and TCAs) and opiates.

Animal studies have not been helpful in the study of the relationship between MDMA, its metabolism and toxicity. Although 5-HT-system neurotoxicity caused by MDMA can be shown in animal models, in mice, this is thought to be due to dopamine-mediated events, as the drug is not metabolized. In rats and monkeys, the profile of MDMA metabolism is markedly different again from man (mostly demethylation), so animal models appear to have limited value in the main objective of this type of research, which is to predict what exposure of MDMA will cause long-term neurological impairment. If anything, animal models have been 'too positive' in underlining the apparent risks of these drugs, which patently flies in the face of the experience of the users. This leads to mistrust of official advice, no matter how well it is intentioned.

The multi-enzymatic complexity of MDMA metabolism and where it takes place in relation to potential sites of neural vulnerability means that accurate predictions of human toxicity may be some way away. However, it may be that factors such as the frequency of use, CYP2D6 status and age of the user might be greater determinants of possible long-term problems than dosage and co-administered drugs. It is likely that future epidemiological studies may determine the ultimate risks of these drugs.

B.6 Cannabis

Introduction

The hemp plant *Cannabis sativa* is the main source of cannabinoids, a group of around 60 terpene psychoactive agents which are probably the most commonly used illicit substances for recreational purposes. In the plant itself, the richest source of the cannabinoids is the resin removed from the leaves of the female plant. The most potent of the cannabinoids is Δ-9 tetrahydrocannabinol (Δ-9 THC), although Δ-8 THC is as psychoactive and is chemically more stable. Cannabinoids are usually prepared from the dried flowering tops and leaves (marijuana, up to 5 per cent Δ-9 THC), the resin itself combined with the flowers (hashish, up to 25 per cent Δ-9 THC) and the industrial strength version, hash oil. This is resin that has been extracted and purified with solvents and concentrated and it can exceed 70 per cent in Δ-9 THC content. These agents are quite potent and a dose of less than 10 mg is required for the standard 'high' effects. Cannabinoids have stimulant, sedative and even hallucinogenic properties and it is now clear that they have more in common with opiates than other drugs of abuse such as cocaine, in that there are specific cannabinoid receptors (CB1 receptors) which are sensitive to THCs within the brain, particularly areas associated with cognition, memory and movement coordination. They are still known as cannabinoid receptors as their endogenous functions are not entirely understood. A separate set of cannabinoid receptors (CB2) are found in the immune system. Endogenous agonists are being found, such as anandamide, and many synthetic agonists and antagonists have been made. The receptors are found in most animals and even insects, which suggests a vital and conserved role for them in homeostasis, probably as neurotransmitters to modulate neural activity. It is possible that more subtypes of cannabinoid receptors will be found and the full medicinal potential of these receptors will emerge in years to come. It appears that cannabinoids are agonists that activate these receptors to modulate cyclic nucleotide cascades to exert their central effects. It seems the main reason that cannabinoids are not very toxic is that unlike, say, opiate receptors, they are not found in vital neural areas which control respiration or heart rate. Fatal overdosage has not been reported so far.

Metabolism

THC-derivative clearance is extensive, with dozens of metabolites formed; indeed, only small amounts of parent Δ-9 THC appear in urine. The half-life of Δ-9 THC in blood is around 20 hours, although the effects from smoking appear within 5–10 minutes. When cannabis products are smoked, Δ-9 THC is cleared within a few minutes to 9-carboxy Δ-9 THC (Figure B.9), which is pharmacologically inactive and is the major urinary metabolite. This metabolite is used to monitor cannabis usage in drug-testing protocols. It is unclear as to which CYP performs this function, although it is believed that CYP3A4 may form oxo-metabolites from 7- and 8-hydroxy derivatives of Δ-8 THC, which retain activity, although 2C9 and 1A1 and 1A2 were also involved. It is interesting that school friends of mine who used the drug in the late 1970s insisted that it was far better consumed orally than smoked and that the effects were longer in duration. Indeed, it is now known that this is the case, as oral dosage promotes the formation of 11-hydroxy Δ-9 THC which is not only more potent than Δ-9 THC, but enters the brain more quickly. There is some evidence that CYP2C9 catalyses this reaction. It is possible that chronic use leads to induction of THC metabolism, but the metabolites are still very lipophilic and accumulate in fatty areas. After around a week, more than one-third of the dose is still in the user. The metabolites' oil

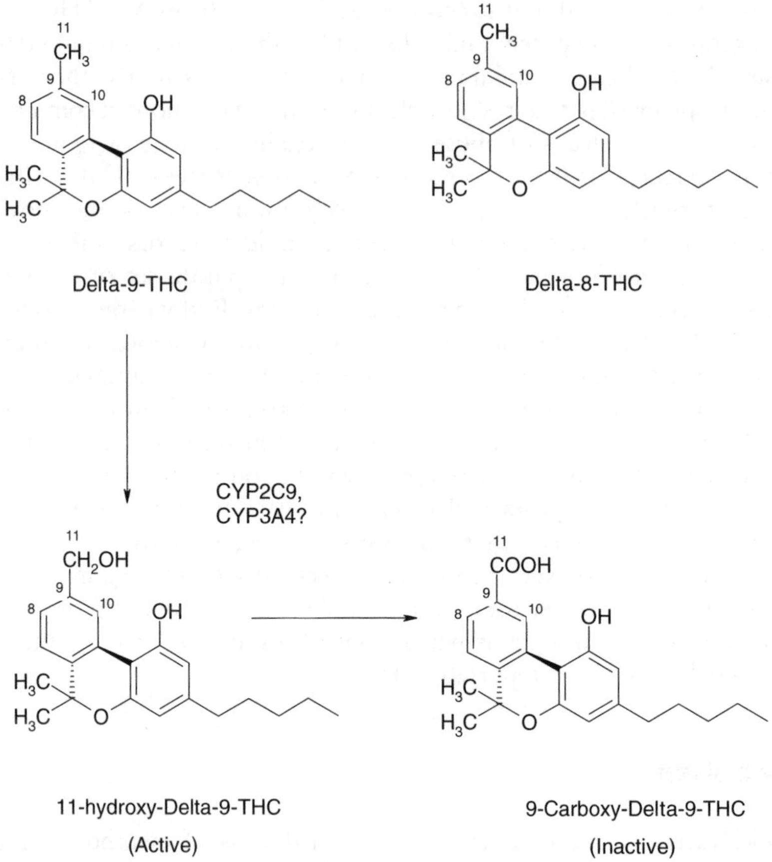

Figure B.9 The main active constitutuents of *Cannabis sativa*, Δ-8 and Δ-9 THC and the clearance of Δ-9 THC to its hydroxyl carboxy products by CYPs 2C9 and possibly 3A4

solubility means that they are consequently difficult to clear into urine and complete excretion of the various metabolites usually occurs in faeces and can take months after high doses. Hence, the consumption of small quantities can lead to the failure of a random drug test several weeks later. Although non-acutely toxic, heavy THC usage can cause intense paranoia and a form of psychosis, which can lead to users being 'sectioned' under the Mental Health Act. This process is exacerbated by the accumulation of active THC derivatives.

Carcinogenic activity of cannabis products

It is hotly debated by various groups as to whether cannabis smoking does lead to increased risks of lung cancer. Logically, it would appear to be very hard to separate the effects of tobacco, a known carcinogen, from the cannabis itself, as they are more often than not co-administered. There is evidence both for and against the possible carcinogenic properties of cannabis; in animal cell-line studies, cannabis was shown to be capable of inducing CYP1A1 activity, thought to be a key factor in lung carcinogenesis. Indeed, Δ-9 THC was shown to act through the Ah receptor system in classical fashion. However, Δ-9 THC was also shown to competitively inhibit the induced CYP1A1; what this might mean for possible carcinogenesis over many years of use is difficult to extrapolate. If Δ-9 THC exposure was fairly constant, then CYP1A1 levels would be maintained in accordance with exposure. It has been suggested that when 1A1 is 'idle', i.e. not oxidizing substrates, it 'leaks' reactive species that lead to DNA damage. Since THC derivatives are so persistent, it is possible that there may not be much time when the isoform is 'idle', so the THC might restrict reactive species formation. Clearly, arguments could be made in the opposite direction and on balance it is unlikely that occasional use would be carcinogenic, just as occasional use of tobacco is much less risky than heavy use. That the issue is not resolved after more than 25 years of study indicates that confounding factors such as the lack of filters on cannabis cigarettes, the variability of dose, the difficulty in estimating concurrent tobacco exposure and the effects of THCs on the immune system may well make it impossible to prove conclusively whether marijuana use is carcinogenic. It is, however, not unreasonable to suggest that heavy use, which is effectively abuse, will increase the risk of lung neoplasms.

B.7   PCP

Phencyclidine (PCP), an arylcyclohexylamine, was developed in the 1950s as a dissociative anaesthetic, where the patient is made motionless, but wakeful. It had a potent analgesic effect, but at clinically effective doses it did not depress respiration or the cardiovascular system. Although initially promising, the drug was withdrawn in the early 1960s after patients experienced extremely unpleasant hallucinations and agitation when they emerged from anaesthesia. Later in that decade, the drug began to be abused, although its effects were so unpredictable and often horrible, it never gained mass popularity. Once it was discovered it could be smoked to exert some rudimentary control of its effects, it gained more adherents, although it remains confined to some large cities in the US, notably Los Angeles and Philadelphia.

The drug is effective orally as well as through smoking PCP oil-soaked tobacco. The 'oil' is an ether extract of the drug when illicitly manufactured. In the pure form it is a white crystalline powder, but the street drug can be anything from a powder or pill to a brownish syrupy gum. The powdered form of the drug ('Angel Dust') is virtually pure PCP and is so lipophilic it can be absorbed through the skin in pharmacologically effective quantities. It enters the brain easily and interacts with so many neurotransmitter systems that it exhibits a very wide range of central stimulant and depressant effects, including paranoid delusions, depression and hallucinations. Those suffering from acute intoxication can be diagnosed by their generally bizarre and violent behaviour, nystagmus (eye oscillations and visual impairment) and a positive urine test for the parent drug. It causes seizures and can be lethal at only 1 mg/kg, often due to a variety of severe reactions, from strokes, respiratory arrest, status elepticus and hyperthermia. The drug is spectacularly addictive on repeated use and users often die violently or commit suicide under its influence.

Metabolism

PCP is extensively metabolized to several main hydroxylated derivatives, including PCHP (1-(1-phenylcyclohexyl)-4-hydroxypiperidine), PPC (4-phenyl-4-(1-piperidinyl)-cyclohexanol) and PCAA (5-[N-(1-phenylcyclo-hexyl)]-aminopentanoic acid; Figure B.10). The drug has a long half-life in

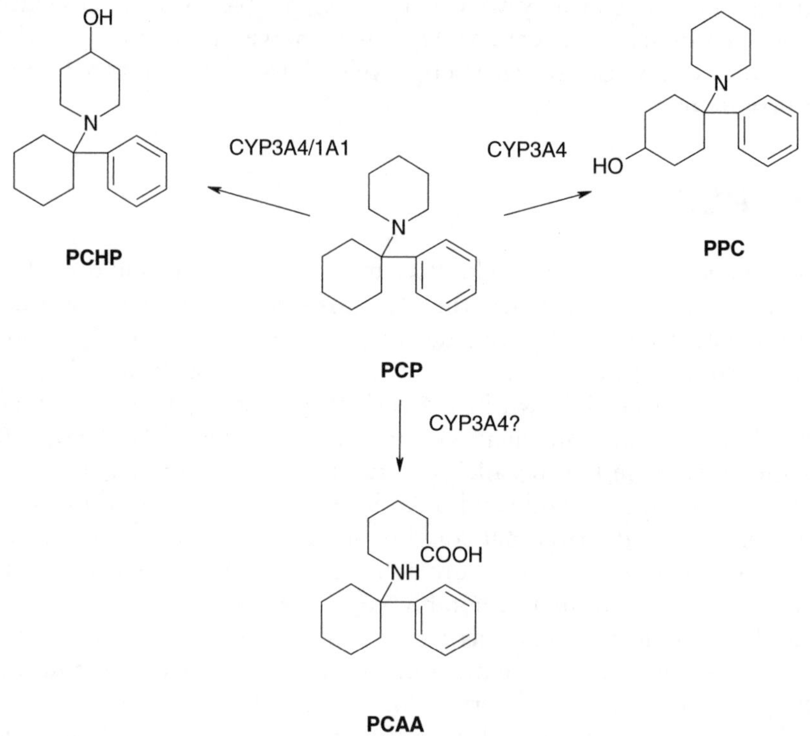

Figure B.10   Major metabolites of PCP in man

man and the effects of one dose can last several days in chronic users. The metabolites are difficult to clear, but are eventually eliminated in the urine and faeces, where they can be detected up to 28 days after drug use. PCP appears to be able to affect CYP expression in animals, although it is unknown whether this might occur in man. The only human liver microsome study carried out showed that PPC and PCHP were cleared by CYP3A4, although there was high inter-individual variation in the pattern of its metabolite formation. These metabolites included at least one tissue reactive unknown structure. PCHP was also formed by CYP1A1. It was also apparent that PCP could inhibit CYP3A4 metabolism. It is likely that CYP3A4 inducers would accelerate its metabolism and the clearance of 3A4 substrates might be disrupted by the drug. There is concern over PCP use in those taking anti-retroviral protease inhibitor combinations, which are potent CYP3A4 inhibitors. It is possible that PCP levels could rise precipitously in those individuals in response to the inhibition of clearance. Essentially, it is more than unwise to take PCP – indeed, it is taken by the kind of people who are bored with jumping off bridges handcuffed to engine blocks.

Were such things here that we do speak about,
Or have we eaten on the insane root that takes
the reason prisoner?

Act 1, Scene 3, *Macbeth*, by William Shakespeare

Appendix C
Examination Techniques

C.1 Introduction

This section does not just apply to drug metabolism, but to almost any life-science subject. Obviously, the type of examination you might be sitting for this subject could be anything from continuous assessment, through to multiple choice or essay-style questions. It is true that the vast majority of students extract from the university system more or less exactly what they put in. Every student, if they are honest, knows that they will get the degree they deserve and most put in enough effort to achieve this. If all you want is a modest degree, then you will not exert yourself, no matter what your lecturers say. However, there will be a fair number of students who would like to obtain the very best degree they can, but are unsure as to how to achieve this. Often, it is possible to emerge from 13 years of school examinations and still be none the wiser as to how to produce a first-class performance, *even though you are capable of it*. So how is it done?

C.2 A first-class answer

This does not consist of simply reproducing, like an elaborate living photocopier, the notes your lecturer gave you – you need much more than this. The detail of the lectures is a starting point, a platform, if you like, for building a first-class answer. If you have learned the course then you can understand and exploit the opportunity for extra reading and graft the extra knowledge onto your existing knowledge. This means you can show that you know and understand more than you were given. The initial source of this extra reading could be a textbook, but at the highest level it is better to use primary knowledge from journals. You may not be able to understand all of a scientific paper, but the introduction and discussion will provide an overview of the

Human Drug Metabolism, Michael D. Coleman
© 2005 John Wiley & Sons, Ltd

subject and if you read a few papers on the subject, you will see that they basically say the same thing. Another essential component in the construction of a first-class answer is the integration of your knowledge, perhaps with different courses and particularly in how you answer the question. Up to now, your answer will be clearly different from the run-of-the-mill student effort, but it still lacks a vital component for top marks. This final component can only appear once you have mastered the previous ones. You need to be 'creative'. Your answer must show depth of thought about a subject that means you have evaluated the available knowledge and come up with your own view and even your own interpretation on it. At the stage of a final degree, the subject is still evolving and 5, 10 or 20 years later, you might look back and see how wrong the prevailing wisdom of the time was, in terms of understanding of a particular phenomenon. So it is right to question the ideas and theories of current scientific literature, providing it is done through logical argument. So the five components are:

- Learn and understand the lecture notes;

- Extra reading of primary literature;

- Demonstrate integration of knowledge;

- Answer the specific question;

- Show originality of thought and analysis.

If you can manage all this, your answer will practically leap off the page and stun your examiner, as the majority of students are either not prepared or not intellectually able to go to these lengths to succeed and this shows in their answers. It is unlikely that most of you can write first-class answers on every subject in your course. However, you should be able to, on courses that you find particularly interesting, as your interest makes the work easier to absorb. On courses that you really do not enjoy or have always had trouble with, work on them to the point where you can get a good second-class answer no matter what the question.

C.3 Preparation

From the above you can see what is *required* to achieve a first-class answer. You may be wondering exactly *how* you might achieve this. Up to university, most students have evolved a method of learning their work which has served them reasonably well, well enough indeed, to actually get to university. This may not be enough to compete at the highest level and the usual problems encountered are:

- Lack of sufficient time devoted to revision;
- Poor 'productivity' from time spent;
- Inability to recall what was learned;
- Exam terror/horror/panic (or worse).

Lack of sufficient time

This is obviously related to commitment and determination. Starting revision two or three weeks before a major examination is startlingly inadequate, even with a photographic memory. To some extent, efforts must be made throughout the academic year to understand and process information accrued through lectures/practicals, etc.; certainly, several months before major examinations, revision should have been started. Many courses tend to communicate the bulk of the work required early in the year, so the majority of the course has usually been covered several months in advance of the finals. It is a case of 'how committed are you?' You may be capable of first-class work, but do not have the inclination to fulfil your potential. Regarding the future outside university, perhaps it is worth considering how much a good degree distinguishes you from 'the pack'. This gives you the widest possible choice in future directions, and in the context of near 50 per cent participation in higher education in the UK, you will need every edge you can get to find a specific job or position.

Poor productivity

It is very easy to sit in front of notes or a book for several hours and then adjourn to the nearest drinking establishment while transported in a haze of self-congratulation at your academic prowess. It is quite another thing to actively test how much you actually learned, by using past exam papers and setting yourself written tests. This can be a little demoralizing at first, but the truth must be found in terms of how much you have retained. Once you have been through your courses, you must start again and again and as many times as you can to commit them to long-term memory. After the second run-through, this is the time to incorporate extra reading and original thought, as you have worked out most of the basics and have something to build on.

Inability to recall

You may have been annoyed by a friend while watching an old film on the TV, who then announces who did it and why, having seen it once before in a drunken haze at party seven years previously. We appear to have almost unlimited space in our brains for storing information; the problem arises when we try to recall it. Obviously, you will remember where you went on holiday last year and have problems remembering what you did at 4.25 pm last Tuesday. The key appears to be some form of indexing system that provides a focus for recall. One way around this is to condense each lecture or parcel of a particular subject to a few lines, memorize them (word perfect), then memorize a list of these short condensates for each course. It is time consuming, but it means that you will be able to recall the entire course in serious detail. One of the keys to good performance in examinations is mastery of detail. This impresses examiners and can be attained with enough commitment. You may find your own way to 'reach' the knowledge you have learned. It is important that you use some method, as otherwise there is little point in learning your work if it cannot be recalled.

Exams – 'The horror . . .'

This accounts for a considerable proportion of lack of fulfilment of potential and often has dogged a student's academic career. There is no easy answer, other than building confidence by using the techniques described above. Often poor examination performance in otherwise good candidates is due to 'rabbit in the headlights' – inexplicably strange choices made in the exam. Consider a crude and not entirely appropriate analogy: you will be aware that members of the armed forces, firefighters and the like, develop fears about what they have to face like anyone else, but they can overcome these fears and function during otherwise terrifying situations by sheer repetition in their training. How often do you read about some heroic individual who usually says something like 'I was staring certain death in the face, then my training kicked in and I saved the day. . . . I didn't have time to scared, we had trained for this for months, etc.'.

If they can do it, you can, by training yourself to face the exam horror by focusing on preparation, building confidence and looking forward to the exam. Before the exam you will have:

- Learned the basic notes from the lectures;

- Supplemented with primary literature;

- Worked in your integration and understanding of the courses;

- Where you can, applied original thought to the work;

- Ensured that even courses which are less than thrilling, you can answer any question to high second-class standard.

This means you have trained yourself to turn a situation you dread into an occasion you actually want to arrive so you can shine.

C.4 The day of reckoning

It is possible to avoid the 'rabbit in the headlights' by using some important tips that should be burned into the consciousness so no amount of panic will erase them:

- Read the question: every word will have been scrutinized by maybe a dozen external and internal academics, so clearly every word, punctuation mark, etc. is essential and cannot be ignored.

- If there is a choice, *do the easiest question first*: you gain confidence with 'money in the bank'. You will save time also, which you can use in tackling harder questions. The questions should be done in order of difficulty.

- Do not write things that you know are not relevant to question: this is double jeopardy, you are getting no marks and losing time that you could have used to answer a question where you might have excelled.

Finally, you have done all you can do. A university/college is the last opportunity in your life where you will receive an absolutely fair deal, whether or not you might have extenuating circumstances or whatever might apply. The staff and the external examiners are guaranteed to give you every consideration so that the degree you received is a fair and accurate reflection of your commitment and aptitude. You will never again encounter a more 'level playing field', so make the most of it.

Appendix D
Summary of Major CYP Isoforms and their Substrates, Inhibitors and Inducers

This is not an exhaustive list and many drugs are metabolized by several CYP isoforms to varying degrees.

CYP	Substrates	Inhibitors	Inducers
1A1	Polycyclic aromatic hydrocarbons (PAHs), organochlorine insecticides	Alpha-naphthoflavone	PAHs, organochlorine
1A2	Amitryptyline, imipramine, caffeine, fluvoxamine, clozapine, haloperidol, mexiletine, ondansetron, propranolol, tacrine, theophylline, verapamil, R-warfarin, zolmitriptan	Amiodarone, cimetidine, furafylline, fluvoximine, ticlopidine	PAH amines in barbecued/ flame-broiled meat, Brussels sprouts, insulin, tobacco
2A6	Coumarins, aflatoxins 1,3, butadiene	Tranylcypramine, methoxalen, grapefruit juice	Phenobarbitone, rifampicin
2B6	Amfebutamone, coumarins, cyclophosphamide, mephenytoin, methadone, methoxychor (pesticide)	Tranylcypramine, thiotepa, ticlopidine	Phenobarbitone, rifampicin
2C8	Amodiaquine, cerivastatin, paclitaxel	Quercetin, glitazone drugs, gemfibrozil	Rifampicin, phenobarbitone
2C9	Amitryptyline, dapsone, fluoxetine, fluvestatin, NSAIDS, phenytoin, sulphonyl ureas, tamoxifen, S-warfarin	Isoniazid, fluvastatin, fluvoxamine, lovastatin, sulphafenazole	Rifampicin, secobarbitone

Human Drug Metabolism, Michael D. Coleman
© 2005 John Wiley & Sons, Ltd

CYP	Substrates	Inhibitors	Inducers
2C19	Barbiturates, citalopram, mephenytoin, proton pump inhibitors e.g. omeprazole, phenytoin, proguanil, R-warfarin	Tranylcypramine, cimetidine, fluoxetine, ketoconazole, ticlopidine	Carbamazepine, norethindrone, prednisone, rifampicin
2D6	TCAs, antipsychotics (haloperidol, etc.), anti-arrhythmics: flecainide, mexiletine, beta-blockers (e.g. timolol, S-metoprolol, bufuralol), MDMA, SSRIs, opiates (e.g. tramadol, codeine), venlafaxine	Amiodarone, cimetidine, ranitidine, histamine H-1 receptor antagonists (e.g. chlorpheniramine), quinidine, SSRIs (e.g. fluoxetine), St John's wort	Not conventionally induced
2E1	Benzene, chlorzoxazone, ethanol, flurane anaesthetics (e.g. halothane), paracetamol	Sulphides (e.g. DDC, diallyl sulphide, disulfiram)	Ethanol, acetone isoniazid
3A4/5	Aflatoxin B1, antihistamines (terfenadine, astemizole), calcium channel blockers (e.g. felodipine), cannabinoids, cyclosporine, macrolides (e.g. erythromycin), opiates (e.g. methadone), PCP, protease inhibitors (e.g. ritonavir), statins (except pravastatin), tacrolimus, paclitaxel	Amiodarone, azoles (ketoconazole fluconazole), cimetidine, grapefruit juice, macrolides, steroids, protease inhibitors	Barbiturates, carbamazepine, glucocorticoids, glitazones, nevirapine, phenytoin, rifampicin, St John's wort

Suggested Further Reading

This section is intended for those interested in looking at some of the source literature that I consulted when I wrote the text. By the time you read this, many more up-to-date reports will be available which can be found easily using electronic systems. These fresh reports will probably contradict some of the conclusions in the text as knowledge develops. As part of your study, real understanding of many life-science processes is often difficult to acquire. In many cases, it will be necessary to read several authors' versions of an explanation before it is possible to form an understanding that makes sense to you. This is not an instant process and you must give yourself time to absorb the arguments and explanations made in scientific literature. Sometimes, there are conflicting data available and leading authors come to different conclusions. In this case, have confidence in your own ability to follow the logic of the arguments and even if you feel that you lack experience in this field, you still bring the ability to follow a well-written argument. If you cannot follow it, then it is possible that it is not as logical as it appears and your interpretation of the process could be more valid. Remember that senior figures in science certainly have vastly superior knowledge of the field, but in terms of raw intelligence they may not necessarily be any cleverer than yourself!

Drug Biotransformational Systems: Origins and Aims

van Grevenynghe J et al., Polycyclic Aromatic Hydrocarbons Inhibit Differentiation of Human Monocytes into Macrophages J. Immunol. 170: 2374–2381, 2003.

Josephy PD et al., 'Phase I' and 'Phase II' metabolism: terminology that we should phase out? Drug Met Rev 37: 575–580, 2005.

Pombo M and Castro-Feijoo L, Endocrine disruptors. J Ped Endocrinol Met 18: 1145–1155, 2005.

How Oxidative systems metabolize substrates

Burk O and Wojnowski L, Cytochrome P450 3A and their regulation. *N-S Arch. Pharmacol.* **369**: 105–124, 2004.

Gonzalez FJ, Role of cytochromes P450 in chemical toxicity and oxidative stress: studies with CYP2E1. *Mutation Res.* **569**: 101–110, 2005.

Guengerich FP, Cytochrome p450: what have we learned and what are the future issues? *Drug Met. Rev.* **36** (2): 159–197, 2004.

Guengerich FP et al., Evidence for a role of a perferryl–oxygen complex, FeO^{3+}, in the N-oxygenation of amines by cytochrome P450 enzymes. *Mol. Pharmacol.* **51**: 147–151, 1997.

Hu Y and Kupfer D, Metabolism of the endocrine disruptor pesticide-methoxychlor by human P450s: pathways involving a novel catechol metabolite. *Drug Metab. Disp.* **30**: 1035–1042, 2002.

Luo G, CYP3A4 induction by xenobiotics: biochemistry, experimental methods and impact on drug discovery and development. *Curr. Drug Met.* **5**: 483–505, 2004.

Nebert DW, Role of aryl hydrocarbon receptor-mediated induction of the CYP1 enzymes in environmental toxicity and cancer. *J. Biol. Chem.* **279** (23): 23847–23850, 2004.

Nishikawa A, Cigarette smoking, metabolic activation and carcinogenesis. *Curr. Drug Met.* **5**: 363–373, 2004.

Ridderström M et al., Analysis of selective regions in the active sites of human cytochromes P450, 2C8, 2C9, 2C18, and 2C19 homology models using GRID/CPCA. *J. Med. Chem.* **44**: 4072–4081, 2001.

Werck-Reichhart D and Feyereisen R, Cytochromes P450: a success story. *Genome Biology* 2000 (http://genomebiology.com/2000/1/6/reviews/3003).

Williams PA et al. Crystal structure of human cytochrome P4502C9 with bound warfarin. *Nature* **424**: 464–468, 2003.

Induction of Cytochrome P450 systems

Baird P, Beware cytochrome P450 inducers; prescribing tips to prevent drug–drug interactions. *Curr. Psychiatry Online*1(11)2002 (http://www.currentpsychiatry.com/2002_11/1102_hepatic.asp).

Bolt HM, Rifampicin, a keystone inducer of drug metabolism: from Herbert Remmer's pioneering ideas to modern concepts. *Drug Met. Rev.* **36**: 497–509, 2004.

Handschin C and Meyer UA, Induction of drug metabolism: the role of nuclear receptors. *Pharmacol. Rev.* **55**: 649–673, 2003.

Kliewer SA et al., The nuclear pregnane X receptor: a key regulator of xenobiotic metabolism. *Endocrine Rev.* **23**: 687–702, 2002.

Mannel M, Drug interactions with St John's Wort – mechanisms and clinical implications. *Drug Safety* **27**: 773–797, 2004.

Markowitz JS, Effect of St John's Wort on drug metabolism by induction of cytochrome P450 3A4 enzyme. *JAMA* **290**: 1500–1504, 2003.

Patsalos PN *et al.*, The importance of drug interactions in epilepsy therapy. *Epilepsia* **43**: 365–385, 2002.

Plant NJ and Gibson GG, Evaluation of the toxicological relevance of CYP3A4 induction. *Curr. Opin. Drug Dis. & Dev* **6**: 50–56, 2003.

Ramaiah SK, Cytochrome P4502E1 induction increases thioacetamide liver injury in diet-restricted rats. *Drug Metab. Disp.* **29**: 1088–1095, 2001.

Savas U *et al.*, Molecular mechanisms of cytochrome P-450 induction by xenobiotics: an expanded role for nuclear hormone receptors. *Mol. Pharmacol.* **56**: 851–857, 1999.

Woodcroft KJ and Novak RF, Xenobiotic-enhanced expression of cytochromes P450 2E1 and 2B in primary cultured rat hepatocytes. *Drug Metab. Disp* **26**: 372–378, 1998.

Zhang S, Flavonoids as aryl hydrocarbon receptor agonists/antagonists effects of structure and cell context. *Environ. Health Perspect.* **111**: 1877–1882, 2003.

Cytochrome P450 enzyme inhibition

Coleman MD and Taylor CT, Effects of dihydrolipoic acid (DHLA), α-lipoic acid, N-acetyl cysteine and ascorbate on xenobiotic-mediated methaemoglobin formation in human erythrocytes in-vitro. *Env. Tox. Pharmacol.* **14**: 121–127, 2003.

Coleman MD and Tingle MD, The use of a metabolic inhibitor to reduce dapsone-dependent haematological toxicity. *Drug Dev. Res.* **25**: 1–16, 1992.

Coleman MD *et al.*, The use of cimetidine to reduce dapsone-dependent methaemoglobinaemia in dermatitis herpetiformis patients. *Brit. J. Clin. Pharmac.* **34**: 244–249, 1992.

Didziapetris R *et al.*, Classification analysis of P-glycoprotein substrate specificity. *J. Drug Tar.* **11**: 391–406, 2003.

Dresser GK and Bailey DG, The effects of fruit juices on drug disposition: a new model for drug interactions. *Eur. J. Clin. Invest.* **33**: 10–16 Suppl., 2003.

Egashira K *et al.*, Pomelo-induced increase in the blood level of tacrolimus in a renal transplant patient. *Transplantation* **75**: 1057, 2003.

Fallowfield L *et al.*, Quality of life of postmenopausal women in the Arimidex, Tamoxifen, Alone or in Combination (ATAC) Adjuvant Breast Cancer Trial. *J. Clin. Oncol.* **22**: 4261–4271, 2004.

Greenblatt DJ *et al.*, Time course of recovery of cytochrome P450 3A function after single doses of grapefruit juice. *Clin. Pharm. & Ther.* **74**: 121–129, 2003.

Howell A *et al.*, Results of the ATAC (Arimidex, Tamoxifen, Alone or in Combination) trial after completion of 5 years' adjuvant treatment for breast cancer. *Lancet* **365** (9453): 60–62, 2005.

Jalava KM *et al.*, Itraconazole greatly increases plasma concentrations and effects of felodipine. *Clin. Pharm. & Ther.* **61**: 410–415, 1997.

Kang BC *et al.*, Influence of fluconazole on the pharmacokinetics of omeprazole in healthy volunteers. *Biopharm. & Drug Disp.* **23**: 77–81, 2002.

Sagir A *et al.*, Inhibition of cytochrome P450 3A: relevant drug interactions in gastroenterology. *Digestion* **68**: 41–48, 2003.

von Richter O *et al.*, Cytochrome P450 3A4 and P-glycoprotein expression in human small intestinal enterocytes and hepatocytes: a comparative analysis in paired tissue specimens. *Clin. Pharmacol. Ther.* **75**: 172–183, 2004.

Yasuda K, Interaction of cytochrome P450 3A inhibitors with P-glycoprotein. *J. Pharm. Exper. Ther.* **303**: 323–332, 2002.

Zhou SF *et al.*, Herbal bioactivation: the good, the bad and the ugly. *Life Sci.* **74**: 935–968, 2004.

Conjugation and Transport processes

Ethell B *et al.*, Effect of valproic acid on drug and steroid glucuronidation by expressed human UDP glucuronosyl transferases. *Biochem. Pharmacol.* **65**: 1441–1449, 2003.

Gagné JF *et al.*, Common human *UGT1A* polymorphisms and the altered metabolism of irinotecan active metabolite 7-ethyl-10-hydroxycamptothecin (SN-38). *Mol. Pharmacol.* **62**: 608–617, 2002.

Gamage NU *et al.*, Structure of a human carcinogen-converting enzyme, SULT1A1 – structural and kinetic implications of substrate inhibition. *J. Biol. Chem.* **278**: 7655–7662, 2003.

Hein DW, Molecular genetics and function of NAT1 and NAT2: role in aromatic amine metabolism and carcinogenesis. *Mutation Res.* **506–507**: 65–77, 2002.

Huang W. *et al.*, Induction of bilirubin clearance by the constitutive androstane receptor (CAR). *PNAS* **100**: 4156–4161, 2003.

Kreis P *et al.*, Human phenol sulfotransferases hP-PST and hM-PST activate propane 2-nitronate to a genotoxicant. *Carcinogenesis* **21**: 295–299, 2000.

Laffon B *et al.*, Effect of epoxide hydrolase and glutathione S-transferase on the induction of micronuclei and DNA damage by styrene 7,8 oxide *in vitro*. *Mutation Res.* **536**: 49–59, 2003.

Leslie EM *et al.*, Toxicological relevance of the multidrug resistance protein 1, MRP1 (ABCC1) and related transporters. *Toxicology* **167**: 3–23, 2001.

Mizuno N *et al.*, Impact of drug transporter studies on drug discovery and development. *Pharmacol. Rev.* **55**: 425–461, 2003.

Raftogianis RB *et al.*, Human phenol sulfotransferases SULT1A2 and SULT1A1. *Biochem. Pharmacol.* **58**: 605–616, 1999.

Schultz M *et al.*, Inhibitors of glutathione-S-transferases as therapeutic agents. *Adv. Drug Del. Rev.* **26**: 91–104, 1997.

Sheehan D *et al.*, Structure, function and evolution of glutathione transferases: implications for classification of non-mammalian members of an ancient enzyme superfamily. *Biochem. J.* **360**: 1–16, 2001.

Tabrett CA and Coughtrie MW, Phenol sulfotransferase 1A1 activity in human liver: kinetic properties, interindividual variation and re-evaluation of the suitability of 4-nitrophenol as a probe substrate. *Biochem. Pharmacol.* **66**: 2089–2097, 2003.

von Dippe P *et al.*, Cell surface expression and bile acid transport function of one topological form of m-epoxide hydrolase. *Bio. Biophys. Res. Comm.* **309**: 804–809, 2003.

Yueh MF *et al.*, Involvement of the xenobiotic response element (XRE) in Ah receptor mediated induction of human UDP glucuronosyltransferase 1A1. *J. Biol. Chem.* **278**: 15001–15006, 2003.

Factors affecting drug metabolism

Blanco GJ *et al.*, Human cytochrome P450 maximal activities in pediatric versus adult liver. *Drug Metab. Disp.* **28**: 379–382, 2000.

Brockton N *et al.*, N-acetyltransferase polymorphisms and colorectal cancer. *Am. J. Epidemiol.* **151**: 846–861, 2000.

Ginsberg G, Evaluation of child/adult pharmacokinetic differences from a database derived from the therapeutic drug literature. *Toxicol. Sci.* **66**: 185–200, 2002.

Hattis D, Russ A, Banati P, Kozlak M, Goble R and Ginsberg G, Development of a Comparative Child/Adult Pharmacokinetic Database Based Upon the Therapeutic Drug Literature. Report to *USEPA, Assistance Agreement* 827195–0, Oct. 2000 (Childrens Pharmacokinetic database: http://www2.clarku.edu/faculty/dhattis).

Isbister GK *et al.*, Paracetamol overdose in a preterm neonate. *Arch. Dis. Child Fetal Neonatal Ed.* **85**: F70–F72, 2001.

Kearns GL *et al.*, Cisapride disposition in neonates and infants: in vivo reflection of cytochrome P450 3A4 ontogeny. *Clin. Pharm. & Ther.* **74**: 312–325, 2003.

Keshava C *et al.*, CYP3A4 Polymorphisms-Potential Risk factors for breast and Prostate cancer. A HuGE Review. *Am. J. Epidemiol.* **160**: 825–841, 2004.

Lampe JW, Health effects of vegetables and fruit: assessing mechanisms of action in human experimental studies. *Am. J. Clin. Nutrition* **70**: 475S–490S, 1999.

Leung AYH *et al.*, Genetic polymorphism of exon 4 of cytochrome P450 CYP2C9 may be associated with warfarin sensitivity in Chinese patients. *Blood* **98**: 2584–2587, 2001.

Loi MC *et al.*, Aging and drug interactions. III. Individual and combined effects of cimetidine and ciprofloxacin on theophylline metabolism in healthy male and female nonsmokers. *Pharmacol and Exper. Ther.* **280**: 627–637, 1997.

Murray S *et al.*, Effect of cruciferous vegetable consumption on heterocyclic aromatic amine metabolism in man. *Carcinogenesis* **22**: 1413–1420, 2001.

Pirmohamed M and Park BK, Cytochrome P450 enzyme polymorphisms and adverse drug reactions. *Toxicology* **192**: 23–32, 2003.

Shann F, Paracetamol: use in children. *Aust. Prescr.* **8**: 33–35, 1995.

Song N *et al.*, CYP1A1 polymorphism and risk of lung cancer in relation to tobacco smoking: a case-control study in China. *Carcinogenesis* **22**: 11–16, 2001.

Stamer UM, Rapid and reliable method for cytochrome P450 2D6 genotyping. *Clinical Chem.* **48**: 1412–1417, 2002.

Strassburg CP, Development aspects of human hepatic drug glucuronidation in young children and adults. *Gut* 50: 259–265, 2002.

Weathermon R and Crabb DW, Alcohol and medical interactions. *Alcohol Res. and Health* 23: 40–54, 1999.

Role of metabolism in drug toxicity

Arlt VM *et al.*, Human enzymes involved in the metabolic activation of the environmental contaminant 3-nitrobenzanthrone: evidence for reductive activation by human NADPH: cytochrome P450 reductase. *Cancer Res.* 63: 2752–2761, 2003.

Arlt VM *et al.*, 3-aminobenzanthrone, a human metabolite of the environmental pollutant 3-nitrobenzanthrone, forms DNA adducts after metabolic activation by human and rat liver microsomes: evidence for activation by cytochrome P450 1A1 and P450 1A2. *Chem. Res. Toxicol.* 17: 1092–1101, 2004.

Buetler TM *et al.*, Oltipraz-mediated changes in aflatoxin B-1 biotransformation in rat liver: implications for human chemointervention. *Cancer Res.* 56: 2306–2313, 1996.

Coleman MD, Dapsone mediated agranulocytosis: risks, possible mechanisms and prevention. *Toxicology* 162: 53–60, 2001.

Coleman MD and Coleman NA, Drug-induced methaemoglobinaemia. *Drug Safety* 14: 394–405, 1996.

Funk C *et al.*, Cholestatic potential of troglitazone as a possible factor contributing to troglitazone-induced hepatotoxicity: in vivo and in vitro interaction at the canalicular bile salt export pump (Bsep) in the rat. *Mol. Pharmacol.* 59: 627–635, 2001.

Galisteo G *et al.*, Hepatotoxity of tacrine: occurrence of membrane fluidity alterations without involvement of lipid peroxidation. *J. Pharmacol. Exp. Ther.* 294: 160–167, 2000.

Green MD and Tephly TR, Glucuronidation of amine substrates by purified and expressed UDP-glucuronosyltransferase proteins. *Drug Metab. Disp.* 26: 860–867, 1998.

Honma W *et al.*, Phenol sulfotransferase, ST1A3, as the main enzyme catalyzing sulfation of troglitazone in human liver. *Drug Metab. Disp.* 30: 944–949, 2002.

Kassahun K *et al.*, Studies on the metabolism of troglitazone to reactive intermediates in vitro and in vivo. Evidence for novel biotransformation pathways involving quinone methide formation and thiazolidinedione ring scission. *Chem. Res. Toxicol.* 1: 62–70, 2001 .

Kitteringham NR *et al.*, Protein expression profiling of glutathione S-transferase pi null mice as a strategy to identify potential markers of resistance to paracetamol-induced toxicity in the liver. *Proteomics* 3(2): 191–207, 2003.

Lankat-Buttgereit B and Tampé R, The transporter associated with antigen processing: function and implications in human diseases. *Physiol. Rev.* 82: 87–204, 2002.

Mansouri A *et al.*, Tacrine inhibits topoisomerases and DNA synthesis to cause mito-chondrial DNA depletion and apoptosis in mouse liver. *Hepatology* **38**: 715–725, 2003.

Naisbitt DJ *et al.*, Immunopharmacology of hypersensitivity reactions to drugs. *Curr. Aller. Asth. Rep.* **3**: 22–29, 2003.

Pichler WJ. Delayed drug hypersensitivity reactions. *Ann Int. Med.* **139**: 683–693, 2003.

Roychowdhury S and Suensson CK. Mechanisms of doug-induced delayed type hypeaseusitivity reactions in the skin. *AAPS J.* **7**: E834–E846, 2005.

Sheen CL, Paracetamol toxicity: epidemiology, prevention and costs to the health-care system. *Q. J. Med.* **95**: 609–619, 2002.

Stachlewitz RF *et al.*, Development and characterization of a new model of tacrine-induced hepatotoxicity: role of the sympathetic nervous system and hypoxia-reoxygenation. *Drug Metab. Disp.* **282**: 1591–1599, 1997.

Talaska G, Aromatic amines and human urinary bladder cancer: exposure sources and epidemiology. *J. ENV. Sci. Health Part C – Env. Carc. & Ecotox. Rev.* **21**: 29–43, 2003.

Turesky RJ, The role of genetic polymorphisms in metabolism of carcinogenic heterocyclic aromatic amines. *Curr. Drug Met.* **5**: 169–180, 2004.

Uetrecht JP, Is it possible to more accurately predict which drug candidates will cause idiosyncratic drug reactions? *Curr. Drug. Metab.* **1**: 133–141, 2000.

Wolf CR, The Gerhard Zbinden memorial lecture – Application of biochemical and genetic approaches to understanding pathways of chemical toxicity. *Toxicol Lett.* **127**: 3–17, 2002.

Appendix A Methods in drug metabolism

Buratti FM *et al.*, Kinetic parameters of OPT pesticide desulfuration by c-DNA expressed human CYPs. *Env. Tox. Pharmacol.* **11**: 181–190, 2002.

Coleman MD and Kuhns MK, Methaemoglobin formation by 4-aminopropriophenone in single and dual compartmental systems. *Env. Tox. Pharmacol.* **7**: 75–80, 1999.

Fujita K and Kamataki T, Role of human cytochrome P450 (CYP) in the metabolic activation of N-alkylnitrosamines: application of genetically engineered Salmo-nella typhimurium YG7108 expressing each form of CYP together with human NADPH-cytochrome P450 reductase. *Mut. Res.* **483**: 35–41, 2001.

Stiborová M *et al.*, Sudan I is a Potential Carcinogen for Humans: evidence for its metabolic activation and detoxication by human recombinant cytochrome P450 1A1 and liver microsomes *Cancer Research* **62**: 5678–5684, 2002.

Tingle MD *et al.*, Investigation into the role of metabolism in dapsone-induced methaemoglobinaemia using a two-compartment *in vitro* test system. *Brit. J. Clin. Pharmac.* **30**: 829–838, 1990.

Wojkcikowski J *et al.*, Contribution of human cytochrome P-450 isoforms to the metabolism of the simplest phenothiazine neuroleptic promazine *Brit. J. Pharma-col.* **138**: 1465–1474, 2003.

Appendix B Metabolism of major illicit drugs

Antoniou T and Tseng AL, Interactions between recreational drugs and antiretroviral agents. *Ann. Pharmacother.* **36**: 1598–1613, 2002.

Casey Laizure S *et al.*, Cocaethylene metabolism and interaction with cocaine and ethanol: role of carboxylesterases. *Drug Metab. Disp.* **31**: 16–20, 2003.

de la Torre R and Farré M, Neurotoxicity of MDMA (ecstasy): the limitations of scaling from animals to humans. *Trends Pharm. Sci.* **25**: 505–508, 2004.

Oda Y and Kharasch ED, Metabolism of methadone and *levo*-α-acetylmethadol (LAAM) by human intestinal cytochrome P450 3A4 (CYP3A4): potential contribution of intestinal metabolism to presystemic clearance and bioactivation. *Pharm. Exper. Ther.* **298** (3): 1021–1032, September 2001.

Sun H *et al.*, Cocaine metabolism accelerated by a re-engineered human butyrylcholinesterase. *Pharm Exper. Ther.* **302** (2): 710–716, August 2002.

Xie W *et al.*, An improved cocaine hydrolase: the A328Y mutant of human butyrylcholinesterase is 4-fold more efficient. *Mol. Pharm.* **55** (1): 83–91, January 1999.

Index

Human Drug Metabolism, Michael D. Coleman
© 2005 John Wiley & Sons, Ltd